DREAM RESEARCH

This edited volume shows the relationship between dream research and its usefulness in treating patients. Milton Kramer and Myron Glucksman show that there is support for searching for the meanings of dreams as experiences extended in time. Dreams reflect psychological changes and are actually an orderly process, not a random experience. This book explores interviewing methodologies that will help clients reduce the frequency of their nightmares and thus contribute to successful therapy.

Milton Kramer, MD, is emeritus professor of psychiatry at the University of Cincinnati. He has produced seven books, the most recent being *The Dream Experience,* along with writing 181 articles, 155 abstracts, and 68 book reviews and discussions having to do primarily with dreams, sleep disorders, and other health-related issues.

Myron Glucksman, MD, is a clinical professor of psychiatry at New York Medical College, as well as a training and supervising analyst on the faculty of its psychoanalytic institute. He is the author of many papers, has co-edited two books, and most recently authored *Dreaming: An Opportunity for Change.*

DREAM RESEARCH

Contributions to Clinical Practice

*Edited by Milton Kramer and
Myron Glucksman*

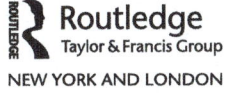

First published 2015
by Routledge
711 Third Avenue, New York, NY 10017

and by Routledge
27 Church Road, Hove, East Sussex BN3 2FA

Routledge is an imprint of the Taylor & Francis Group, an Informa business.

© 2015 Taylor & Francis

The right of the editors to be identified as the authors of the editorial material, and of the authors for their individual chapters, has been asserted in accordance with sections 77 and 78 of the Copyright, Designs and Patents Act 1988.

All rights reserved. No part of this book may be reprinted or reproduced or utilized in any form or by any electronic, mechanical, or other means, now known or hereafter invented, including photocopying and recording, or in any information storage or retrieval system, without permission in writing from the publishers.

Trademark notice: Product or corporate names may be trademarks or registered trademarks, and are used only for identification and explanation without intent to infringe.

Library of Congress Cataloging-in-Publication Data
Dream research : contributions to clinical practice / [edited by]
  Milton Kramer, Myron Glucksman.
    pages cm
  1. Sleep—Research. 2. Sleep disorders. 3. Dreams—Psychological aspects. 4. Clinical medicine. I. Kramer, Milton, 1929– editor.
II. Glucksman, Myron L., editor.
  RA786.D74 2010
  616.8′498072—dc23
  2014044532

ISBN: 978-1-138-79299-9 (hbk)
ISBN: 978-1-138-79300-2 (pbk)
ISBN: 978-1-315-76164-0 (ebk)

Typeset in Bembo
by Apex CoVantage, LLC

Printed and bound in Great Britain by
TJ International Ltd, Padstow, Cornwall

To Matan: Our hope for the future
Milton Kramer

To my patients
Myron Glucksman

CONTENTS

Contributors List		ix
Introduction: The Contribution of Dream Research to the Clinical Enterprise		xi
1	Establishing the Meaning of a Dream *Milton Kramer*	1
2	Teaching Dream Interviewing for Clinical Practice *Loma K. Flowers*	14
3	The Continuity Between Waking and Dreaming: Empirical Research and Clinical Implications *Michael Schredl*	27
4	Dream Incubation: Targeting Dreaming to Focus on Particular Issues *Gayle Delaney*	38
5	Finding Gender Differences in Dream Reports *Stanley Krippner*	56
6	Friends and Friendliness: Could They Be the Clue in Psychiatric Patients' Dreams? *G. William Domhoff*	67

7 Dreams: Thinking in a Different Biochemical State   80
   Deirdre Barrett

8 The Digital Revolution in Dream Research   95
   Kelly Bulkeley

9 The Manifest Dream Report and Clinical Change   106
   Myron L. Glucksman and Milton Kramer

10 The Hill Cognitive–Experiential Model: An Integrative Approach to Working With Dreams   123
   Patricia T. Spangler and Clara E. Hill

11 Posttraumatic Nightmares: From Scientific Evidence to Clinical Significance   135
   Lutz Wittman and Thérèse de Dassel

12 Nightmare Therapy: Emerging Concepts From Sleep Medicine   149
   Barry Krakow

13 Positive Aspects of the Classic Nightmare   161
   J. F. Pagel

14 The Contrasting Effects of Nightmares, Existential Dreams, and Transcendent Dreams   174
   Don Kuiken

15 Cross-Cultural Aspects of Extraordinary Dreams   188
   Jacquie Lewis and Stanley Krippner

16 Lucid Dreaming: Metaconsciousness During Paradoxical Sleep   198
   Stephen LaBerge

17 Reality: Waking, Sleeping, or Virtual?   215
   Jayne Gackenbach, Hannah Stark, Arielle Boyes, and Carson Flockhart

Index   *225*

CONTRIBUTORS LIST

Deirdre Barrett, Harvard Medical School

Arielle Boyes, MacEwan University

Kelly Bulkeley, Graduate Theological Union in Berkeley, California

Thérèse de Dassel, International Psychoanalytic University, Berlin, Germany; The Royal Brisbane and Women's Hospital, Brisbane, Australia

Gayle Delaney, Codirector of the Delaney & Flowers Dream and Consultation Center

G. William Domhoff, University of California, Santa Cruz

Carson Flockhart, MacEwan University

Loma K. Flowers, Clinical Professor of Psychiatry, University of California, San Francisco

Jayne Gackenbach, MacEwan University

Myron L. Glucksman, Clinical Professor of Psychiatry, New York Medical College, Valhalla, N.Y.

Clara E. Hill, University of Maryland

Barry Krakow, Sleep and Human Health Institute

Milton Kramer, Emeritus Professor of Psychiatry, College of Medicine, University of Cincinnati

Stanley Krippner, Saybrook University

Don Kuiken, University of Alberta

Stephen LaBerge

Jacquie Lewis, Saybrook University

J. F. Pagel, Associate Clinical Professor University of Colorado School of Medicine—Southern Colorado; Family Medicine Residency Program—Pueblo, Colorado; and Medical Director—Sleep Disorders Center of Southern Colorado, Parkview Medical Center, Pueblo, Colorado

Michael Schredl, Central Institute of Mental Health, Medical Faculty Mannheim/Heidelberg University, Germany

Patricia T. Spangler, Uniformed Services University of the Health Sciences

Hannah Stark, MacEwan University

Lutz Wittman, International Psychoanalytic University, Berlin, Germany

THE CONTRIBUTION OF DREAM RESEARCH TO THE CLINICAL ENTERPRISE

Introduction

Interest in the dream experience goes back to ancient times. The earliest reference to dream interpretation is in the Gilgamesh myth, 10th to 13th century BCE. The Beatty Papyrus, an Egyptian dream book, dates to 1800 BCE and contains dream interpretations directed at predicting the future. According to Oppenheim, the initial focus of dream understanding in the ancient Near East (primarily the Sumerian and Akkadian civilizations from 2700 to 2200 BCE) was focused on royalty receiving messages from the gods. The ancient Greeks—Plato, for example, in 400 BCE—saw in dreams the raw sexual and destructive desires of humankind. The Babylonian Talmud, written between 200 and 500 CE, says that "a man is shown in his dreams only what is in his own thoughts." In the fifth century, Artemidorus provided a dream interpretation manual that took into account the dreamer's personal circumstance. The application of dream interpretation to the clinical situation was established in the modern era with Freud's publication of *The Interpretation of Dreams* in 1900. The extensive outpouring of depth psychological dream literature—Freudian, Jungian, and Adlerian—that followed was essentially all anecdotal.

As Cartwright has pointed out, it was only with Aserinsky and Kleitman's 1952 discovery of REM sleep that we became able to collect adequate samples of dreams at a given point in time, which is necessary to perform meaningful scientific studies of dreaming. Hall and Van de Castle published *The Content Analysis of Dreams* in 1966, providing us with a reliable method of quantifying the dreams we studied. In 1979 Winget and Kramer published *Dimensions of Dreams*, which described more than a hundred methods to quantify dream content.

Dream research is the effort to describe the sources, construction, function, and meaning of the dream experience. The data for study are not the experiences themselves but rather the reports of those experiences. These data are either gathered in the laboratory from sleep awakenings, both REM and non-REM, or gathered by asking subjects to report their dreams. The reports are taken from previously reported dreams (e.g., dream diaries) or from population surveys that include questions about dreams. The fundamental assumption in dream research is that dreaming is an altered form of consciousness under the special conditions of sleep. We believe, on the basis of considerable supporting evidence, that the dream report reflects the psychology of the dreamer, including both long-term and concurrent aspects of the dreamer's emotional condition, both trait and state related.

After more than 60 years of scientific dream study, we are certainly at a point to ask dream researchers how their work has contributed to the clinical enterprise of treating emotionally troubled patients. In this volume we explore this contribution. We have recruited 22 dream researchers who have written 17 chapters summarizing their research and indicating its potential value to treating emotionally troubled patients.

In Chapter 1, Kramer explains how meaning can be found in the dream. He describes evidence that the dream exists as an experience extended in time, and he shows content differences where one would expect to find psychological differences (e.g., in demographic variables). Dreams are orderly, not random, events such that the possibility they have meaning exists. Kramer illustrates an associative method called *dream translation* that yields a meaning for a dream report.

Chapters 2, 3, and 4 (by Flowers, Schredl, and Delaney, respectively) summarize work that focuses on interview techniques in which collecting the dream report results in exposing the meaning of a dream. Schredl also looked at the continuity relationship of waking and sleeping mentation. Delaney uses incubation techniques to reveal the dynamics of a dreamer's particular life problem. Flowers uses an interview technique to establish the meaning in a dream.

Chapters 5 and 6 use aspects of the Hall–Van de Castle dream content scoring system to enhance our understanding of dreaming. In Chapter 5, Krippner points out large cross-cultural gender differences in dream reports and calls attention to variability in aggression that is cultural rather than ethnocentric. In Chapter 6, Domhoff finds that dreams of mental patients include fewer friendly interactions and fewer people. This friendless world, the world of mentally ill, changes in a positive direction with effective treatment.

A group of studies focus on identifying the dreamers' problem as revealed in their dreams, showing that changes in dreaming co-varied with improvement and demonstrating how to work with dreams in psychotherapy. In Chapter 7, Barrett shows how dreams help people to solve problems and recover from trauma. In Chapter 8, Bulkeley uses digital tools to illustrate how patterns of dream content reflect both the emotional problems of dreamers and their resources for healing. In Chapter 9, Glucksman and Kramer show that dream changes (or failure to change) from early to late in treatment in mental patients reflect improvement or lack of improvement. Changes in dream affect and dream narrative from negative to positive, from first to last dream report, reflect improvement in the dreamer's emotional condition. The first dream reported in therapy can reveal the patient's core psychological problem.

In Chapter 10, Spangler and Hill report their research on establishing how to work on a patient's dreams effectively in therapy.

A major concern for dream researchers has been severe dream disturbances, namely nightmares. In Chapter 11, Wittman and de Dassel summarize the research on posttraumatic nightmares and illustrate clinical applications of treatment. In Chapter 12, Krakow describes imagery rehearsal therapy, an effective approach for treating nightmares. Krakow also explores a possible link between nightmares and sleep apnea. In Chapter 13, Pagel explores the positive aspects of nightmares by discussing how creative individuals—including authors, painters, and musicians—use their nightmare experience in their creative endeavors.

Researchers describe a group of extraordinary dreams that includes existential dreams, lucid dreams, creative dreams, and initiation dreams. In Chapter 14, Kuiken points out that there are at least two types of negative-affect dreams, nightmares and existential dreams. These types of dream should not be conflated as they have different precipitants and aftereffects. In Chapter 15, Lewis and Krippner found in a large, unsystematic collection of cross-cultural dream material that includes lucid dreams, creative dreams, initiation dreams, and many other types worth examining. In Chapter 16, LaBerge provides a detailed examination of lucid dreams and their possible therapeutic value. Gackenbach and her colleagues have studied how virtual reality experiences such as playing video games affect subsequent dreaming. In Chapter 17 they describe their findings, including simple dream incorporation, increased lucid dreams, and especially increase in the control of dreaming. These factors offer the possibility of protection when dealing with distressing dreams.

Milton Kramer, MD, and
Myron Glucksman, MD, 2014

1

ESTABLISHING THE MEANING OF A DREAM

Milton Kramer

EMERITUS PROFESSOR OF PSYCHIATRY
COLLEGE OF MEDICINE, UNIVERSITY OF CINCINNATI

The dream process is an experience that the dreamer has during sleep that cannot be observed while it is occurring. Therefore, content-related dream research is not research of the dream experience but of the dreamer's report of that experience. In this essay I summarize my research; I do not review the work of others in the various areas covered, as I did in my book *The Dream Experience* (Kramer, 2007).

The first question that should be asked is, does the dream exist? I will report the four studies (Kramer, Czaya, Arand, & Roth, 1974; Kramer, Winget, & Roth, 1975; Taub, Kramer, Arand, & Jacobs, 1978; Kramer, Kinney, & Scharf, 1983) that my colleagues and I have done support the existence of the dream as a valid experience that occurs during sleep and is extended in time. We collected reports from REM sleep awakenings at six time points into the REM period. In the first study, subjects rated the dream on a number of variables (Kramer et al., 1974); in the second study, independent judges did so (Kramer et al., 1975). Both ratings showed a significant effect of time for four variables: recall, emotion, anxiety, and pleasantness. A trend analysis showed they were all linear. However, emotion showed a quadratic (stepwise) change: 10 minutes was different than 5; 20 minutes was not different than 10, but was from 30. There was an intensity increase up to 10 minutes, a plateau between 10 and 20, and then a rise to 30 minutes. We replicated (Johnson, Kramer, Bonnet, Roth, & Jansen, 1980) a study by Azerinsky (1971) that showed a 20-minute eye movement cycle during REM sleep. This suggests a relationship between eye movement distribution and reported dream content intensity.

The third study supporting the existence of the dream as an experience during sleep involved comparing a report of a dream and a nightmare from the same subjects (Taub et al., 1978). A similar group of subjects gave a report of what they thought a nightmare was like (a confabulated nightmare). The experienced dream reports were mainly similar but on some dimensions significantly different. The dreams were friendlier, and they had less apprehension and fewer misfortunes than the nightmares. Confabulated nightmares compared to experienced nightmares had more aggression, movement activity, intensity and misfortune, and they had less friendliness. Subjects reported confabulated nightmares in half the words of both experienced nightmares and ordinary dreams. The similarity of experienced dreams and their difference from a confabulated dream further suggests an experience is occurring.

In the fourth study, we provided a stimulus during REM sleep in an attempt to have it incorporated into the dream experience (Kramer et al., 1983). During REM sleep we played either a familiar or unfamiliar name in the subject's own recorded voice. We found that the familiar name was incorporated into the subjects' dream reports more often than the unfamiliar name. The familiar name was five times more likely to be incorporated than the unfamiliar (59% vs 11%). The name was mentioned in the dream report about as far into the report as the time into REM sleep when the stimulus was given. The subjects did not report hearing the name. Apparently during sleep an ongoing experience is occurring that the dreamer is reporting on awakening.

The second question to be asked is, does the dream report give a reasonable approximation of the dream experience? We did a number of dream studies that support the veridical nature of the dream report. The first and second studies described earlier (Kramer et al., 1974, 1975) found that the rise and fall of affect across the REM period coincides with the pattern of eye movement cycles during REM sleep (Azerinsky, 1971; Johnson et al., 1980). In a group that slept 20 consecutive nights in the laboratory, we were able to distinguish those dream reports collected early in the series from those collected toward the end of the series (Kramer, Roth, & Cisco, 1977). We were also able to show a greater incorporation of known names into dream reports and also show that the names appeared at approximately the correct time into the dream report (Kramer et al., 1983). We also found that dream intensity across the REM period has a time pattern identical to that of the eye movement cycles, that external influences (starting and stopping an activity) can be distinguished in dream reports, and that stimuli are incorporated into the dream report at approximately the time during the REM period when it was introduced. These findings all support the view that the dream report does reflect the dream experience.

Now we know that the dream is an experience during sleep that is extended in time and that the dream report does adequately reflect the experience. If we are to explore dreaming scientifically, we need to be able to collect the dream report and establish that it can be reliably and validly evaluated.

The factors that influence the collection of dreams are (1) the place where the dream is experienced and reported, (2) the method of awakening, (3) the interpersonal nature of the reporting, (4) the style of collection, (5) the stage of sleep, and (6) the type of subject reporting (Kramer, Winget, & Roth, 1975). We did a study of dream recall that showed the following classical factors influencing recall even in schizophrenic patients: recency, primacy, length, and dramatic intensity (Trinder & Kramer, 1971).

We wanted to compare the reliability of quantifying dream report content to scoring sleep physiology to see if they were discordant or comparable. We did a reliability study by having two judges score seven parameters of sleep physiology every 30 seconds for eight hours of two sleep records (polysomnograms) for 11 subjects for 15 consecutive nights (Roth, Kramer, & Roehrs, 1977). The average reliability for sleep physiology across all parameters scored was 92.5%. The mean successive night-to-night correlation of sleep stages for time data was 0.28 and for percentage data was 0.44. Next, we had 14 college-age subjects sleep for 20 consecutive nights and awakened them for dream report collection from the first four REM periods of each night (Kramer & Roth, 1979). The blinded reports were scored by two judges on the characters, activities, and descriptive elements scales of the Hall–Van de Castle system (Hall & Van De Castle, 1966). The overall percentage agreement on each dream report was 91% on all three scales. The mean dream content of each night of sleep was correlated with the successive night's sleep. The average overall correlation was 0.46. It is striking that the reliability of scoring of sleep and dream reports is essentially the same: 92.5% and 91%, respectively. The stability of measurement across 2 weeks is also nearly identical: 0.44 and 0.46. The choice to study sleep physiology versus dreaming is one of interest, not that one is science and the other is not. We found the frequency of items on the Hall–Van de Castle dream scoring system that were scored on laboratory-collected reports to be the same as on reports that were not collected in the laboratory (Sandler, Kramer, Fishbein, & Trinder, 1969; Sandler, Kramer, Trinder, & Fishbein, 1970). In addition, the frequency of items showed excellent validity (Kramer, Roth, & Palmer, 1976). We summarized a total of 123 dream content scoring systems and provided tables illustrating what has been found using them (Winget & Kramer, 1979). We also demonstrated the validity of dream reports in our finding of content differences where we believed there were psychological differences for demographic variables, for example, or for gender, age, marital status, and social class (Winget, Kramer, & Whitman, 1972), or for mental illness variables such as schizophrenia and major depression (Kramer, Baldridge, Whitman, Orenstein, & Smith, 1969).

For dreams to have the possibility of having meaning, dream reports should reflect content differences where we have reason to believe psychological differences exist. Indeed, that is the case both at a group and individual level. There are group differences among demographic variables, namely sex, age social class, race, and marital status (Winget et al., 1972). The dreamer's sex is the major organizer of dream content. In a later study, we found 35 non-laboratory studies that showed male/female differences in dream content (Winget & Kramer, 1979). Men reported more unpleasant dreams, including dreams of mutilation, and women reported more intimacy. The Hall–Van de Castle (1966) dream content norms were derived from 500 dreams from 100 college-age males and 500 from

100 college-age females, and they compare the frequency and proportions of various categories. The systematic and large number of male/female content differences is striking. Women have more characters in their dreams; men have more males in their dreams, while women have an equal percentage of characters of each sex. Men have more physically aggressive encounters, women more friendly interactions. Sexual interactions are not common in dreams, but when they do occur they are three times as common in men's dreams as in women's. Emotions are found more often in women's dreams. Women's dreams are set indoors, and men's are set outdoors. A laboratory study of 20 consecutive nights of 11 men and women who had their REM dreams collected (594 from the former and 596 from the latter) found that 11 of 45 scales showed significant differences between men and women (Kramer et al., 1983). Women had more thinking and intensity references; men had more male characters, strangers, auditory activity, achromatic colors, large sizes, and crooked or curved references. In our population study based in Cincinnati, Ohio, we asked a stratified, random sample of subjects to tell a dream (Winget et al., 1972). We found nine content differences between male and female subjects. Women had more dreams with characters, friendly social interactions, emotions, indoor settings, and references to home and family. Men had increases on the following scales: aggression, achievement striving with success, castration anxiety, and overt hostility. The four studies that I have just reviewed clearly support dream content differences between men and women. Interestingly, many of the differences are replicated across studies.

We found 20 non-laboratory dream content studies that deal with the **age** of the dreamer showing changes across the lifespan from 2 to 92 (Winget & Kramer, 1979). Unpleasant dreams decrease in frequency between the ages of 1 and 4, and again between the ages of 9 and 12. Children's dreams include less aggression than adults. Anxiety decreases with age, while sex differences in aggression increase with age. Adolescents have more destructive themes, castration threats, and concern with personal safety than do adults. Dream content changes between ages 3 and 15 mirror waking cognitive development. Older adults, over 65, have more dreams involving lost resources, helplessness, or weakness. In our Cincinnati population survey, we found that references to death and death anxiety were directly correlated with age (Winget et al., 1972). Guilt anxiety was highest among young adults aged 21–34. Young adults are concerned with right and wrong while the elderly are concerned with decline and dying. Nonetheless, age appears to be less important in determining dream content than the sex of the dreamer as described earlier.

We calculated the socioeconomic class of our population sample based on the education and income of the respondents and then divided the group into three classes: lower, middle, and upper middle (Winget et al., 1972). We found that the dreams of upper-middle class respondents had fewer characters, less death anxiety, and fewer premonitions. Misfortune was more common in the dreams of the lower two classes. For white respondents in the upper-middle class there was less total anxiety and fewer dreams with home and family themes than for other respondents. In this survey, the upper-middle class has a less troubled dream life than the lower classes.

We found very few dream content differences related to the race or marital status of the dreamer (Winget et al., 1972). The dreams of black men included more castration anxiety and penis envy. The dreams of white respondents had more covert hostility directed outward. The dreams of widows had the most death anxiety. Subjects who were formerly married and were widowed, divorced, or separated dreamed more of family members from the family of marriage rather than their family of origin, and they had more premonition dreams.

From a demographic point of view, the main determinant of dream content is the sex of the dreamer, with a moderate contribution from age and social class, and only a minimal contribution from their race or marital status. The frequencies in our population study (Winget et al., 1972) are similar to what Hall and Van de Castle (1966) reported from their study of college-age dreamers. The differences from Hall–Van de Castle may be attributable to the population study having shorter dreams and a wider age range.

We would expect to find dream content differences at the group level for dreamers who suffer from major psychiatric illnesses such as schizophrenia, depression, or dementia. This would further support that dreams may be seen as meaningful and that a search for meaning can be seen as a more reasonable undertaking.

We collected and examined the most recent dream reports from 40 schizophrenic patients, 40 psychotically depressed, and 40 medical patients in a Veterans' Administration hospital; all were male (Kramer, Baldridge, Whitman, Ornstein, & Smith, 1969). The dream reports were examined for plausibility, hostility direction, and major character type. The typical dream report of the paranoid schizophrenic patient finds him in an implausible situation in which he is being attacked by a stranger. The psychotically depressed patient typically reports dreaming of a family member, usually in a plausible situation. Hostility is present about half the time, and this is as likely to be addressed toward others as toward the dreamer. The nonpsychotic medical patient reports dreaming of being with a friend in a plausible situation that is rarely hostile. If it is hostile, he is as likely to be the expresser as the recipient of the hostility.

The dreams of patients with depression (Kramer, Whitman, Baldridge, & Lansky, 1966; Kramer, Whitman, Baldridge, & Orenstein, 1968) and schizophrenia (Kramer, Clark, & Day, 1973; Kramer & Roth, 1973; Kramer, Trinder & Roth, 1972; Kramer et al., 1969) show systematic changes concomitant with improvement in their waking condition. Depressed patients with improvement show a decrease in hostility and anxiety and an increase in heterosexuality and motility scale scores. When improved, the schizophrenic patients showed more concise and better organized dreams with proportionally fewer aggressive interactions compared with friendly ones, fewer emotions, and more success and good fortune. In our REM dream studies, the most frequent characters in the dreams of depressed patients were family members, and in the dreams of schizophrenics were strangers (Kramer et al., 1969). These results were similar to our non-laboratory studies. We also found that schizophrenics had more groups of people in their dreams than depressed patients. Both groups showed change in their dreams as they improved clinically.

We compared small groups of mildly, moderately and severely brain damaged subjects in the laboratory and collected reports of their REM dreams (Kramer & Roth, 1975). Our only statistically significant finding is that patients with severe brain damage had more characters in their dreams than did patients with mild brain damage. In addition, age and severity of damage decreased recall of dreams. Compared to the Hall–Van de Castle norms, the dreams of the middle-aged group with brain damage had more family members, more friendly social interactions, and fewer aggressive interactions. They also did not include emotions. Age and brain damage are associated with changes in dream content.

The studies I have reviewed so far show that dreams have differences at the group level in situations that we know have psychological difference. I will proceed to demonstrate differences that exist at the individual level (Kramer, Hlasny, Jacobs, & Roth, 1976). Judges were able to correctly sort a group of 75 REM dream reports into five groups of 15—one group for each normal subject. They did the same for 65 REM dream reports from five schizophrenic subjects, sorting them correctly into groups of 13. This supports the view that dreams of different individuals are indeed distinguishable from each other. We then gave our judges 15 REM dream reports, three from each of five nights, from each of 10 college students and from five schizophrenic patients. The judges were asked to sort each packet of dreams into sets of three dreams each. They were able to do this successfully for the students and the patients. This showed that dreams were different night to night for each individual. Finally, we asked our judges to properly order the position of the REM dreams within a night, using 50 sets of three dreams from the college students and 34 sets of three dreams from the patients. This attempt was not successful.

During the same study we were able to use group data to show a positional effect within the night. We examined the first four REM dreams of 22 subjects, each of whom slept in the laboratory for 20 consecutive nights. The dream report word counts showed that REM I was shorter than REM II, and REM III was shorter than REM IV, but REM II and REM III were not different. With word length held constant, we found nine content differences across the night: four between REM I and REM II, and five between REM II and REM III, but none between REM III and REM IV. The findings suggest a positional difference across the night.

Where we know there are psychological differences between groups, we find meaningful differences in their dreams. In addition, the dreams of individuals are different from each other—as are the dreams of one night different from those of another. Even within one night, the content of a REM period could depend on its position in the series of dreams. Within one REM period there is the orderly development of dream content.

The emotional preoccupation of the dreamer (his or her immediate current concern) significantly influences the content of the subsequent dreams. It is the more intense emotional experience of the day that appears in dreams (Piccione, Jacobs, Kramer, & Roth, 1977). Emotionally laden experiences such as beginning and ending a relationship are identifiable in dream reports (Kramer et al., 1977). In addition, the emotional nature of the interpersonal experience between the dreamer and the dream collector helps determine which of the night's dreams is reported (Whitman, Kramer, & Baldridge, 1963b). By varying the sex of the dream collector, we have shown how an emotionally charged situation is elaborated over a series of nights (Fox, Kramer, Baldridge, Whitman, & Ornstein, 1968). The continuing occurrence of sleep laboratory representation in the dreams of the night is evidence that dream content does not adapt across 20 nights (Whitman et al., 1963a). A medication that alters the emotional condition of the dreamer shows concomitant changes in their dream content (Kramer, Whitman, Baldridge, & Ornstein, 1968). Dream content appears to be both stable and variable, and night-to-night content correlation explains 21% of the variance (Roth et al., 1977). The emotional intensity of the pre-sleep experience apparently determines its impact on dreaming.

For dreams to have meaning, they must be orderly and not random, signal not noise. Meaning does not exist in the dream. To establish the meaning of the dream, a meaning system must be applied to the dream content. The Talmud says that the meaning of the dream follows its interpretation. The evidence that dreams are orderly includes (1) the organization of dreams across REM periods (Kramer et al., 1974); (2) the difference in dream content in each REM period of the night (Kramer, McQuarie, & Bonnet, 1980; (3) the differences in dream content from night to night within an individual (Kramer et al., 1976); (4) the correlation of dream content from night to night within an individual (Kramer & Roth, 1970); (5) the differences in dream content among individuals, whether normal or mentally ill (Kramer et al., 1976); and (6) the differences in dream content among groups based on demographic variables (Winget et al., 1972) and mental illness such as schizophrenia and depression (Kramer et al., 1969; Kramer & Roth, 1973). That dreams are structured and show differences where psychological differences are known to exist lends credence to the possibility that dreams have meaning.

Dreams are responsive to the emotional concerns of the dreamer. My colleagues and I have shown that (1) the more emotionally rated experience of the day is found in the night's dream report; (2) judges can distinguish in dreams the reflections of significant immediate (Kramer et al., 1977) and ongoing (Piccione, Thomas, Roth, & Kramer, 1976) emotional events (including the beginning and ending of the laboratory experience and the laboratory experience itself as an ongoing experience); (3) charged interpersonal experiences influence the content and reporting of the dream (e.g., the choice of the dream to be reported) (Whitman et al., 1963b); the impact of the supervisory experience in psychotherapy (Whitman et al., 1963a) and the relationship in the laboratory of the dreamer to the dream collector (Fox et al., 1968); (4) mood altering drugs change dream content (Kramer et al., 1968); (5) the mood-regulatory function of sleep relates the change in the sleepy aspect of mood across the night to the amount of non-REM sleep the sleeper has had, while the change in the unhappy aspect of mood is a function of who one dreams about (Kramer, 1993a); and (6) the dream experience as it is occurring can be influenced by meaningful input such as the differential incorporation of known and unknown names (Kinney, Kramer, & Bonnet, 1981; Kramer et al., 1983; Kinney & Kramer, 1985).

Dreams have the necessary relationships to have psychological meaning. Dreaming is an orderly event that is structured and reflects important psychological differences, responds to immediate emotional concerns, and is related to the waking preoccupations of the dreamer. Meaning does not exist in dreams but is brought to it from some external system of meaning. Examples of meaning systems that have been applied to dreams include the depth psychological systems of Freud, Adler, and Jung (Van de Castle, 1994).

I have described a system to establish the meaning of dreams called *dream translation* (Kramer, 1991, 1993b; Kramer & Roth, 1977). This system is based on treating the dream as a figure of speech, utilizing neo-Freudian interpersonal parameters and assuming a relatively strict determinism in approaching the dream report.

The dream translation method has a series of assumptions, orientations, and rules that serve to guide the translation. There are three deterministic and causal assumptions: (1) the dream report is determined; (2) the order of elements in the dream report is determined; and (3) the order of elements in the report is causal. One must examine all elements in the report and take into account the actual relationships in the report.

Dream reports may be approached by the dream interpreter from three psychological points of view and any of three responsive roles. The three points of view are (1) the interpersonal, in which the dreamer is in relation to other people; (2) the intrapsychic, in which the dream is read as if the elements are all part of the self; and (3) the narcissistic or self-psychological, which focuses on the vagaries of the dreamer's self-esteem. The three responsive roles in which the dream may be seen by the dream interpreter are (1) reflective, simply displays dreamer's preoccupations; (2) reactive, translate and then speculate as to what it is reacting too; (3) anticipatory, translate and speculate on what is being anticipated.

The dream translator assumes the dream is a metaphor and the meaning is other than what a literal reading would yield. The translator substitutes his or her associations for the dreamer's to each element in the dream report. The translator starts at the beginning of the report. Successive associations to each dream element, which are assumed to be causal, serve to constrain the associational breadth and focus the search for meaning. This sequential approach yields a narrative.

The approach of dream translation is based on our common human experience as described by Dilthey and incorporates a cognitive and empathic point of view (Palmer, 1969). The constraining effect of associations to successive dream elements is analogous to the corrective value of dialogue to establish meaning described by Schliermacher (Palmer, 1969). Dream translation is a hermeneutic, yet is better perhaps described an exegesis as it is a search for the meaning of a text, the dream report. The dream translator is searching for an understanding that fits the dreamer's situation and that is helpful. The search for meaning is connotative, associative, and figurative. It explores the metaphoric structuring of our subjective world, as the meaning is in the metaphor (Lakoff & Johnson, 2003). The dream report has to be seen as its own context, and the translator has to get into the dream. The choice between possibilities has to be guided by likelihood, as dreams can have multiple meanings.

Explanatory paradigms from depth psychological schools can be helpful. For example, psychoanalysis suggests that three-person situations may be oedipal; same-sex and opposite-sex pairs may be homosexual or heterosexual; peers may be siblings; and movement towards, attraction and aversion, rejection and dependency may imply on someone for something. The formula "on someone for something" applies to all impulses.

The dream translator must stay close to the text, interpreting only what is in the text. We cannot deal with reversals in the text. However dichotomies always imply the other half of the dichotomy (Chandler, 2002). In providing the substitute text, Occam's law applies. Applications of the methodology are available, one to the dream report of a Vietnam veteran (Kramer & Roth, 1977) and the other to the Irma dream, the so-called dream specimen of psychoanalysis (Kramer, 1999).

We create our own world: a subjective, affective, figurative one. As the Buddha said, "With our thoughts we make the world." This is the world the dream translator tries to capture. How may this approach to dream reports be helpful in the clinical situation?

The psychodynamic theme from a dream translation of the first dream reported can predict the core psychodynamic theme to be found in therapy (Glucksman & Kramer, 2011, 2012). For example, in an initial dream in therapy, a patient reported: "I am in the military and going off to war. I don't want to go and I try to figure out how to get out of it" (Glucksman & Kramer, 2011). The patient's therapist offered this psychodynamic theme: "This dream is about feeling trapped and wanting to escape. However, the dreamer is uncertain as to how he can accomplish this. He feels scared, vulnerable and unable to protect himself." The external rater who only had the dream report offered this theme: "The dreamer is in a situation where he has to go along with a group [work, social, religious] that can make him do things he doesn't want to do. It may be dangerous and he wants out.

However, he could be punished or rejected if he tries to leave." The principal current concern for the dreamer/patient was that he was in a power struggle with one of his peers at work. He felt very threatened and was afraid of being humiliated if his rival prevailed. He thought about leaving his job, but was uncertain about his future if he did so. He felt anxious, vulnerable, and stymied. The similarity is apparent between the two themes offered and is relatable to the current concern of the dreamer. It provides a potentially valuable early clinical insight to how the patient feels and what he is grappling with at the time.

It is likely that changes in dream reports across psychotherapy, such as the change in affective valence and narrative structure of a manifest dream report (MDR) from negative to positive, would reflect improvement. It is clinically helpful to have a sense of whether the therapy has progressed. Change or lack of change from first to last MDR has been shown to co-vary with improvement or lack of improvement in psychotherapy (Glucksman & Kramer, 2004). The first MDR in psychotherapy is more likely to be affectively negative rather than positive, while when clinically improved it is more likely to be positive than negative (Kramer & Glucksman, 2006; Glucksman & Kramer, 2012) as is the dream as a narrative (Glucksman & Kramer, 2012).

At times of a block in psychotherapy the MDR gives clues as to what may be transpiring. A resident reported a patient's dream in which the two of them were squabbling over a piece of cake. The patient finally said, "You can have it." This suggested that the patient felt the resident/therapist was competing with the patient and getting things from the therapy (possibly satisfaction/success) that the patient wanted. It was an alerting insight for the therapist (Personal Communication).

Summary

The dream exists as an experience extended in time that can be captured in the dream report as an excellent approximation of the experience. Dreams can be adequately collected and reliably measured. Dream reports are both stable and variable across time. Dream reports show meaningful content differences in group and individual situations where psychological differences are known to exist. Dreams and waking life are linked and dreams are responsive to the immediate emotional concern of the dreamer. The dream is sufficiently orderly and the search for its meaning is justified. The meaning of the dream experience can be established through various methods that involve working with dreamer through associations or amplification. One such method, dream translation, involves exploring the meaning of the dream report by using the associations of the translator rather than the dreamer. The clinician could use this translation approach to assess whether the patient has improved and to establish the immediate current emotional concern of the patient at initial contact or at points of block in the therapy.

In closing, although the dream report has the characteristics necessary to establish a meaning, does not address the possible functional significance of dreaming.

My colleagues and I have explored this question in a monograph on dream function in which I describe my selective, mood-regulatory function of dreaming (Moffitt, Kramer, & Hoffman, 1993).

References

Azerinsky E. Rapid eye movement density and pattern in the sleep of normal young adults. Psychophysiology. 1971; 8:361–375.

Chandler D. Semiotics: The basics. New York: Routledge; 2002.

Fox R, Kramer M, Baldridge B, Whitman R, Ornstein P. The experimenter variable in dream research. Diseases of the Nervous System. 1968; 29:698–701.

Glucksman M, Kramer M. Using dreams to assess clinical change. Journal of the American Academy of Psychoanalysis and Dynamic Psychiatry. 2004; 32:345–358.

Glucksman M, Kramer M. The clinical and predictive value of the initial dream of treatment Journal of the American Academy of Psychoanalysis and Dynamic Psychiatry. 2011; 39:263–283.

Glucksman M, Kramer M. Initial and last manifest dream reports of patients in psychodynamic psychotherapy and combined psychotherapy and pharmacotherapy. Psychodynamic Psychiatry. 2012; 40:617–634.

Hall C, Van de Castle R. The content analysis of dreams. New York: Appleton-Century-Crofts; 1966.

Johnson B, Kramer M, Bonnet M, Roth, Jansen T. The effect of Ketazolam on ocular motility during REM sleep. Current therapeutic research. 1980; 28:792–799.

Kinney L, Kramer M. Sleep and sleep responsivity in disturbed sleepers. Sleep Research. 1985; 14:178.

Kinney L, Kramer M, Bonnet M. Dream incorporation of meaningful names. Sleep Research. 1981; 10:157.

Kramer M. Dream translation: A non-associative method for understanding the dream. Dreaming. 1991; 1:147–159.

Kramer M. The selective mood regulatory function of dreaming: An update and revision. In: Moffit A, Kramer M, Hoffman R, editors. The functions of dreaming. Albany: State University of New York Press; 1993a. p. 139–196.

Kramer M. Dream translation: An approach to understanding dreams. In: Delaney G, editor. New directions in dream interpretation. Albany: State University of New York Press; 1993b. p. 155–194.

Kramer M. Unresolved problems in the dream of Irma's injection. Journal of the American Academy of Psychoanalysis. 1999; 27:253–263.

Kramer M. The dream experience: A systematic exploration. New York: Routledge, Taylor & Francis; 2007.

Kramer M, Baldridge B, Whitman R, Ornstein P, Smith P. An exploration of the manifest dream in schizophrenic and depressed patients. Diseases of the Nervous System. 1969; 30 Suppl: S126–130.

Kramer M, Clark J, Day N. Dreaming in schizophrenia. In: Zikmund V, editor. The oculomotor system and brain function. London: Butterworths; 1973. p. 439–452.

Kramer M, Czaya J, Arand D, Roth T. The development of psychological content across the REM period. Sleep Research. 1974; 3:121.

Kramer M, Glucksman, M. Changes in manifest dream affect during psychoanalytic treatment. Journal of the American Academy of Psychoanalysis and Dynamic Psychiatry. 2006; 34:249–260.

Kramer M, Hlasny R, Jacobs G, Roth T. Do dreams have meaning? An empirical inquiry. American Journal of Psychiatry. 1976; 133:778–781.

Kramer M, Kinney L, Scharf M. Dream incorporation and dream function. In: Koella W, editor. Sleep 1982. Basel: S. Karger; 1983. p. 369–371.

Kramer M, McQuarie E, Bonnet M. Dream differences as a function of REM period. Sleep Research. 1980; 9:155.

Kramer M, Roth T. A comparison of dream content in laboratory collected dream reports of schizophrenic and depressed patient groups. Comprehensive Psychiatry. 1973; 14:325–329.

Kramer M, Roth T. Dreams and dementia: A laboratory exploration of dream recall and dream content in chronic brain syndrome patients. International Journal of Aging and Human Development. 1975; 6:179–182.

Kramer M, Roth T. Dream translation. Israel Annals of Psychiatry and Related Disciplines. 1977; 15:336–351.

Kramer M, Roth T. The stability and variability of dreaming. Sleep. 1979; 1:319–325.

Kramer M, Roth T, Cisco J. The meaningfulness of dreams. In: Koella W, Levin P, editors. Sleep 1976, Basel: S. Karger; 1977. p. 324–326.

Kramer M, Roth T, Czaya J. Dream development within a REM period. In: Koella W, Levin P, editors. Sleep 1974, Basel: S. Karger; 1975. p. 406–408.

Kramer M, Roth T, Palmer T. The psychological nature of the REM dream report and T.A.T. stories. Psychiatric Journal of the University of Ottawa. 1976; 1:128–135.

Kramer M, Trinder J, Roth T. Dream content analysis of male schizophrenic patients. Canadian Psychiatric Assn J. 1972; 17 Suppl 2: S251–257.

Kramer M, Whitman R, Baldridge B, Lansky L. Dreaming in the depressed. Canadian Psychiatric Assn J. 1966; 11 Suppl: S178–192.

Kramer M, Whitman R, Baldridge B, Ornstein P. Drugs and dreams III. The effects of imipramine on the dreams of depressed patients. American Journal of Psychiatry. 1968; 124:1385–1392.

Kramer M, Winget C, Roth T. Problems in the definition of the REM dream. In: Koella W, Levin P, editors. Sleep 1972, Basel: S. Karger; 1975. p. 149–152.

Lakoff G, Johnson M. Metaphors we live by. Chicago: University of Chicago Press; 2003.

Moffitt A, Kramer M, Hoffman R (Eds.) The functions of dreaming. Albany: State University of New York Press; 1993.

Palmer R. Hermeneutics: Interpretation theory in Schliermacher, Dilthey, Heidegger and Gadamer. Evanston, IL: Northwestern University Press; 1969.

Piccione P, Jacobs G, Kramer M, Roth T. The relationship between daily activities, emotions and dream content. Sleep Research. 1977; 6:133.

Piccione P, Thomas S, Roth T, Kramer M. Incorporation of the laboratory in dreams. Sleep Research. 1976; 5:120.

Roth T, Kramer M, Roehrs T. The consistency of sleep measures. In: Koella W, Levin P, editors. Sleep 1976, Basel: S. Karger; 1977. p. 286–288.

Sandler L, Kramer M, Fishbein H, Trinder J. Interlaboratory reliability of the Hall–Van de Castle character scale. Psychophysiology. 1969; 6:248.

Sandler L, Kramer M, Trinder J, Fishbein H. Interlaboratory reliability of the Hall–Van de Castle characters, social interactions, activities and emotions scales. Psychophysiology. 1970; 7:333.

Taub J, Kramer M, Arand D, Jacobs G. Nightmare dreams and nightmare confabulations. Comprehensive Psychiatry. 1978; 19:285–291.

Trinder J, Kramer M. Dream recall. American Journal of Psychiatry. 1971; 128:296–301.

Van de Castle R. Our dreaming mind. New York: Ballantine Books; 1994.
Whitman R, Kramer M, Baldridge B. Which dream does the patient tell? Archives of General Psychiatry. 1963a; 8:277–282.
Whitman R, Kramer M, Baldridge B. Experimental study of supervision of psychotherapy. Archives of General Psychiatry. 1963b; 106:529–535.
Winget C, Kramer M. Dimensions of dreams. Gainesville: University Press of Florida; 1979.
Winget C, Kramer M, Whitman R. Dreams and demography. Canadian Psychiatric Assn J. 1972; 17 Suppl 2: S203–208.

2

TEACHING DREAM INTERVIEWING FOR CLINICAL PRACTICE

Loma K. Flowers

CLINICAL PROFESSOR OF PSYCHIATRY,
UNIVERSITY OF CALIFORNIA, SAN FRANCISCO

Introduction

Although the practice of dream interpretation has a venerable history worldwide that spans at least four millennia from Babylon and Egypt to China and medieval Islam, the teaching of dream interpretation to novices (Pesant & Zadra, 2004) has been far less extensively explored. Most known written works on dream interpretation focus on the meanings of dreams (Delaney, 1998). However, teaching is essential to assure a pipeline of competent practitioners.

Of the early extant writings, the second century AD Greek text, *Oneirocritica* [The Interpretation of Dreams] is notable for the significant attention Artimedorus devoted to actually teaching dream interpretation. However, those last two of his five books that focused on technique were intended for the sole use of his son, and explicitly not for the public or other practitioners. This deliberate cloak of mystery around deciphering the meaning of dreams foreshadows the proprietary secrets of medieval guilds and possibly contributes to the dearth of literature today.

This gap persisted despite Freud's *The Interpretation of Dreams* in 1900, which established dreams in clinical practice. Subsequently, numerous writers contributed to dream interpretation theory, e.g., Jung (1974), Boss (1977), Ullman and Zimmerman (1979), and Delaney (1981). However, I can find no parallel traditions of teaching outside of the analytic institutes. Moreover, even there, advanced candidates and graduates have reported their training inadequate, leading to "missing opportunities to make productive use dreams in their clinical work" (Levy, 2009).

One earlier exception was the annual meetings of the International Association for the Study of Dreams (IASD), founded in 1983. Those IASD conferences always included workshops primarily led by well-known writers on dreams and designed to demonstrate, teach and/or coach the various methodologies practiced by the diversely trained leaders. The participants were an eclectic group of professionals—from sleep researchers to clinicians—and nonprofessionals devoted to dreams.

Fortunately, interest in teaching the practice of dream interpretation has slowly emerged (Krippner, Gabel, Green, & Rubien, 1994), supported by observations that although clients may not gain significantly from training in dream work (Rochlen, Ligiero, Hill, & Heaton, 1999), trained clinicians were more likely to work with dreams (Crook & Hill, 2003). Nonetheless, opportunities remain limited for formal training in dream interpretation beyond personal initiative, e.g. continuing education and self-study (Keller et al., 1995).

In this era of intense interest in neurobiology, it would be easy to continue to ignore training in dream interpretation. However, with the identification of the deficiency, there is also an opportunity. We can not only remedy the lack but also explore ways to increase our understanding of the psychobiologic mechanisms (Reiser, 2001), and enhance the exploration of dream interpretation as an effective agent for change through a therapeutic approach that is patient, clinician, and—in the long run—probably payer friendly.

I first selected Dream Interviewing (Flowers & Zweben, 1996) as a clinical model for dream interpretation because of two unique factors. First, it has a reproducible transparency that was unique when it was introduced as an interpretative technique (Delaney, 1981) and was also convincing to dreamers, enabling them to more easily accept insights available to them from dreams interpreted in this manner. Secondly, it was precociously culturally competent (Flowers, 1972) in its premise that the therapists' perspectives on the meanings of images, etc., were not necessarily relevant to the dreamer or the dream.

I was persuaded by empirical evidence to use Dream Interviewing for a training model. Early clinical application showed promising observations in both psychosomatic illness (Flowers, 1993) and substance abuse recovery (Flowers & Zweben, 1998). Greater dissemination of competent Dream Interviewers will support further study.

Overview of the Dream Interview Method

Dream Interviewing has been in clinical use for 40 years. In common with all dream interpretation techniques, it shares two assumptions and has a third unique assumption. The first shared assumption is that dreams have meanings that are almost always relevant to the waking life of the dreamer. The second shared assumption is that the meaning of a dream is best understood by treating the dream as a metaphor for a waking life issue.

The third groundbreaking assumption is that the interpreter shares no significant common knowledge with the dreamer about key images or actions in any dream. As a result, all information used to interpret the dream comes exclusively from the dreamer. With this profound shift, the traditional interpreter was unseated from the expert's chair and settled into the interviewer's chair. In this new role therapists use expertise and creativity to formulate questions, and carefully avoid cluttering interactions about dreams with statements about their own beliefs, knowledge, ideas, or interpretations. This interviewing role is facilitated by taking the perspective of an outsider inquiring of the dreamer about local habits, facts, feelings, and beliefs. For beginners this is a relief. For experienced practitioners it is a reminder to continually collaborate to explore, rather than assume.

When a patient agrees to work on a dream, the therapist's initial set of questions are designed to elicit a complete description of the dream narrative itself: the facts, feelings, thoughts, and actions *in the dream*, from start to finish. This seemingly straightforward step is quite difficult. Without specific training, therapists often omit it or struggle to get the dreamer to report dreams chronologically and delineate associations from dream narrative. With precise questioning, therapist and patient can complete the task together. I recommend silently filing the unavoidable tangential associations to other dreams and waking observations related to this dream as "editorial comments," and treat them as useful for the therapy but distinct from the dream being explored.

When asked, patients can almost always distinguish between forgetting parts of a dream and there having been no connection between various parts. These pieces of dreams can also be extremely useful although the resulting interpretations may feel incomplete, of course. But the dreamers' curiosity can then provide motivation to use dream incubation (Flowers, 1995), an invaluable presleep suggestion technique designed to focus a dream on answering a conscious question. For instance, one can ask a question about how to maximize overall health to support recovery of any kind. Clinicians can also incubate, "I need a dream that I will be comfortable interpreting in the dream seminar, nothing too personal." Both of these approaches have worked.

The second set of Dream Interview questions is designed to obtain precise but complete "descriptive definitions" of the major images in the dream. Occasionally, a descriptive definition may also be needed for complex actions, such as "I went shopping" or "we had sex." Novice therapists usually find this step is very complicated. Each description has seven components containing facts (physical description, function or personality, uniqueness, and essence), feelings (positive, negative, and beliefs and opinions), and relevant or powerful associations about those specific images. Insignificant associations are explicitly excluded. This latter differs from Freud (1965), Jung (1974), Ullman (1994), etc., who encourage freer associations and offer their own associations and interpretations to others' dreams. Here is an excerpt from a Dream Interview that illustrates a descriptive definition of Klonopin by a physician, an experienced dreamer who dreamed of that medicine.

DREAMER [COMPLETING HER ACCOUNT OF HER DREAM]: . . . to get my afternoon dose of Klonopin . . .
INTERVIEWER: What's Klonopin?

DREAMER: It's a medicine that you take for anxiety, and seizures and insomnia. It calms you down; it can lead to injuries, and can be addictive and you can abuse it. It works well.

The third interpretive or bridging step requires summarizing the dream in small segments, substituting the descriptive definitions for the images, and then asking the dreamer to scan his or her waking life for a match to the dream as a metaphor. Here is an example of bridging that followed the Klonopin definition quoted earlier.

INTERVIEWER: Is there anywhere in your life that you take something for anxiety etc. that calms you down but can be . . . ?
DREAMER: That's yoga and I do sometimes overdo it . . . I don't take medication.

The final reflection step of Dream Interviewing on the implications for action, both intrapersonal and external/interpersonal, is also found in Hill's Cognitive-Experimental Model.

Choice of Dream Interviewing for Training Purposes

There are a number of other features that make Dream Interviewing suitable—and desirable—for widespread training. The transparent assumptions and stepwise process are easy for a clinician to briefly explain to clients/patients. The interview process is also simple to reproduce consistently across interviewers, so students can learn from watching one another in a seminar or workshop and patients can learn the process fairly quickly by working with a few dreams. Dream Interviewing can also be self-reinforcing because even limited skills can yield useful information and repeated practice can increase the productive bridges from dreams.

Clinical experience with Dream Interviewing has confirmed that both the plot (actions) and the feelings in a dream remain constant in the waking life bridge or interpretation (Flowers, 1993). There may be variation in intensity, but not quality. In fact, the actions and feelings described in the interview form the basis of what is essentially a psychodynamic formulation of the waking-life issue addressed in the dream. This makes Dream Interviewing an invaluable tool blending elements of both cognitive behavioral therapy [CBT] and psychodynamic psychotherapy [PDT]. Here is a summary of one dreamer's experience with two sequential Dream Interviews, including his resulting insights and their relevance to changing behavior.

> One man had a repetitive dream in which he was repeatedly doing the same [unrealistic] action, and getting more and more frustrated and angry when it did not work. After his first bridge and some therapeutic work on the interpretation, his next dream had a similar plot but the feelings had changed to

boredom. In treatment, he finally began speculating about discontinuing the old repetitive and frustratingly unproductive behavior that he was loathe to relinquish.

For training, beginning Dream Interviewers often prefer to work in pairs to interview a dreamer simultaneously, helping each other out when posing questions to the dreamer. Most dreamers tolerate this well. They often appreciate the differences in wording because the variations help them find and articulate the answers needed to compose their definitive descriptions. As a result, the trainees learn effective questioning skills from each other, becoming more conscious of their unconscious biases and projections, as well as broadening their repertoires to encompass an ever-widening diversity of dreams and dreamers.

When a dreamer offers the same dream, sequentially, for two different theoretically based interpretative processes, the first interpretation tends to contaminate the second. However, since the Dream Interview process is still often new to patients, I present it as an opportunity to see if there is anything *more* that we can learn from their dream using a second approach, and they decide. Dreamers then table their first interpretation to answer the descriptive Dream Interview questions. At the end, when they summarize their own understanding of each interpretation as part of the final wrap up, identifying the bridges they made from each image to their waking life, they begin consolidating insights, reflecting on the implications for action, both intrapersonal and external/interpersonal, and noting what was not understood. This allows an opportunity for reconciliation of both interpretations.

Experience in Training Clinicians in Dream Interpretation

In 30 years of experience in training clinicians in Dream Interviewing, I found that most established practitioners have customary ways of approaching their clinical work, which may or may not include dreams. Consequently, they have little interest in exploring further in dream tutorials. One exception was a self-selected group of experienced mental health clinicians who invited me to teach a professional dream seminar. They commented that in this seminar they felt safe to expose themselves and their clinical work to the degree necessary to learn the technique with their colleagues. We met regularly for a number of years. In contrast, senior practitioners attending the open group that included residents and early career psychiatrists only came for a few sessions and some residents mentioned that they were relieved by their absence.

One Dream Interviewing seminar began as a midday elective psychiatric residency course on campus and evolved into pro-bono, open-group, professional training sessions held in my office at 6 p.m. It consistently attracted a small number of participants, with no active recruiting beyond email and word-of-mouth information about time and place. Most of those who returned to the training course did so after having been intrigued by a demonstration of the precise process and the resulting powerful interpretations.

This seminar continued for more than 10 years. The participants were an evolving group of clinical trainees and early career clinicians (psychiatrists, psychologists, social workers, and marriage and family therapists), and one religious leader. They came from a radius of 30 miles around and attendance ranged from 15 at the beginning of a new academic year to one or two, with a usual turnout of around four or five participants. While they were all very interested in dreams, their commitments were often limited by time and energy. Early career psychiatrists who were eager to understand dream interpretation and include it in their developing practices were the most consistent attenders.

Teaching the Dream Interview Training Course

To set the tone for learning and actually practicing skills within each hour and a half session, the email orientation to the training course reminded learners to bring a dream—their own or a patient's. Trainees were given access to two written protocols in advance, one for the dreamer's preparation (Flowers, 2007a) and one for the actual Dream Interview itself (Flowers, 2007b). They were encouraged to use these outlines as necessary in their Dream Interviews and were continually reassured that their practice sessions were "not a quiz," and expertise was not expected. They were also repeatedly reminded in the first session and afterwards that the conceptualization of Dream Interviewing is simple, but mastery of interviewing skills—articulating the basic and follow-up questions in the necessary sequence—is a lengthy process that requires continual practice. In addition, references were made available for newcomers at their first attendance, or via email or online afterwards. This delay was deliberate to emphasize that no "expertise" was needed beyond the ability to ask questions and listen to the answers.

Rotating interview practice in the group allowed trainees the opportunity to reinforce their own and their colleagues' visible progress. In addition, the instructor would periodically assume the interviewer role to demonstrate a whole Dream Interview or a particular technique, or to pull together a fragmented Dream Interview. Students also requested help from their colleagues or the trainer to rescue a floundering interview and could resume their role after a breather.

The most productive training sessions require the dreamer to be present (i.e., a trainee amongst the group offers to share his or her personal dream) rather than bringing in a dream with descriptive definitions from a clinical session with a patient. This is important because inevitably key information is missing from any beginner's first Dream Interview with a patient. It is also helpful for trainees' learning to be able to discuss their experiences outside the Dream Interview training group, so we agreed upon partial parameters (i.e., dreamer's anonymity and confidentiality about the overall bridge from the dream) to protect colleagues' privacy. Then trainees made their own choices about sharing, and limits.

Some trainees are not comfortable sharing their own dreams. I occasionally shared parts of my professional development dreams as a way to normalize the process; for example, I shared a dream about a particular car I had when I began my psychiatric residency that I bridged to my independence. Trainees commented that this helped to build trust. In addition, I also explained that covert withholding is destructive to the Dream Interview process and the integrity of the group, so trainees were encouraged to *openly* withhold sharing a bridge if they understood a dream but did not want to share their waking life experience. Moreover, whenever I sensed that pending bridges might be too sensitive to share, I reminded the dreamers of their choice.

There was always one session on how to introduce clients to the idea of dream work in their therapy or to patients in other settings, such as medical or surgical inpatient units, because clinicians often find this surprisingly difficult. As their skills progressed, group members were used as consultants on individual work with clients'/patients' dreams. This served both to reinforce their application of Dream Interviewing to clinical practice and also to hone their skills.

Without theoretical assumptions of meaning (content) the course teaching necessarily focused on process, following the steps of the Dream Interview process, and training learners how to follow this replicable outline. Interviewers were encouraged to collaborate; this was reinforced by rotating the responsibility for orientating newcomers among the returning members of the group. Common challenges mentioned by trainees were routinely addressed and, like Crook-Lyon et al. (2009), I found that individual feedback fostered trainees' improvement.

For instance, the first challenge that trainees often comment on is the difficulty of getting a clear story of the whole dream. People generally do not speak linearly, so it is the clinicians' responsibility to get an accurate chronology of the dream narratives, usually by taking detailed notes. As one trainee said, "The notes remind [the clinician] of the dreamer's words and help keep [them] from slipping into their own vocabulary."

The second challenge in that process is obtaining *all* the feelings of the dreamer and the various characters in the dream, double-checking that each sentence has associated feelings. The temptation to *assume* feelings and details when listening to a dream is almost irresistible. Fortunately, these errors often show up later in a thorough interview process.

A third challenge for clinicians is to keep the dreamer emotionally and intellectually engaged throughout this preliminary process. Unfortunately this is particularly challenging for novices because the clarifications are often prolonged by their lack of expertise. They are reminded that it is better to lose a detail than to lose the dreamer's interest.

A fourth challenge is for clinicians to listen carefully to the answers to questions seeking a descriptive definition, without selecting, distorting, rephrasing, or "translating" in their mind. This requires entering the dreamer's vocabulary and speech style, respecting the dreamers' choice of words (even if they are "wrong" to the interviewer). This process also often necessitates clarifications of seemingly "obvious" meaning. For example, if a dreamer dreams of a platform, the answers to "What's a platform?" may vary depending upon whether the dreamer is a construction worker, a politician, or a programmer. Clinicians are required to convert any hypotheses into specific questions that test their hypotheses—without leading the dreamer to agree or disagree. The patients' answers will usually confirm or disprove the clinician's theories. Here is an example from a CME lecture, demonstrating this point by eliciting descriptive definitions from more than one participant, which is taboo in a real Dream Interview situation.

TRAINER: What's an SUV?
CLINICIAN #1: Wonderful roomy vehicles, great for carpooling and you are high up so you can see and be safe.
CLINICIAN #2: Abominations! They should not be allowed on the road! They guzzle gas, and their arrogant, entitled drivers almost force other cars like mine off the road all the time . . .

In an actual Dream Interview situation, the Interviewer would follow up with an inquiry about any other feelings about SUVs.

The trainer's input from observing the interaction is very important. Video recording can also help trainees see what they missed, since nonverbal communications—from body language to tone—are vital clues to the patients' feelings, censoring, and openness.

A fifth challenge is to synthesize even the most rambling description into a concise summary or recapitulation in the dreamer's words, retaining the key elements, which the dreamer often repeats. Checking that a dreamer thinks your recapitulation is accurate for each description is crucial, as is editing or amending together as needed until the dreamer unreservedly agrees with the description. The goal is thoroughness, without obsessing.

By the time the earlier parts of the Dream Interview are completed, the sixth challenge of the interpretative step, known as *bridging*, is usually eagerly awaited. Bridging involves matching the dream plot, feelings, and descriptive definitions with waking parallels. It is most easily accomplished with a relaxed, interested dreamer who is intrigued to discover what he or she can learn from their hard work in the previous five steps. The bridge question is, "Is there anywhere in your life that . . . ?" The clinician's task is to provide a receptive atmosphere, and time and space for the dreamer to search their conscious awareness. A Day Note—a recording of the important events and feelings of the day prior to the dream—can help jog a patient's memory.

Resistance to seeing or accepting a bridge can last days. One clinician trainee joked that he never understood any of his bridges until training was over and he was walking to his car alone. He realized he was avoiding vulnerability and updated the group next session.

Reflection on the dream, including writing out the interview questions and answers, helps consolidate insight. Subsequent dreams often pick up where the insight left off, and can even indicate a positive emotional development step.

Teaching Interpretive Shortcuts

Limited time is an insurmountable reality when working with clients, so once a clinician has the basic skills mastered, shortcuts can be helpful. Here are three.

First, bridging the setting in the dream usually delineates the area of life to which the dream refers, allowing the dreamer to focus subsequent bridge searches on that area of life. This saves time by not having to cast about the dreamer's whole life to find the closest fit for a bridge from each image. In the following example, *durable* described the essence of the Volvo dream image we were exploring, a key component for accurate bridging.

TRAINEE: I am riding in the back seat of an old four-door Volvo...
INTERVIEWER: Tell me about old four-door Volvos. What are they like?
TRAINEE: A sturdy, square sedan, a *durable* form of transportation—gets you from point A to B—pretty spacious for everyday transportation, can accommodate a small group, comfortable, reliable, not fancy, reminds me of another age, 60s and 70s, a sense of freedom.
INTERVIEWER: Where in your life are you traveling in a durable, pretty spacious, old, comfortable . . . way from point A to B?
TRAINEE: That's my professional life. . . . It's not a jeep!

Second, if the plot is distinctive, you can sometimes just bridge from the plot and feelings alone, without describing any of the images. Here is a dream that illustrates this well.

> A dreamer recalled a childhood dream in which he and a few other guys were pinned down under enemy fire. They were hiding in a ditch in some trees, scared. One by one they ran into the open to escape the trap. He watched each one get hit before reaching safety. He was the last to go.

INTERVIEWER: Think back to the time when you were as old as you were in the dream. Was there anywhere in your life then, where you were with some guys, pinned down by enemy/hostile fire and you watched them all get hit as they tried to run for safety?
DREAMER: Yes. My dad. My brothers were always getting shot down by my dad. My brothers tried to escape but they were all shot down. I was the youngest, so I watched it all happen.

A third shortcut, extremely valuable to intermediate and experienced interviewers, is to limit the descriptive definitions to the pivotal images in a dream.

I define a *pivotal image* as one around which the plot makes a major turn. For example, if the character in the dream is running down a mountain trail when suddenly a mountain lion springs out onto him, the lion is a pivotal image. Regardless of what happens next, that action will be subsequent to, and likely in response to, the attack by the lion. Getting the descriptive definition of the lion, or an even more pivotal image, adds a third reference point to bridging directly from a complicated plot and feelings. This addition increases the likelihood of an accurate bridge.

Interviewers can always test the accuracy of a shortcut bridge by obtaining the definition of a second pivotal or intriguing image that occurs in the course of the dream. If the shortcut dream bridge is accurate, all subsequent bridges developed from other descriptive definition will also match. When the second bridge does not make sense, something is amiss with the overall interpretation. The interviewer needs to go back to the full dream process and fill in the missing definitions, starting as usual with the setting.

Common Issues in Application of Dream Interviewing to Clinical Practices

In Glen Gabbard's words (2014), first quoting Hippocrates, "'It is more important to know what sort of person has a disease than to know what sort of disease a person has.' . . . Indeed, the core of psychodynamic psychiatry is to look at each individual as a person with highly individual, even idiosyncratic features." This perspective is supported by Dream Interviewing, which has been used with patients with multiple diagnoses from anxiety and depression to posttraumatic stress disorder (PTSD), including sexual abuse, and psychosis in remission. It has also been used in multiple settings from private practice and community clinics, to inpatient, consultation-liaison services and prisons.

Notwithstanding differing viewpoints on the use of dreams in spiritual care (Stranahan, 2011), individuals in religious life have also been trained in Dream Interviewing. In addition, a psychopharmacology practice could be very amenable to the use of Dream Interviewing. For instance, short dreams could provide a quick insight into compliance issues that often plague treatment. Since Dream Interviewing requires cognitive functioning to answer questions appropriately it is contraindicated for people with serious cognitive disorders, but educational level need not be considered.

Any dreamers with computer and printer access can download the instructions and complete much of the dream work prior to the session. The therapists' job is then to review the descriptive definitions—because it is easy to omit key parts when working alone—and then to ask the bridge questions. This collaboration saves time, leaving the bulk of the session for additional dreams or other therapeutic work, such as consolidating the insight with the general life issues and discussing alternative courses of action. It is possible that widespread expertise in Dream Interviewing or other interpretive techniques (Ullman, 1994) could lead to self-help dream groups, a free community resource parallel to the 12-step tradition with no cross talk, just questions.

Because Dream Interviewing can be very absorbing it can challenge the therapist's ability to manage the allocation of time. Skill is also needed to balance the focus between insights available from dreams and the overall treatment goals agreed upon together by patient and therapist. Additionally, even an experienced therapist can be overtaxed by the focused multitasking that Dream Interviewing requires. I recommend the usual therapeutic strategies of structure, focus, and boundaries.

Dreams as resistance is a well-known phenomenon, and an "inability" to bridge will stymie the best therapists. I recall one scene in a dream that a very insightful patient could not bridge. It remained unresolved until two years later, when it became clear in the therapy.

Conversely, in my experience denial is not always a reliable protection. The clarity of insight from Dream Interviewing can sometimes be daunting. As a result, trainees and patients can sometimes unintentionally overexpose themselves by bridging without adequate care for their own fragility. Therefore the bridging step of Dream Interviewing needs to be approached cautiously when the clinician suspects a patient may have difficulty handling an abrupt increase in either self-awareness or exposure. Therapists must manage these situations constructively. Trainers normalize them for trainees, possibly including a private conversation—after the training session—and appropriate recommendations for therapy if indicated.

Impact on the Professional Development of Clinicians

Since dreams reflect the dreamer's verbal, cognitive, and personality styles, they often challenge clinician interviewers' interpersonal communication skills, empathy, and ability to emotionally connect and create therapeutic alliances. As a result trainees are encouraged to practice repeatedly with a wide range of dreams and dreamers in many settings. Dream Interviewing training can also enhance trainees' precision in conceptual thinking and avoidance of assumptions, in addition to improving skills in questioning, attentive listening, hearing, and understanding nuances, as well as verbal communication using precise, client/patient-friendly wording while continually eliciting and integrating emotions appropriately. In addition, Dream Interviewing skills can also significantly expand cultural competence.

Additionally, trainees who opt to use their own dreams in the Dream Interviewing training seminar can benefit from insights furthering professional development, and sharing responses to similar stresses with other trainees. Since professional training is inevitably a time of considerable personal and professional growth for future therapists, the impact is addressed at multiple levels in dreams of trainees (Olsson, 1991). Here's a trainee example from an initial training session demonstration.

DREAMER: I was reclining in a chair, my hands resting on my belly. I was gently rubbing, feeling movement. I then noticed my stomach change size, a child growing inside of me. I continued to rub my belly, engaged in conversation. I felt very comfortable and relaxed, a new feeling but I was not surprised, it felt familiar.
TRAINER: So, tell me about a child growing inside you. What's that about?
DREAMER: [recapitulated] . . . a naïve, young new life that is a product of my nature and my environment and lifestyle. It's a self-product with a genetic and complete attachment, not separate; dependent. I felt a connection, love, enjoyment, and pleasure.
TRAINER: Is there anywhere in your life where you have "a naïve, young, new life . . . growing inside of you?"
DREAMER: [looked startled, then grinned] My professional work!

These "ah ha!" moments are very seductive to Dream Interviewers and dreamers alike. It is always worthwhile to test such bridges and establish that the supportive evidence is also there to confirm the accuracy and rule out the alternative hypothesis of an actual pregnancy.

TRAINER: I have to ask: Could this be literal, are you pregnant?
DREAMER: [shakes her head firmly] No. No, I'm not pregnant. The idea of a fetus is so removed from my life right now! No. It's my work. I am feeling very comfortable about my new professional skills and continuing growth.
TRAINER EDITORIAL: Prior to this dream, the trainee was less than half way through her program, and conscious of her inadequacies, This dream provided a more balanced perspective (Flowers, 1988), emphasizing the other aspects of her steep learning curve.

Discussions following such interpretations also lay the groundwork for the development of professional sensitivity to colleagues' stress. This can be invaluable for a lifetime of self-awareness and mutual awareness of and responsibility for professional impairment among peers.

References

Boss, M. (1977). *I Dreamt Last Night . . .* New York, NY: Gardner Press. Transl. S. Conway.
Crook, R. E., & Hill, C. E. (2003). Working with dreams in psychotherapy: The therapists' perspective. *Dreaming, 13*(2), 83–93.
Crook-Lyon, R. E., Hill, C. E., Wimmer, C. L., Hess, S. A., & Goates-Jones, M. K. (2009). Therapists training, feedback and practice for dream work: A pilot study. *Psychological Reports, 105*(1), 87–98.
Delaney, G.M.V. (1981). *Living Your Dreams.* New York, NY: Harper & Row.
Delaney, G. M. (1998). *All About Dreams.* San Francisco, CA: HarperOne.
Flowers, L. K. (1972). Psychotherapy: black and white. *Journal of the National Medical Association, 64*(1), 19–22.

Flowers, L. K. (1988). The morning after: A pragmatist's approach to dreams. *The Psychiatric Journal of the University of Ottawa, 13*(2), 66–71.

Flowers, L. K. (1993). The dream interview method in a private outpatient psychotherapy practice. In G.M.V. Delaney (Ed.), *New Directions in Dream Interpretation* (pp. 241–288). Albany, NY: SUNY Press.

Flowers, L. K. (1995). The use of presleep instructions and dreams in psychosomatic disorders. *Psychotherapy & Psychosomatics, 64*(3–4), 173–177.

Flowers, L. K. (2007a). *19 dreamer's preparation steps*. Retrieved from www.lomaflowersmd.com.

Flowers, L. K. (2007b). *19 dream interviewer's steps*. Retrieved from www.lomaflowersmd.com.

Flowers, L. K., & Zweben, J. E. (1996). The dream interview method in addiction recovery. A treatment guide. *Journal of Substance Abuse Treatment, 13*(2), 99–105.

Flowers, L. K., & Zweben, J. E. (1998). The changing role of "using" dreams in addiction recovery. *Journal of Substance Abuse Treatment, 15*(3): 193–200.

Freud, S. (1965). *The Interpretation of Dreams*. Transl. Strachey, J. New York, NY: Avon Books.

Gabbard, G. (2014). The person with the diagnosis. *Psychiatric News*. doi:10.1176/appi.pn.2013.3b19.

Jung, C. (1974). *Dreams*. Princeton, NJ: Princeton University Press.

Keller, J. W., Brown, G., Maier, K., Steinfurth, K., Hall, S., & Piotrowski, C. (1995). Use of dreams in therapy: A survey of clinicians in private practice. *Psychological Reports, 76*(3 Pt 2), 1288–1290.

Krippner, S., Gabel, S., Green, J., & Rubien, R. (1994). Community applications of an experiential group approach to teaching dreamwork. *Dreaming, 4*(4), 215–222.

Levy, J. (2009). Studying *The Interpretation of Dreams* in the company of analytic candidates. *Journal of the American Psychoanalytic Association, 57*(4), 847–870.

Olsson, G. (1991). The supervisory process reflected in dreams of supervisees. *American Journal of Psychotherapy, 45*(4). 511–526.

Pesant, N., & Zadra, A. (2004). Working with dreams in therapy: What do we know and what should we do? *Clinical Psychology Review, 24*, 489–512.

Reiser, M. F. (2001). The dream in contemporary psychiatry. *American Journal of Psychiatry, 158*(3), 351–359.

Rochlen, A. B., Ligiero, D. P., Hill, C. E., & Heaton, K. J. (1999). Effects of training in dream recall and dream interpretation skills on dream recall, attitudes, and dream interpretation outcome. *Journal of Counseling Psychology, 46*(1), 27–34.

Stranahan, S. (2011). The use of dreams in spiritual care. *Journal of Health Care Chaplaincy, 17*(1–2), 87–94.

Ullman, M. (1994). The experiential dream group: Its application in the training of therapists. *Dreaming. 4*(4), 223–229.

Ullman, M., & Zimmerman, N. (1979). *Working with Dreams*. New York, NY: Delacorte Press.

3

THE CONTINUITY BETWEEN WAKING AND DREAMING

Empirical Research and Clinical Implications

Michael Schredl

CENTRAL INSTITUTE OF MENTAL HEALTH, MEDICAL FACULTY
MANNHEIM/HEIDELBERG UNIVERSITY, GERMANY

Introduction

Trying to understand the meaning of dreams has a long history period. The first comprehensive dream book, compiled by Artemidorus of Daldis, was published in the second century (Papamichael & Marketos, 1995). Systematic use of dreams within the context of therapy was undertaken by Sigmund Freud (1991) and extensive empirical dream research followed the discovery of REM sleep by Eugene Aserinsky and Nathaniel Kleitman (1953) published in 1953 and the groundbreaking work of Calvin S. Hall starting in the late 1940s (Hall, 1951). Empirical studies (Crook & Hill, 2003; Schredl, Bohusch, Kahl, Mader, & Somesan, 2000) indicate that working with dreams is currently part of psychotherapeutic sessions in private practice, even though cognitive-behavioral therapists have little or no training in the techniques for this kind of work.

After introducing basic definitions, this chapter reviews briefly the findings regarding the interaction between waking life and dream content, i.e., how waking life is reflected in dreams and how dreams affect waking life. Based on that research, it is suggested that a simple approach can be used in the clinical setting to understand how the dream relates to the client's problems. In addition, the technique of imagery rehearsal, a very effective method for coping with nightmares, also very nicely fits into the framework of the continuity hypothesis as imagery exercises carried out in the waking state directly transfer to the dreaming world.

Definitions

The following definition is widely used in the field of dream research: "A dream or a dream report is the recollection of mental activity which has occurred during sleep" (Schredl, 2010a).

First, it is important to notice that dreaming as a mental activity during sleep is not directly measurable: the person has to wake up (sleep-wake transition) and has to remember the subjective experiences that occurred during sleep. This leads to the problem of validity: is the dream report an appropriate account of the actual dream experience? Modern dream research using, for example, external stimuli during sleep that are sometimes incorporated into dreams (Schredl, 2010a), indicated that dream reports reflect experiences during sleep but also that the dream report often did not include all the information about the dreaming experience (Schredl & Erlacher, 2003). The second important implication of this definition is to differentiate between dreaming as subjective experience and sleep defined as distinctive patterns in brain activity. Although subjective experiences are related to biological processes (Erlacher & Schredl, 2008), dreaming cannot be explained by physiology. Another advantage of this broad definition is that no *a priori* assumptions regarding content or characteristics of dreaming (like bizarreness, etc.) are necessary.

The term *continuity hypothesis* was coined by Hall and Nordby (1972), who stated that overt behavior (doing something) and covert behavior (thoughts, feelings, and fantasies) in waking life are continuous with dreaming. Over the years different aspects of waking life—like concerns, conceptions, emotions, and preoccupations—were studied within the framework of the continuity hypotheses (Schredl, 2012). One of the major problems with the continuity hypothesis is that the definition is vague; to address this, the current author (Schredl, 2003) formulated a mathematical model to include factors like time interval between waking-life experience and the subsequent dream and the type of waking-life activity into the concept of continuity.

Measuring Continuity Between Waking and Dreaming

Different methodological approaches for studying the relationship between waking life and dreaming have been adopted by dream researchers: analyzing temporal references of dream elements, experimental manipulation of the pre-sleep situation, field studies looking at intra-individual fluctuations, and inter-individual differences. One approach is to ask the participants—after reporting the dream—about the temporal references of their dream elements to waking-life experiences (Strauch & Meier, 1996). The major drawback of this approach is the limited memory capacity of the subjects; it is difficult to remember completely all waking-life experiences, let alone all thoughts, feelings, and fantasies that occurred during the preceding days, weeks, or months. Using this retrospective approach, Sigmund Freud (1991) used the term *day-residue* for the connection of the dream to the previous day. The experimental approach manipulates the pre-sleep situation, for example, by showing an exciting film (Schredl, 2010a). Dreams in the night after such a film are then compared to a control condition (e.g., a neutral film). Interestingly, the effect of films—even if they are strongly negatively toned—on subsequent dreams is quite small (overview: Schredl, 2010a). Because of this problem of the very small effect of experimental manipulation on dream content, studying the effect of waking life on the dream life of individuals (within-subject design) was investigated in field studies. For example, the effect of "real" stress (like intense psychotherapy sessions or awaiting a major surgery) on dreaming is much stronger compared to showing films (Breger, Hunter, & Lane, 1971). The strong effect of traumata such as war experiences, kidnapping, or sexual abuse on dreams even years later also indicates that the emotional intensity of the experience affects the incorporation rate of waking-life events into dreams (Schredl, 2010a).

Another approach for studying the relationship between waking life and dreaming is to correlate inter-individual differences in waking life with inter-individual differences in dream contents. For example, as the waking worlds of men and women differ (e.g., proneness to physical aggression, amount of sexual fantasies) there should be—according to the continuity hypothesis—corresponding differences in dream content (more physical aggression and more sexual dreams among males). Another study design is to correlate the amount of time spent in a particular waking-life activity (e.g., sports or reading) with number of occurrences of these elements within dreams.

In addition to the issue concerning how continuity between waking and dreaming is studied, it should be kept in mind that other methodological issues can affect the results of dream studies: for example, what kind of dream is used (most recent dreams, diary dreams, or laboratory dreams) or what kind of dream content analytic scales are employed. For a more detailed discussion of these issues see Schredl (2010b).

Effect of Waking Life on Dreaming

This section reviews briefly the studies looking at the effect of waking-life experiences on subsequent dream content. For example, the studies regarding gender differences in dream content (Schredl, 2007a) showed that men dream about sex and physical aggression more often than women; findings that are in line with differences in waking reality (more frequent sexual fantasies and higher proneness to physical aggression in men). The amount of time spent with a particular activity (sports, reading, driving a car) during waking is directly correlated with the frequency of the activity appearing in dreams, i.e., showing a continuity on a thematic level (Schredl & Erlacher, 2008; Schredl & Hofmann, 2003). The following review is systematized according to the factors of the continuity model formulated by the current author (2003).

Many studies have shown an exponential decrease of the incorporation rate of waking-life experiences into dreams, with elapsed time between experience and the subsequent dream (Schredl, 2003). However, one has to keep in mind that several studies are based on retrospective assessment of the temporal references. In addition to the day-residue effect (highest occurrence of a waking-life topic in the dreams the first night after the incidence) some diary studies found a so-called *dream lag effect,* e.g., an increase of incorporations 4 to 6 days later that is inconsistent with a simple exponential decrease over time (Blagrove, Henley-Einion, Barnett, Edwards, & Seage, 2011). Further research is needed to clarify the differential time course of incorporating daytime events into dreams.

Carrying out a prospective diary study, the current author (Schredl, 2006) reported that emotional intensity, but not emotional tone, of the waking-life experience was related to chance to be incorporated into subsequent dreams. The differences in effects of experimental stress (small effect on dream content) and "real" stress and trauma research indicate that emotional involvement during waking life affects the incorporation rate. Several studies (Hartmann, 2000; Schredl & Hofmann, 2003) have shown that focused thinking activity (reading, working with a computer) in dreams occurs less frequently than unfocused activities such as talking with friends, etc. These results also indicate that the type of activity is of importance for the continuity between waking life and dreaming.

The time of the night or the time interval between sleep onset and the dream affects the incorporation rate of waking-life experiences; dreams of the second part of the night comprise more elements of the distant past while dreams of the first part of the night incorporate mostly recent daytime experiences (Grenier et al., 2005; Verdone, 1965).

One factor, which has been rarely studied, is a possible interaction between personality traits and the incorporation of waking-life experiences into dreams (Baekeland, Resch, & Katz, 1968; Schredl, Kleinferchner, & Gell, 1996). It seems plausible that personality dimensions such as field dependence or thin boundaries moderate the magnitude of continuity between waking and dreaming.

Interestingly, lucid dream research also supports the continuity hypothesis: skilled lucid dreamers are able to carry out tasks they set for themselves prior to sleep onset (Stumbrys, Erlacher, Johnson, & Schredl, 2014). Also, an overview (Schredl, 2008) of the lab studies indicating that dreams obtained from awakenings in the sleep laboratory often include lab references is also in line with the continuity hypothesis.

In summary, the findings in this area clearly indicate that topics that are relevant in the dreamer's waking life play a role in his/her dreams. Interestingly, there seems to be a second-order continuity such that dreams that are affected by the preceding day have a higher chance to have an effect on the subsequent day—even if emotional intensity is statistically controlled (Schredl & Reinhard, 2009–2010). This means that there are topics that are processed both by day and in the night.

Dreams and Psychopathology

Two motifs have intrigued dream researchers regarding the relationship between dreaming and mental disorders. First, the dream state itself was conceptualized by several theorists as a mental disorder (Hobson, 1997) and, in reverse, hallucinations of schizophrenic patients have been thought of as breakthroughs of dreams into the waking state (Kramer & Roth, 1978). Second, many clinicians since Freud have used dreams in the diagnosis and treatment of their patients (Pesant & Zadra, 2004). The continuity hypothesis (Schredl, 2003) predicts that dreamers' specific waking symptomatology and daytime problems are reflected within the dreams of patients with mental disorders.

Literature reviews (Kramer & Nuhic, 2007; Kramer & Roth, 1978; Skancke, Holsen, & Schredl, 2014) have shown that the majority of empirical studies support the continuity hypothesis; i.e., dream content is affected by the psychopathological symptoms that patients experience in the waking state. Dreams of schizophrenic patients, for example, are typical for this disorder; i.e., the dreams are more bizarre, and are characterized by aggression and negative emotions (Michels et al., 2014; Schredl & Engelhardt, 2001). For depressive patients, an increased amount of "masochistic" themes in their dreams have been found (Beck & Hurvich, 1959). Subsequent studies (Kramer & Nuhic, 2007) confirmed that dreams of depressive patients are more negatively toned and include unpleasant experiences more often than healthy controls (this resembles the definitions of "masochistic" dream content in the earlier studies). The current author and a colleague (Schredl & Engelhardt, 2001) were able to demonstrate that the severity of depressive symptomatology was directly correlated with the intensity of negative dream emotions, irrespective of the patients' diagnoses, supporting a dimensional and not a categorical relationship between waking-life symptoms and dream content; i.e. the dream characteristics were not determined by the diagnoses themselves but the severity of the specific daytime symptoms.

Overall, the research in this area clearly indicates that dreams reflect the daytime psychopathology of the patients.

Effect of Dreams on Waking Life

Whereas a large number of studies looked at the effect of waking life on dreams, research investigating the effect of dreams on waking life is quite rare. In this section two topics will be addressed: (1) the effects of dreams and nightmares on daytime mood and (2) creative inspiration by dreams.

The most frequently reported effect of dreams on waking life is their effect on mood (Kuiken & Sikora, 1993). In one study (Schredl, 2009) it was estimated that about 16% of all dreams affect the mood of the subsequent day, especially if the dreams are emotionally intense and/or negatively toned. Furthermore, Köthe and Pietrowsky (2001) reported that days after experiencing a nightmare are rated much higher on scales of anxiety and lower on scales of concentration and self-esteem than days after non-nightmare nights. The hypothesis of Kathryn Belicki (1992), which states that persons with high neuroticism scores overestimate the effects of nightmares on waking life, has not been supported (Schredl, Landgraf, & Zeiler, 2003). The major factor contributing to nightmare distress is nightmare frequency, even though persons with thin boundaries are more likely to experience effects of their dreams on their daytime mood (Schredl, 2009; Schredl et al., 2003).

Many examples of creative inspiration from dreams have been reported over the years: *Wild Strawberries* (a film by Ingmar Bergmann), the story of Dr. Jekyll and Mr. Hyde by Robert Louis Stevenson, the pop song "Yesterday" by Paul McCartney, and the paintings of Salvador Dali all provide excellent examples (Barrett, 2001). In a large-scale study in an unselected student sample, and in an online survey, about 7.8% of the recalled dreams included creative aspects (Schredl & Erlacher, 2007). Reports include dreams stimulating art, giving an impulse to try something new (approaching a person, traveling, etc.) or helping solve a problem (e.g., mathematical problems, etc.). The factors that are associated with the frequency of creative dreams in this study (Schredl & Erlacher, 2007) were dream recall frequency, the "thin boundaries" personality dimension, a positive attitude towards creative activities, and visual imagination.

Dreams and Psychotherapy

Although dream work is quite common in modern psychotherapy (Schredl et al., 2000) and despite the extensive literature on case reports since Freud's *The Interpretation of Dreams,* systematic research on the efficiency of dream work is limited to the research efforts of one group. For more than ten years, Clara Hill and her coworkers carried out studies to measure the effectiveness of single dream interpretation sessions, dream groups over 6 weeks, and dream interpretation within short-term psychotherapy (Hill & Knox, 2010). The basis for their work is a cognitive-experiential model of dream interpretation that includes three stages: exploration, insight, and action. Reviewing the research, Hill and Goates (2004) cited three sources of evidence for the beneficial effects of dream work: (a) clients have reported on post-session measures that they gained insight, (b) judges rated clients' levels of insight in written dream interpretations as higher after dream sessions than before, and (c) clients identified gaining awareness or insight as the most helpful component of dream sessions. Similar studies for other therapeutic approaches to work with dreams are overdue.

Clinical Implications

What are the clinical implications of the findings regarding the continuity hypothesis of dreaming? This author would like to argue that the strong links between dreaming and waking life with regard to different areas (thematic links, emotions, problems, etc.) can inform the way clinicians work with the dreams of their clients. Hall and Nordby (1972) state, "We remain the same person, the same personality with the same characteristics, and the same basic beliefs and convictions whether awake or asleep" (p. 104). This is indicative for the idea to approach dreams in the same way as waking issues.

If you have a problem in waking life that bothers you, there are typically two basic approaches: (1) the wish to understand why this happened and (2) the wish to do something different in the future in order to cope with the problem. This simple, everyday-life approach can be adopted for working with dreams. First, working with dreams looks at the question of why this particular dream has occurred at this particular point in the life of the dreamer ("understanding the dream"). The continuity hypothesis clearly indicates that the major topics relevant in waking life are often found in dreams, but there are also dreams that do not seem directly connected to waking life; research (Fosse, Fosse, Hobson, & Stickgold, 2003) has shown that dreams are not replays of waking-life episodes. How can one reconcile these, at first glance, conflicting findings? The approach used in the method of working with dreams proposed in this chapter (see Table 3.1) focuses on the basic pattern of the dream: How does the dreamer react to the circumstances that s/he is confronted with within the dream? What kinds of emotions come up? What kinds of coping strategies does the dream ego use? This is in line with the statement of Hall and Nordby (1972): the person is the same, feels and acts in the same ways as in waking life, even if the scenario is not a direct reflection of the current waking life. Take for example the dream of being chased by a monster. Clearly, the monster is not part of the dreamer's waking life, but being afraid and trying to get away from a threat is a quite common behavior in waking life that one can call *avoidance behavior*; i.e., the dream of being chased is not continuous regarding the dream figure (monster) but regarding the basic pattern of avoiding something.

Another idea is to use the waking-life imagination to create ideas of how one can cope with the problematic situation within the dream—based on the wish to do better in the future. For nightmares, a specific method called Imagery Rehearsal Therapy (IRT) has been developed by Barry Krakow and coworkers (Krakow & Zadra, 2010). Patients write down a recent (less intense) nightmare, and then they are asked to change the dream in any way they wish and to write down the altered version. Finally, they are instructed to rehearse the new "dream" once a day over a 2-week period. Numerous randomized controlled trials of IRT performed with chronic nightmare sufferers showed the efficiency of this approach, also in long-term follow-ups. Interestingly, this approach also fits nicely within the framework of the continuity hypothesis: the imagination exercises carried out during the day affect subsequent dream life.

If the findings of the continuity between waking and dreaming are taken seriously, the method of working with dreams should not rely on interpretations from another person or dictionaries of symbols but invite the dreamer to identify the links between his/her waking life and the topics of the dream. In order to apply these principles in practice, this author (Schredl, 2007b) developed a six-step model for working with dreams (see Table 3.1).

TABLE 3.1 Listening to the Dreamer—A Six-Step Approach to Working with Dreams

1	Clarify the dream in order to help the dreamer to reexperience the dream: e.g., ask, "What kind of emotions did you experience during the dream while encountering *X*?"
2	Ask the dreamer what kind of waking-life memories are associated with the dream characters, animals, objects, surroundings, etc., that occurred in the dream.
3	Ask the dreamer about the basic action patterns and basic emotions in the dream. Ask her/him to retell the actions and interactions in the dream without using the particular images of the dream (abstract/general level): e.g., "I am scared and I am running away."
4	Ask the dreamer whether s/he sees any parallels between the basic dream pattern and her/his current waking life.
5	Ask the dreamer whether s/he would like to do something different now, act differently from what s/he did within the dream.
6	Ask the dreamer whether some of the insights into the dream situation can be used for changing waking behavior.

The name of the approach is *listening to the dreamer* as the main ingredients are open-ended questions in order to stimulate the dreamer to think about his/her dream and its connections with waking life.

Step 1 of the approach sets the stage and helps the dreamer reexperience the dream, especially the emotions of the dream. Step 2 is based on the continuity findings. If a person, an animal, objects, or settings show up in the dream, this might be related to topics that are relevant for the dreamer. Instead of being asked for associations that might come up in the session, the dreamer is specifically asked whether there are any incidents in waking life regarding this dream character, object, and so on. As already pointed out, Step 3 of the model concentrates on the basic pattern of the dream, not on the dream elements. In the example of the monster dream, the general pattern is: "I am scared and I am running away" (i.e., reflecting some kind of avoidance behavior). In Step 4, the dreamer is asked whether s/he can make any connections with current waking-life issues, focusing not on the dream elements but on the basic pattern of the dream. The clinical experience of the author indicates that these relationships are easier to detect than relationships between dream characters, objects, and waking life, especially in bizarre dreams. Step 5 encourages the dreamer to use his/her imagination in waking life to fantasize a constructive coping strategy for the difficult dream situation. If the dreamer produced avoidance strategies like fleeing or hiding, or very aggressive behavior like killing the monster, s/he will be asked whether there are any other options for coping with the situation. In the long run, active and constructive strategies seem to be better suited for benefiting the dreamer, especially with regard to Step 6. The basic idea of Step 5 is that training during the day affects your dreams in a positive way. The last part of the work with dreams, Step 6, explores whether any insights of the working with the dream can be transferred into waking life: e.g., if the fantasized solution of the dream problem includes helpers, an option would be to think about whether the waking problem associated with the dream would also be solved more easily if the dreamer asks a close person for help. Interestingly, this 6-Step approach can also be applied to positively toned dreams. The question would be: "What can you do in your waking life to experience these positive feelings you had within the dream?"

Conclusions

The findings regarding the continuity between waking and dreaming have implications concerning how to work with dreams in a clinical setting. However, much research in the future is needed to understand what approaches to working with dreams are the most beneficial for clients.

References

Aserinsky, E., & Kleitman, N. (1953). Regularly occurring periods of eye motility and concomitant phenomena during sleep. *Science, 118*, 273–274.
Baekeland, F., Resch, R., & Katz, D. (1968). Presleep mentation and dream reports: I. Cognitive style, contiguity to sleep and time of the night. *Archives of General Psychiatry, 19*, 300–311.
Barrett, D. (2001). *The committee of sleep: How artists, scientists, and athletes use dreams for creative problem-solving—and how you can too*. New York: Crown.
Beck, A. T., & Hurvich, M. S. (1959). Psychological correlates of depression: I. frequency of "masochistic" dream content in a private practice sample. *Psychosomatic Medicine, 1*, 50–55.
Belicki, K. (1992). Nightmare frequency versus nightmare distress: Relation to psychopathology and cognitive style. *Journal of Abnormal Psychology, 101*, 592–597.
Blagrove, M., Henley-Einion, J., Barnett, A., Edwards, D., & Seage, C. H. (2011). A replication of the 5–7 day dream-lag effect with comparison of dreams to future events as control for baseline matching. *Consciousness and Cognition, 20*(2), 384–391.
Breger, L., Hunter, I., & Lane, R. W. (1971). *The effect of stress on dreams*. New York: International Universities Press.
Crook, R. E., & Hill, C. E. (2003). Working with dreams in psychotherapy: the therapists' perspective. *Dreaming, 13*, 83–93.
Erlacher, D., & Schredl, M. (2008). Do REM (lucid) dreamed and executed actions share the same neural substrate? *International Journal of Dream Research, 1*, 7–14.
Fosse, M. J., Fosse, R., Hobson, J. A., & Stickgold, R. J. (2003). Dreaming and episodic memory: a functional dissociation? *Journal of Cognitive Neuroscience, 15*, 1–9.
Freud, S. (1991). *The interpretation of dreams* (Org.: Die Traumdeutung, 1900). London: Penguin Books.
Grenier, J., Cappeliez, P., St-Onge, M., Vachon, J., Vinette, S., Roussy, F., Mercier, P., Lortie-Lussier, M., & De Koninck, J. (2005). Temporal references in dreams and autobiographical memory. *Memory and Cognition, 33*, 280–288.
Hall, C. S. (1951). What people dream about? *Scientific American, 184*(5), 60–63.
Hall, C. S., & Nordby, V. J. (1972). *The individual and his dreams*. New York: New American Library.

Hartmann, E. (2000). We do not dream of the 3 R's: implications for the nature of dream mentation. *Dreaming, 10*, 103–110.
Hill, C. E., & Goates, M. K. (2004). Research on the Hill cognitive-experiential dream model. In C. E. Hill (Ed.), *Dream work in therapy: facilitating exploration, insight, and action* (pp. 245–288). Washington: American Psychological Association.
Hill, C. E., & Knox, S. (2010). The use of dreams in modern psychotherapy. *International Review of Neurobiology, 92*, 291–317.
Hobson, J. A. (1997). Dreaming as delirium: a mental status examination of our nightly madness. *Seminars in Neurology, 17*, 121–128.
Köthe, M., & Pietrowsky, R. (2001). Behavioral effects of nightmares and their correlations to personality patterns. *Dreaming, 11*, 43–52.
Krakow, B., & Zadra, A. (2010). Imagery Rehearsal Therapy: Principles and Practice. *Sleep Medicine Clinics, 5*, 289–298.
Kramer, M., & Nuhic, Z. (2007). A review of dreaming by psychiatric patients: an update. In S. Pandi, R. Ruoti & M. Kramer (Eds.), *Sleep and psychosomatic medicine* (pp. 137–155). New York: Taylor and Francis.
Kramer, M., & Roth, T. (1978). Dreams in psychopathologic patient groups. In R. L. Williams & I. Karacan (Eds.), *Sleep disorders: diagnosis and treatment* (pp. 323–349). New York: John Wiley & Sons.
Kuiken, D., & Sikora, S. (1993). The impact of dreams on waking thoughts and feelings. In A. Moffitt, M. Kramer & R. Hoffmann (Eds.), *The functions of dreaming* (pp. 419–476). Albany: State University of New York Press.
Michels, F., Schilling, C., Rausch, F., Eifler, S., Zink, M., Meyer-Lindenberg, A., & Schredl, M. (2014). Nightmare frequency in schizophrenic patients, healthy relatives of schizophrenic patients, patients at high risk states for psychosis, and healthy controls. [Nightmares; schizophrenia; distress]. *International Journal of Dream Research, 7*, 9–13.
Papamichael, E., & Marketos, S. G. (1995). Artemidorian Oneirocrisia. *History of Psychiatry, 6*, 125–131.
Pesant, N., & Zadra, A. (2004). Working with dreams in therapy: what do we know and what should we do? *Clinical Psychology Review, 24*, 489–512.
Schredl, M. (2003). Continuity between waking and dreaming: a proposal for a mathematical model. *Sleep and Hypnosis, 5*, 38–52.
Schredl, M. (2006). Factors affecting the continuity between waking and dreaming: emotional intensity and emotional tone of the waking-life event. *Sleep and Hypnosis, 8*, 1–5.
Schredl, M. (2007a). Gender differences in dreaming. In D. Barrett & P. McNamara (Eds.), *The new science of dreaming—Volume 2: Content, recall, and personality correlates* (pp. 29–47). Westport: Praeger.
Schredl, M. (2007b). *Träume—Die Wissenschaft entschlüsselt unser nächtliches Kopfkino*. Berlin: Ullstein.
Schredl, M. (2008). Laboratory references in dreams: Methodological problem and/or evidence for the continuity hypothesis of dreaming? *International Journal of Dream Research, 1*, 3–6.
Schredl, M. (2009). Effect of dreams on daytime mood: the effects of gender and personality. *Sleep and Hypnosis, 11*, 51–57.
Schredl, M. (2010a). Characteristics and contents of dreams. *International Review of Neurobiology, 92*, 135–154.
Schredl, M. (2010b). Dream content analysis: Basic principles. *International Journal of Dream Research, 3*, 65–73.

Schredl, M. (2012). Continuity in studying the continuity hypothesis of dreaming is needed. *International Journal of Dream Research, 5*, 1–8.
Schredl, M., Bohusch, C., Kahl, J., Mader, A., & Somesan, A. (2000). The use of dreams in psychotherapy: a survey of psychotherapists in private practice. *Journal of Psychotherapy Practice and Research, 9*, 81–87.
Schredl, M., & Engelhardt, H. (2001). Dreaming and psychopathology: dream recall and dream content of psychiatric inpatients. *Sleep and Hypnosis, 3*, 44–54.
Schredl, M., & Erlacher, D. (2003). The problem of dream content analysis validity as shown by a bizarreness scale. *Sleep and Hypnosis, 5*, 129–135.
Schredl, M., & Erlacher, D. (2007). Self-reported effects of dreams on waking-life creativity: An empirical study. *Journal of Psychology, 141*, 35–46.
Schredl, M., & Erlacher, D. (2008). Relationship between waking sport activities, reading and dream content in sport and psychology students. *Journal of Psychology, 142*, 267–275.
Schredl, M., & Hofmann, F. (2003). Continuity between waking activities and dream activities. *Consciousness and Cognition, 12*, 298–308.
Schredl, M., Kleinferchner, P., & Gell, T. (1996). Dreaming and personality: thick vs. thin boundaries. *Dreaming, 6*, 219–223.
Schredl, M., Landgraf, C., & Zeiler, O. (2003). Nightmare frequency, nightmare distress and neuroticism. *North American Journal of Psychology, 5*, 345–350.
Schredl, M., & Reinhard, I. (2009–2010). The continuity between waking mood and dream emotions: Direct and second-order effects. *Imagination, Cognition and Personality 29*, 271–282.
Skancke, J., Holsen, I., & Schredl, M. (2014). Continuity between waking life and dreams of psychiatric patients: A review and discussion of the implications for dream research. *International Journal of Dream Research, 7*, 39–53.
Strauch, I., & Meier, B. (1996). *In search of dreams: results of experimental dream research.* Albany: State University of New York Press.
Stumbrys, T., Erlacher, D., Johnson, M., & Schredl, M. (2014). The Phenomenology of Lucid Dreaming: An Online Survey. *The American Journal of Psychology, 127*(2), 191–204.
Verdone, P. (1965). Temporal reference of manifest dream content. *Perceptual and Motor Skills, 20*, 1253–1268.

4

DREAM INCUBATION

Targeting Dreaming to Focus on Particular Issues

Gayle Delaney

CODIRECTOR OF THE DELANEY & FLOWERS DREAM
AND CONSULTATION CENTER

Dream work can be a powerful tool in psychotherapy if efficiently used and if the resulting dreams are accurately, or at least heuristically, explored and understood by therapist and dreamer (Moffitt, Kramer, & Hoffman, 1993; Hill, 2013). This is true, of course, only if the client is motivated to recall and present dreams, and is able to overcome resistance to new points of view and insights that will move the therapeutic goals forward.

When clients first successfully incubate a dream on a particular topic, such as "What keeps me from finding satisfying work?" or "Is this man a good fit for me as a husband?" or "What is really going on between me and my son?" their motivation to recall and bring dreams into therapy soars. Rather than recalling apparently random or vague dreams that trouble or torment, at last, a dream enters one's inbox that responds to the question from the night before! The dreamer's curiosity about the meaning of the asked-for dream can markedly assist in overcoming resistance.

Dream incubation increases a sense of partnership between the dreamer and his or her dreams. If the therapist can help the dreamer understand his or her dream in a nondogmatic way that is transparent, efficient, and effective, this sense of partnership with the dream can be reflected in the partnership between the therapist and the client, thus reducing resistance and increasing trust as well as courage in discovering and integrating new insights generated by the dream work and the therapy in general. The clients who actively solicit dreams on their issues feel they are doing more than complaining; they are creating and contributing dreams that help them to understand and resolve their problems.

White and Taytroe (2003) conducted an experiment on the effect of using Phrase-Focusing dream incubation on personal problem solving and found that

"Night dream incubation participants were particularly likely to report reduced problem distress, greater problem solvability, and improvement in their focal problem" (White & Taytroe, 2003, p. 193). This paper describes at length the difficulties in researching the effectiveness of dream incubation and points out that several studies have been hampered by the challenges of getting dreamers sufficiently interested in solving abstract puzzles that many research designs suggest. Their study asked participants to choose their own personally relevant target problems. As Barrett (1993), Hartmann (1998), Cartwright and Lamberg (2001), and others have noted, the processes in dreams or sleep that help us solve problems are likely to fully engage only when the problem really matters to the dreamer. I have certainly found this to be the case in my training work.

Incubating a dream is easy; understanding the resultant dreams can be challenging and time consuming. Usually, responses to incubation questions are not literal, but metaphorical. A novice dreamer who asked for a dream on why she keeps picking men who are dead ends thought her dream about shopping for yet another rescue dog had missed the mark. When her therapist asked her to describe rescue dogs as if the therapist had never heard of such things, the metaphoric link was obvious: she had the habit of selecting men who, exactly as she described the dogs in the dream, were "lonely, abandoned, unloved, and needed to be rescued." Her therapist had only to ask for one description in order for the client to make the metaphoric bridge and interpret her own dream.

Dream incubation has a long history born in shamanistic and religious cults that employed pre-sleep rituals and group experiences led by a priest or shaman. Henry Reed (1976) and others have revived and enacted similar practices from the 1970s to the present. In 1971—being of a more humanist bent—I developed a modern, secular, therapeutically oriented approach to incubation aimed at teaching people to use it alone, at home, for use in psychotherapy, personal growth, and creative problem solving. This Phrase-Focusing dream incubation (Delaney, 1996, 1998) is entirely secular in nature and does not require belief in any religion or philosophy. It is simply a method for focusing one's intention to dream about a particular issue with the aim of understanding it better or of solving a problem.

People around the world have been "sleeping on" problems for centuries, and most of us have had at least one experience of waking with the partial or full solution to a problem that had occupied us the night before. Sometimes we awake with the solution in mind and have no recall of a dream. The clarity is just there. Other times, when we sleep on a problem, or when we formally or informally incubate a dream, we awake with a dream that is so nearly literal, that there is almost no interpretation necessary—as when a newly engaged woman dreamt that her fiancé gave her a fake diamond engagement ring. But many recalled dreams, both incubated and spontaneous, escape all understanding of the dreamer, who is unable to find any relation between the dream and current life issues. In 40 years of working with thousands of dreamers, I have found that teaching them how to spot metaphors has revealed how many of their dreams offer previously unrecognized metaphors that shed brilliant light on the dynamics of their problems.

Formalizing the setting of the intention, moving from hoping to have a helpful dream to clearly setting one's intention to do so and being prepared to record the dream the following morning, simply capitalizes upon a natural human ability to problem solve in sleep. It develops this ability to gain higher reliability through clearer intention setting in writing, improving the chances of recalling a dream that might answer the incubation question, and learning how to interpret the resultant dream to extract a more detailed understanding than one could without recalling and understanding the dream. After presenting simple directions on how to incubate a dream, I shall describe this interpretive approach, the Dream Interview method (Delaney, 1991), and combine its use with dream incubation focusing on particular issues in clinical settings.

Phrase-Focusing Dream Incubation

The directions for this form of dream incubation are so simple, they can be handed to the patient on a sheet of paper, or even outlined over the phone before the first session if appropriate—for example, with former clients coming back to work on a particular issue. The directions that follow may be copied and given to your individual or group clients.

Dream Incubation: Steps for Maximizing the Chances of Eliciting a Dream on a Given Topic

1. Day notes: In your electronic or paper dream journal, write three to four lines about the emotional highlights of the day.
2. Incubation discussion: Write three to four lines about the issue you want a dream to help you better understand or resolve.
3. Incubation phrase: Write a one-line phrase clearly stating your question or request.
4. Repeat this exact phrase silently over and over as you fall asleep. If your mind wanders, return to repeating your incubation phrase. This turns off your worrying and puts you to sleep surprisingly quickly.
5. When you wake, whether in the middle of the night or in the morning, think backwards and ask yourself, "What was I just thinking?" Write down whatever comes to mind without judgment as to whether it is relevant, complete-enough a dream, or even if it was a dream at all. This teaches you how to recall dreams more easily and often offers surprisingly relevant memories or dream fragments that are rich in themselves and sometimes turn into full dreams as you write.
6. Bring your dream into your next session or start a Dream Interview on your own and we can work together on anything that remains unclear.

Short Form of Dream Incubation

1. As you fall asleep, repeat your incubation phrase over and over.
2. When you awake, write down whatever is in your mind, with no judgment as to whether your incubation was successful.
3. Interview yourself about your dream before you decide if it answered your query.

Dream recall for most people is considerably enhanced by recording day notes and by recording the dream immediately upon awakening. Because the dream often appears to shape its manifest story line and metaphors in line with the exact phrasing of the incubation question, it is tremendously useful for the dreamer to write it out before sleep. If the day notes or the incubation phrase are written down the morning after the dream, the material is of a different nature (interpretive, hindsight/day-residue cluttered) and generally less useful in the understanding of the dream.

Some clients are stunningly able to simply set the intention to incubate a dream at any time during the day—but these are few. In my four decades of teaching incubation, success is enhanced when more of the steps are executed before sleep. Even experienced dreamers who make the effort to spend three to five minutes before sleep to set up the incubation find that their clarity of recall and success in eliciting relevant dreams are significantly enhanced.

What if the incubation does not work? Some incubations fail utterly. Recall fails or the resultant dream treats another topic. Awakening with no recall is a disappointment. I suggest the dreamer try again for three nights. If there is still no response, we consider if the dreamer is asking a question that he or she does not dare to have answered. Hot questions like, "Was I sexually abused?" or "Am I gay or straight?" often draw blanks, or the dreamer awakes with dreams about issues at work, or a new way to hold her golf club! At such times, the therapist can deal with the anxiety around the question and suggest the dreamer "step down" the intensity of the question. "Am I gay or straight?" could become, "What are the traits of a good partner for me?" The issue of uncovering early sexual or physical abuse is so intense and can involve such fallout that, in my opinion, it should not be broached via incubation unless the client is in ongoing therapy, and ideally, in group therapy as well.

Wouldn't the dreamer have had the dream anyway? Does incubation really make a difference? We dream about the concerns of our entire lives and especially of our current concerns. It is impossible to say what the dreamer would have dreamt that night had he or she not incubated a dream. I would guess that incubating a dream often increases the dreamer's motivation to work with a particular issue, perhaps one of several on his or her psychological plate, and increases clarity of recall—that the dreamer would indeed have dreamt of one of his or her current issues in any case. However I have heard so many incubated dreams that not only excite the dreamer with a sense of having hit a bull's-eye, but also have recurred several times only on the disjunctive nights the dream was repeatedly incubated, that I and my students believe that incubating dreams effectively directs our dreaming brains to deal with chosen topics. In waking, we can choose to focus on a particular issue; in dreaming we seem able to order up a dream for delivery in the morning.

How do you know if the incubated dream is relevant to the question posed? In rare instances, the resulting dreams are almost literal, metaphorically transparent, as in the dream of a man who dreamt of having fun at a party with former drinking buddies, taking a drink, then realizing, within the dream, that he was once again lost to his addiction to alcohol. His incubation question: "What is the most dangerous threat to sobriety?"

Most dreams are visual and emotional metaphors about waking concerns and need to be recognized before they can be bridged to the client's life. In a dreamer's enthusiasm about incubation there is a tendency to force the dream to fit the question. This can lead to a double loss: the incubation question is poorly or wrongly answered, and the dream that was recalled is robbed of its own meaning. First, one needs to see what the dream *is* about, before considering if the dream answers the incubation question or if it is treats another topic entirely.

Interpreting the Incubated Dream

The pitfalls of force-fitting a dream into a theoretical framework, into the dreamer's wish for an answer or an escape, or into a superstitious or tradition-defined meaning, are many. Not only does one risk misinterpretation that leads in the wrong direction, but also one also misses the insights the dream actually offers. It is easier to see this when observing interpretations made by therapists of orientations different from your own.

I shall present here a transparent, secular method of interpretation, the Dream Interview method that I began to use in 1971 and have developed with Loma Flowers, MD, over the last three decades. Dr. Flowers, a psychiatrist, has made extensive use of this method in her San Francisco private practice, her teaching at University of California, San Francisco Medical School, and elsewhere (Flowers, 1988, 1993, 1995; Flowers & Zweben, 1998).

Outline of the Dream Interview Method

The goal of the Dream Interview is to reduce (to a minimum) interpretive intrusions from the therapist, be they based on his or her psycho-theoretical, spiritual, or religious beliefs, or upon his or her intuitions, erudition, or wisdom. This is in order to allow the client's dream to speak in its own language, reflecting the dreamer's unique conceptualization of life. Only after this is perceived, after the interpretation is found, does the therapist help the client reinforce and integrate the resulting insights and new points of view.

While minimizing therapist projections and formulations onto the dream interpretation, the Dream Interview method provides very specific tools to actively and methodically unveil and connect the dream metaphors to the waking life of the dreamer. One can avoid being directive and intrusive by simply asking, "What do you think your dream means?" or "What does this dream bring to mind for you?" Such nondirective questions can indeed bring up useful material. But most all dreams offer much more information about the dynamics and possible resolution of life issues if they are methodically explored in a way that takes advantage of the specificity of the dream images and their dynamic meaning when linked to the context of the entire dream.

In this approach, the therapist, peer dream analyst, or group member is asked to take the role of interviewer rather than that of interpreter. The aim of the interviewer is to ask the right questions to get at the meaning of a dream and to make it easy for the dreamer to connect the dots as the metaphors are identified and bridged to waking life. The interviewer is very active, and is charged with keeping in mind the dramatic structure of the dream, so that each metaphoric bridge is seen in the context of the entire dream rather than in isolation. The therapist must put aside his or her preconceptions about the meaning of any image or dream theme and take pride in not having the answer, but in having the right question. To this end, the Dream Interviewer asks the dreamer to pretend that the therapist comes from another planet and has very little knowledge of life on earth. This pivotal device reminds the therapist that it is the dreamer's perceptions, associations, and judgments that count in deciphering the dream that the dreamer built. It also frees the dreamer to describe with feeling almost any action or element of a dream without fear of being corrected or overruled. It further brings forth descriptive and associative material that is highly relevant and less tangential than that elicited by more general invitations to give associations. And importantly, in speaking to a newcomer to the planet, the dreamer often enthusiastically reveals feelings and judgments that in other contexts would be withheld or remain unrecognized.

Thus, while a dream about a cat might make the *interpreter* think of time-honored interpretations of cats as mother, or as a symbol of the feminine principle, the *interviewer* eschews these tempting symbol substitutions and says to the dreamer: "Pretend that I come from another planet and have never seen a cat before. What are cats like?" Here is a brief example from a young woman:

> I dreamt that a black cat was sitting on my windowsill. It came into my room, ran all over, raised a ruckus, and left.

INTERVIEWER: Theresa, for now, pretend I have just come from another planet and have never seen a cat. Tell me, what are cats like?

THERESA: They are beautiful creatures, sleek and agile. They are distant and aloof, they love you when they want to and leave you when they want to.
I: What was the cat in your dream like?
T: Just like that. The one in my dream was black and just gorgeous!
I: Do you know which room the cat came into?
T: My bedroom.
I: How did you feel when it was in the room and when it left?
T: At first I was thrilled, then when it left, I was in tears at the loss.
I: Is there anything, anyone, or any part of yourself that is like a beautiful, sleek, agile, gorgeous black cat that is distant and aloof, loves you when it wants to, leaves you when it wants to, raises a ruckus in your bedroom, thrills you, then leaves you in tears?
T: Yes! My boyfriend. And he is black too! He is just like the cat: distant and aloof, loves me when he wants to, leaves me when he wants to, and breaks my heart!

Theresa's rush to confirm the same cat-like traits in her boyfriend is typical of dreamers who have made a strong bridge to a waking issue. Even when the interpretation is not good news, the pleasure of seeing something from a new point of view and of deciphering the dream so convincingly is exciting. If the therapist had "given" the same interpretation, resistance would have been higher and the thrill of discovery would have been stolen from her.

Three minutes after this interview, Theresa said, "You know, *all* my boyfriends have been cats. What I need is a *dog!*" The dream and the interview process had done what dreams do so well: they helped the dreamer recognize a pattern in her choice of mates to which she had been blind, and for which she had suffered much. A therapist could help the dreamer integrate this new insight and even suggest the client incubate a dream asking, "Why am I so attracted to cat men?" Or ask a simple question in this or the next session like, "When was the first time you wanted love from a cat-man who was distant, aloof, etc.?" The therapist could assist the dreamer in recognizing the degree to which her habitual patterns have influenced her life and how she came to develop them, then help her learn new patterns. What would have happened if the interviewer had heard the dream and begun to share her understanding of mother goddesses, mother complexes, or the feminine principle within the dreamer?

The Four Basic Steps of the Dream Interview

The basic steps of the interview, description, recapitulation, and bridge and test, are applied to the major image or all the images of the dream. The last step, linking and summary, is applied partway through or at the end of the dream.

A Dream Interview can be conducted by two people, by a group in which one person tells a dream and the group members take turns playing the role of interviewer, or by a solo dreamer playing both roles. For teaching purposes, I shall divide the roles between the therapist/interviewer and the dreamer. It is helpful if the dreamer as well as the therapist know the basic steps and structure of the Dream Interview. Detailed instructions in the method are found in several of my books (Delaney, 1991, 1993, 1997, 1998).

1. Description: After hearing the dream, the interviewer asks the dreamer to describe the first main image as if he or she had never heard of such a place, thing, person, feeling, or action. In the beginning, the interviewer reminds the dreamer that he or she comes from another planet: "Remember, I come from another planet. We don't have [Teslas, taxis, Texans, Mafia men, giraffes, banksters, Republicans, etc.] on Mars. What are they like?" The interviewer resists every impulse to help the dreamer find the right descriptive words, because the words the dreamer uses—even if it's a struggle to find them—are the ones that will trigger the metaphoric leap.

   When working with certain images, especially animals and people, it is important to ask for a generic description (Generic D) first, then for the specific description (Specific D) of how the image appears in the given dream. This way, if the dreamer portrays the image in a manner uncharacteristic of his or her usual perception of the image, the unusualness and the specificity of the image can be described and captured in the recapitulation and the bridge. For example, asking the dreamer, "What is a Jaguar XKE like?" may elicit the response, "The most elegantly designed car body ever! My favorite car when I was in college." Asking, "What was the XKE in your dream like?" might elicit the al-important dream-specific description: "It was old, outmoded, lacking vital safety engineering, and should not be allowed on the road. Unsafe at any speed, as Ralph Nader would say!" Now the interviewer is in a good position to recapitulate and ask for a bridge with a blending of these descriptions: "Is there anything, anyone, any part of you that is like an XKE, the most elegantly designed car body ever . . . and is outmoded, lacking in vital safety engineering and . . . unsafe at any speed?"

   When working with objects, it is usually helpful to ask not only "What is a Z?", but also "What is the function of a Z?" (D of function) as well as "What sorts of people ride, use, or like Zs?" With experience, interviewers learn to use follow-up questions that stay with the alien point of view and keep close to the scent of the images and the dramatic thrust of the action and plot of the dream.

2. Recapitulation: The interviewer restates the dreamer's description, using only the dreamer's words and intonations, while editing out repetitions and fillers to keep the pace interesting for the dreamer. The interviewer invites the dreamer to correct any misstatements, add to, change, or emphasize any part of the description. This step helps the dreamer and the interviewer assess the richness and adequacy of the description. If it needs more elaboration, the interviewer withholds descriptions, as well as resists any tendency to correct

or elaborate, and asks follow-up description questions. (See the Cue Card that follows.)

3. Bridge and test: We have arrived at the first level of interpretation of the dream element (before it is placed in the dramatic context of the whole dream). The interviewer asks the dreamer if there is anything, any part of himself or herself, or anyone in his or her life like the thing described, then briefly repeats the recapitulation. Surprisingly, this is usually the first time the dreamer really hears his or her own description. The dreamer often exclaims: "Oh! Now that you put it that way, that is just like my wife [or boss, brother, etc.]!" The interviewer then asks, "How so?" inviting the dreamer to see if the traits/qualities of the description match well the traits of the person, place, situation, etc. to which the dreamer bridged the dream image. This is called *testing the strength of the bridge* and is essential to avoid red herrings. If the bridge is weak, the interviewer returns immediately or later to the image and elicits a richer description. The bridge question is then repeated. Often, after a few more images have been described and bridged, the dreamer has more contextual clues and can make a stronger bridge.

4. Linking and summary: Here, either the dreamer or the interviewer links the bridges made partway through, or at the end of the interview. This is the second level of interpretation in which all the images are seen in the context of the dramatic plot of the dream story. If there remain images or elements that don't make sense in the context of the dream, the interviewer asks if the dreamer would like to return to the description step, or go home and reflect upon the dream for a couple of days and then take a fresh look. Since 1991, I have asked dreamers to write a half-page summary and email it to me within the next few days. This written summary describes how the dreamer understands the dream and what parts remain unclear. I have found that this exercise has a tremendous effect on the dreamer's ability to integrate the dream insights and to develop skills in working with his or her own dreams. As a client becomes more skillful, he or she can come to therapy with part of the interview started and work much more quickly with the therapist on a given dream.

Cue Card: Questions That Execute the Steps of the Dream Interview

Questions tailored to each dream element (Settings, People, Animals, Objects, Feelings, Actions/Plots) are used to elicit rich descriptions, the key step in the interview. The use of these questions requires a lively discipline. The interviewer restrains any impulse to "lead the witness" with questions or tones of suggestion and is patient in letting the dreamer find his or her own words in response. These words are powerful triggers that the dreamer will recognize as he or she bridges to a matching life situation. Having spent decades refining the wording of these questions, I suggest the interviewer try them first, then modify to his or her liking. The Cue Card questions are applied to each step of the process: description questions vary most according to the target image; the other steps use questions that vary little. This list is brief; follow-up questions (always asked from the POV of an alien) will come as the interviewer gains experience.

Describe and Recapitulate Questions

Settings

1. Describe the opening [or the next] setting of the dream as if I came from another planet and need to know its nature, function, and how you feel about the place. (description step, or D)
2. What is this place like in your dream? [Using the word *like* is very helpful.] (D)
3. How does it feel to be there? (D)
4. So this place is [recapitulate the description]. Have I got that right? (recapitulation step, or R)
5. Does this setting, which you describe as [recapitulate the description again] remind you of anything, any situation, or any area of your life? (bridge step, or B)
6. How so? (test the bridge, or Test)

People

1. Who is X? Pretend I [come from another planet and] have never heard of [him/her] before. (D)
2. What is X like in waking life? Describe [him/her] with three to four adjectives. [Adjectives require specificity of articulation and are efficient metaphor links.] (D)
3. What is X like in your dream and what is [he/she] doing? (D)
4. Do you like X or not? Elaborate. (D)
5. So X is [recapitulate the description]. Right? (R)
6. Does X, who is [recapitulate the description again], remind you of anything, any part of yourself, or of anyone in your life? (B)
7. How so? (Test)

Animals

1. What is a Z like? (Generic D)
2. How would you describe the personality of a Z? (D)
3. What is the Z like in your dream and what is it doing? (Specific D)
4. So this Z is [recapitulate]. Have I got that right? (R)

5. Does this Z that is [recapitulate again] remind you of anything, anyone, or any part of yourself? (B)
6. How so? (Test)

Objects

1. What is a Y like? (Generic D) [Pretend that I come from another planet and have never heard of such a thing. (Keep saying this when a reminder is needed.)]
2. Why do humans have or use Ys and how do they work? (D of function)
3. How do you feel about Ys in general? (D) [Rich descriptions always include feeling or judgment.]
4. What is the Y in your dream like? (Specific D)
5. How do you feel about the Y in your dream? Like or dislike it? Why? (Specific D)
6. So the Y in your dream is [recapitulate]. Right?
7. Is there anything, anyone, or any part of yourself that is like the Y, which is [recapitulate again]? (B)
8. How so? (Test)

Feelings

1. What are you feeling at this moment in the dream? (D)
2. Yes, it can be difficult to find words for feelings. Take your time. [The less time pressure the dreamer feels, the better and more quickly he or she can work.] (D)
3. [If the dreamer gets stuck, the interviewer can guess several general words, including very unlikely ones.] Were you pleased, displeased? Anxious, relieved, frustrated, sad, lonely, thrilled? [If the dreamer accepts another word, ask for elaboration to be sure it really fits and that the dreamer can find no word that better describes his or her feelings.] (D)
4. In what way were you [pleased, frustrated, etc.]? (Specific D)
5. Let me see if I have this right; you were feeling [recapitulate]. Is that close? (R)
6. Does this feeling of [recapitulate again] remind you of anything or any time of your life? (B)
7. How so? (Test)

Actions/Plots

1. Describe the action in this part of the dream. Pretend I come from another planet and tell me if and why humans usually do this [play tennis with a baseball bat, go to church half naked, drive cars wearing blindfolds, etc.]? (D)
2. How do you feel about this action? [like, dislike, approve, disapprove] Would you do this? What kind of human would do this? (D)

3. So the action here is [recapitulate]. Right? (R)
4. Is there any situation in your life that is like [recapitulate]? (B)
5. How so? (Test)
6. [This question can be asked at the beginning, or anytime up to the end of the dream.] Would you describe the major theme or plot of your dream? (D)
7. Is this normal on Earth? Tell me why or why not. (D)
8. How does it feel for a human to be in such a situation? (D)
9. So in your dream you (or someone) [recapitulate theme or plot]. Right? (R)
10. Is there any situation in your life that is like this theme of [recapitulate again]? (B)
11. How so? (Test)

Linking and Summary Questions

1. Okay. How would you like to summarize your interview so far? Or would you like me to do it as you listen and add or modify at any point?
   [Here the dreamer or interviewer tells the story of how the interview progressed, outlining the descriptions given and the bridges made. "I (or you) were in your sister's house, which you described as and bridged to . . ." Then I felt . . . which I described as and bridged these feelings to . . ." This summary is helpful in many ways, but takes some time and skill and may be skipped.]
2. Could you tell me how you understand your dream now, and what parts remain unclear?

Because I believe the major cause of far-fetched, inaccurate, and vague interpretations to be either the dreamer's or the interpreter's tendency to jump to associative tangents and interpretive conclusions based upon traditional or theoretical projections, I think the most important device in the interview is that of asking questions from the perspective and with the naïve curiosity of someone from another planet. This gives both dreamer and interviewer the chance to know the jumping-off side of the metaphor before it is bridged to waking life. Elaborations based on particular metapsychological frameworks and the therapist's understanding of psychodynamics can most profitably be introduced *after the Dream Interview has revealed its client-centered web of bridges.*

Dream Incubation in Individual and Group Therapy, Medical Practices, and Hospice Settings

Individual Therapy

Many therapists are hesitant to work with dreams because they have not learned an efficient interpretive method, or because they fear the patient will resist or that they will look inadequate if they can not arrive at a meaning for the dream. Suggesting that the patient "sleep on" a particular issue is an easy introduction to the idea of incubating a dream. If the patient is interested, the therapist can offer a handout with tips on how to do it. Or the therapist can simply say: "If you write out your question before sleep, repeat it to yourself as you fall asleep and write down whatever is in your mind upon awakening. It might just work."

When the patient brings in an incubated or spontaneous dream, the therapist can conduct a partial or full Dream Interview, focusing on the elements around which the major feelings and actions of the dream turn. Often working with just a few images in the context of the dream theme can produce significant insights that could take months to achieve in therapy. The dreamer can then go home and continue the interview alone if so motivated. The Dream Interview is devised to be efficient. With practice, the interviewer learns not to use unnecessary words and becomes fluent in moving from one step to another. With practice, the dreamer learns to give more concise and rich descriptions, rarely needs to be reminded that the interviewer pretends to come from another planet, and catches on more quickly to the bridging process.

As the therapist repeatedly demonstrates skill in asking good questions and his or her desire for the dreamer to guide his or her recapitulations and testing of the bridges, the patient's trust of the therapist and respect for her or his own input will increase. The dream work can greatly enhance the therapeutic alliance.

Asking for suggestions or suggesting topics the dreamer could incubate is an optimistic moment in therapy where the therapist communicates confidence that the patient can contribute important clues and information that can produce insight and resolve problems. The incubations can target almost any issue and can be especially helpful in breaking through impasses in the therapy. They can also target unfinished business from dreams that were inaccurately or incompletely understood.

Lincoln, an IT engineer in his 40s, incubated a dream about his dissatisfaction with his job. He titled his dream "The Cave of the Secret Experiments." A slightly shortened dream account and highlights from our interview follow. To conserve space, I have omitted several recapitulations that were productive in the session.

> I'm driving my parents out of the city to the hills and tell them it's a 45-minute drive. I take an exit that puts us on a two-lane dirt road. I figure that the road is being prepared for paving.
>
> Now we are riding a motorcycle through a dark tunnel on dried mud. I focus on staying in the groove of a single tire track lit by the motorcycle's headlamp in order to stay upright. At the end of the tunnel is an entrance to a cave.
>
> A park ranger who looks like J.K. is unlocking the door to give the tour group access.
>
> Inside the cave, is a finished area containing a laboratory where secret experiments were once conducted. On part of the unfinished cave wall someone scrawled a word in large letters using chalk. I think the word is

German and interpret it to mean that the experiments were psychological in nature.

A man dressed in black clothes is standing at the far side of the lab looking at a laptop computer and speaking into a cell phone. He says that he has everything he needs from the lab. I think the he is implying that the lab can be destroyed now.

INTERVIEWER: Does the 45-minute drive out of town with your parents remind you of anything?
LINCOLN: That is the exact time and direction I am willing to commute to my city job. My parents treat me like a child and encourage me to stay in my job. I am reminded of my search for property to build on. My parents live in the suburbs. I don't like suburbs, and their presence in the dream suggests that they are still influencing my decisions.
I: Did your parents influence your career decision?
L: They absolutely decided my career for me, by economic force.
I: What is it like to ride your motorcycle in the dream?
L: Difficult. I need to balance both parents on my back, and stay upright. This is a burden. Driving though the tunnel staring at the tire track lit by the headlamp reminds me of working at a computer all day long. The area where I work at my company is actually labeled "The Cave" because the software engineers prefer to keep the lights off and the blinds down to reduce glare on the computer monitors. I really hate that dark, sunless environment of cubicles.
I: Who is J.K. and what is he like?
L: He is a good leader, like a helpful park ranger who knows how to teach you about the environment.
I: Can you describe the lab with the German word and the nature of the experiments that used to be carried out there?
L: The lab seems to have electronic equipment not flasks and burners. The scrawled word being in German suggests a connection to the medical experiments that Nazis did in the concentration camps.
I: What were the Nazis like?
L: They were evil. But they set up a whole mythology in a very short time. They were agile, efficient, effective. They wanted a pure race, were into control, and did psychological experiments to control people better. They were meticulous, mechanical, orderly.
I: Does this lab with experiments by agile, efficient, effective, meticulous, mechanical, orderly Nazi types who are into controlling people and who set up a whole mythology in a short time remind you of anyone, of anything, or of any part of your self or of your life?
L: This is the IT world and my career in it. It is all those things, efficient, effective, mechanical, orderly, meticulous, and in just a few decades it has created a new

world mythology. It has its evil side in its tendency to control people and I feel very controlled and trapped in my "Cave."
I: What is the man in the black clothes like? What is he doing?
L: He looks like me. He is not invasive, nor is he hiding. He is matter-of-factly reporting that the lab can be destroyed now; he has gotten what he needs from it.
I: How do you feel about him and his actions?
L: Fine. I was relieved that the lab could now be destroyed. I suspect that I am that guy. I've gotten all I need from this job/career and can move on now. My parents may still be influencing how I think about work and where I live. Time to move on.

Helping the Dreamer Choose an Incubation Phrase

Some clients don't know how to choose an incubation topic and some have trouble choosing only one topic per night. A few suggestions can be very helpful. Questions like "What shall I do with the rest of my life?" and "Should I divorce my husband?" are either too general or place the client in the position of asking for a hotline to an all-knowing and ever attentive Supreme Being or font of wisdom. They rarely elicit helpful dream responses. Better phrasing is as specific as possible and reflects the dreamer's willingness to take responsibility for and agency in improving her or his situation. Here are some common incubation phrases that work well for most people:

What keeps me from [finding a good mate, getting along with my daughter, finding a better job, speaking up at work, etc.]?

What are the pros and cons of my present options in [my career, girlfriend search]?

Why am I so anxious when . . . ?

What are the dynamics underlying my conflicts with . . . ?

Why am I so hatefully envious of . . . ?

Why am I stuck in my life, project, career and what can I do about it?

Once a client starts incubating dreams, the few minutes writing the incubation discussion will usually suffice to create a deeply felt incubation question.

Group Therapy

There are several ways to work with dreams in group therapy (Hill, 1995; Krippner, Gabel, Green, & Rubien, 1994; Perls, 1992; Ullman & Zimmerman, 1979). The use of incubated dreams would work with all those I know of. Whether or not the dreamer reveals to the group the topic of his or her incubation may influence the result. The danger in revealing the incubation topic is that the group members may be tempted to force the interpretations into an answer to the incubation. Resisting the temptation to "lead the witness" is harder than most people think.

This is especially true of group dream work methods that invite projections from the group members, as in Ullman's method in which members are invited to say, "If this were my dream, it would mean . . ."

For this reason, if the dreamer simply presents the dream and only after the interpretive work is done reveals the question posed, one is more likely to get cleaner results. The dreamer can then ask herself or himself if the dream she or he has worked on answered the question or if it treats another subject.

In groups using the phenomenological, nonprojective Dream Interview, the group members take turns interviewing the dreamer while withholding their projections, intuitions, and interpretations. But even here, knowing the target of the incubation is still difficult to ignore. The temptation to lead the witness with questions overly influenced by the incubation phrase is great. When working with people new to the method, especially with therapist group members who have the most difficulty in adopting a naive point of view, I usually suggest we not hear the incubation phrase until the interview is ended.

Medical Practices

In the rushed climate of medical clinics, HMOs, and even private practice, what does one do when suddenly a patient blurts out a terrifying or repetitive dream that is troubling him or her? Referring the patient to a therapist may not be the answer for financial, bureaucratic, or other practical reasons.

First, do no harm. Dismissing the upsetting dream or interpreting it without adequate training or information are mistakes for obvious reasons. If, however, the physician can ask a couple of well-aimed questions, and then present a questioning hypothesis about the possible meaning of the dream, much can be learned and accomplished (Delaney, 2010; Flowers, 1995; Flowers & Zweben, 1996).

While such contexts do not lend themselves to suggesting an incubation to be discussed at a future date, asking one or two general interview questions can uncover situations that may need immediate attention from a physician or psychotherapist. For example, a man who volunteers a dream about shooting himself in the head or one about the great relief of blending into a great black nothingness, or a woman who dreams about being strangled by her husband, could be offering a key to locked door. By asking an Actions/Plots question such as, "Is there some way you are shooting yourself in the head in your life? Or "Tell me about that sense of relief. Do you long for it?" Both these dream themes are common among people who are thinking about suicide. Asking the woman, "Do you sometimes feel your husband is strangling you?" could lead to a timely referral.

Pediatricians who hear dreams from their patients about sexual themes paired with coercion, or of witnessing or experiencing sexual activity or physical abuse, may consider further investigating the family relationships or referring the child to a therapist. Every adult I have seen who was abused as a child recalls such dreams dating from the early abuse.

Hospice and Other End-of-Life Care Settings

Working with the dreams of the dying can bring both insight and comfort. Dreams of dying loved ones can also become interesting topics of conversation among sympathetic family members. Some pre-death dreams are extraordinarily beautiful and generate feelings of love, hope, and peace. Visiting physicians, hospice workers, and family members who know how to mind their interviewing manners—remaining modest, gentle, and curious only upon invitation—can help the dreamer work through anxiety, loss, family conflict, and existential issues. When hospice patients can successfully incubate dreams, they feel satisfaction in having learned a new skill even in the last months or weeks of life.

Samuel, a man of 70 years, was a few months from dying and had a heavy heart. His younger brother, a therapist, had visited him earlier that day. Samuel's son, also a therapist, suspected that unfinished business with the brother was weighing on his father. He suggested that Samuel incubate a dream asking what was getting him down. His father said his approaching death should be a sufficient explanation for that—still, he agreed to "sleep on it" and see what happened.

Samuel awoke with a dream about his younger brother upstaging him in a school play. Then in the dream he realized his brother was such a novice that he had not meant to do it. He approached the brother and, to his surprise, felt a torrent of love for him. They hugged as the dream ended.

No interview was needed for this dream. The dreamer understood that his lifelong resentment for his brother, who had been the star of the family, had held him at a distance for much of their lives. In the dream, Samuel had the vivid experience of letting go of his resentment and feeling forgiveness and love for his brother. The brothers had a long-overdue discussion the next day.

Nicole Gratton and Monique Séguin (2009) have described end-of-life dreams and included accounts of striking "contact" dreams in which dreamers feel strongly they have had contact with deceased loved ones. The dreamers recount that these dreams are a great comfort. I have not worked much with this population, and have heard none of these dreams. However, I have often heard survivors recount dreams of having vivid, meaningful visits from their deceased loved ones. What the underlying reality of these dreams is, I do not know—but they are so impactful they deserve more study.

Dreams, whether spontaneous or incubated, offer zip lines to the core of issues influencing patients in therapy. Incubating dreams, using an efficient and transparent method of interpretation that can be learned by the patient, clarifies dynamics and speeds progress while enhancing the therapeutic alliance as well as adding the pleasure of figuring out a puzzle to sometimes trying therapy sessions.

Works Cited

Barrett, D. (1993). The "committee of sleep": A study of dream incubation for problem-solving. *Journal of the Association for the Study of Dreams*, Vol. 3, 115–122.

Cartwright, R., & Lamberg, L. (2001). *Crisis dreaming: Using your dreams to solve your problems.* Bloomington, IN: iUniverse.
Delaney, G. (1991). *Breakthrough dreaming: How to tap the power of your 24-hour mind.* New York: Bantam Books.
Delaney, G. (1993). The dream interview. In G.M.V. Delaney (Ed.), *New Directions in Dream Interpretation* (pp. 195-240). Albany, NY: SUNY Press.
Delaney, G. (1996). *Living your dreams.* San Francisco: HarperCollins.
Delaney, G. (1997). *In your dreams.* San Francisco: Harper San Francisco.
Delaney, G. (1998). *All about dreams.* San Francisco: HarperCollins.
Delaney, G. (2010). Everyday dream work: Using dreams to identify stress factors in medical practice. *San Francisco Medicine, Journal of the San Francisco Medical Society.* Vol. 83, No. 10, 35–36.
Flowers, L. K. (1988). The morning after: A pragmatist's approach to dreams, *The Psychiatric Journal of the University of Ottawa,* Vol. 13, No. 2, 66–71.
Flowers, L. K. (1993). The dream interview method in a private outpatient psychotherapy practice. In G. Delaney (Ed.), *New directions in dream interpretation* (pp. 241–288). Albany, NY: State University of New York Press.
Flowers, L. K. (1995). The use of presleep instructions and dreams in psychosomatic disorders. *Psychotherapy & Psychosomatics,* Vol. 64, 173–177.
Flowers, L. K., & Zweben, J. E., (1996). "The dream interview method in addiction recovery, a treatment guide." *Journal of Substance Abuse and Treatment,* Vol. 13, No. 2, 99–105.
Flowers, L. K., & Zweben, J. E., (1998). "The changing roles of 'using' dreams in addiction recovery." *Journal of Substance Abuse and Treatment,* Vol. 15. No. 3, 193–200.
Gratton, N., & Séguin, M. (2009). *Les rêves en fin de vie.* Québec: Flammarion.
Hartmann, E. (1998). *Dreams and nightmares: The new theory on the meaning and origin of dreams.* New York: Plenum.
Hill, C. E. (1995). Effectiveness of dream interpretation groups for women undergoing a divorce transition. *Dreaming,* Vol. 5, No. 1, 29–42.
Hill, C. E. (2013). *Dream work in therapy: facilitating exploration, insight, and action.* American Psychological Association. Kindle Edition.
Krippner, S., Gabel, S., Green, J., & Rubien, R. (1994). Community applications of an experiential group approach to teaching dreamwork. *Dreaming,* Vol. 4, No. 3, 215–222.
Moffitt, A., Kramer, M., & Hoffman, R. (1993). *The functions of dreaming.* Albany, NY: State University of New York Press.
Perls, F. S. (1992). *Gestalt therapy verbatim.* Gouldsboro, ME: Gestalt Journal Press.
Reed, H. (1976). Dream incubation: A reconstruction of a ritual in contemporary form. *Journal of Humanistic Psychology,* Vol. 16, 53–69.
Ullman, M. & Zimmerman, N. (1979). *Working with dreams.* Los Angeles: Tarcher.
White, G. L., & Taytroe, L. (2003). Personal problem-solving using dream incubation. *Dreaming,* Vol. 13, No. 4, 193–209.

5
FINDING GENDER DIFFERENCES IN DREAM REPORTS

Stanley Krippner

SAYBROOK UNIVERSITY

For centuries, human beings have been intrigued with the topic of psychological gender differences. When scientific psychology emerged around 1879, there was no consensus on this issue; some psychologists maintained that gender differences were large and others claimed that they were small (Hyde, 2014). This is an important issue because it affects education (e.g., single-gender schooling), military service (e.g., front-line assignments), and job selection (e.g., faculty appointments, corporate hiring, wage differentials), among other factors.

Gender differences in dream reports have been studied extensively over the years and these investigations have raised a number of issues in regard to their findings. For example, investigators realize that the dream as directly experienced is not studied; dream reports might be incomplete, poorly remembered, or completely fabricated. In addition, the dream report might change or undergo revision depending on the social or temporal context of the recall. Domhoff (2009) pointed out that such studies have the potential to evoke the tensions that accompany any discussion of gender in a world where gender discrimination—and conflicts between men and women on many personal issues—are pervasive.

Dreams reports are usually gathered from questionnaires, dream diaries, or laboratory awakenings, and the source of the reports may influence the way in which dreams are shared with researchers. There are variations in gender roles from culture to culture as well as major individual differences in the way that dream diaries are kept by men and women, which also prevents any large generalizations from being definitive.

The most systematic empirical data on gender and dream content come from a comprehensive system for studying dream content developed by Hall and Van de Castle (1966). The most frequently used categories concern characters, social interactions, misfortunes and good fortunes, activities, emotions, and settings. The categories rest on the "nominal" level of measurement, which means there is a simple counting of frequencies for the content categories, such as "men" or "women," or "indoor" or "outdoor" setting. Content analysis employs an explicit, organized plan for assembling data, quantifying them to measure the concepts under study, examining their patterns and interrelationships, and interpreting quantitative comparison of verbal reports produced by research participants (Tartz, Baker, & Krippner, 2006–2007).

Domhoff (1999) pointed out that the findings of the Hall and Van de Castle system are most useful and readily understood when they are conveyed as percentages and ratios, because they lend themselves to the form of statistical analysis—nonparametric statistics—that is most appropriate for data from nominal categories. According to Domhoff (2009), the failure of some dream researchers to take these methodological problems seriously has led to several misunderstandings and disagreements concerning gender similarities and differences in dream content. Another problem arises when dreamers and external judges disagree in their scoring, perhaps because of the demand characteristics that arise when dreamers are assigned rating tasks. For example, dreamers tend to rate the emotions in their dreams as more pleasant than do outside judges (e.g., Tonay, 1990–1991). Tartz, Baker, and Krippner (2006–2007) added that dream length needs to be considered when making gender comparisons: one gender's dreams might contain more words than the comparison gender, providing more of an opportunity for a content item to appear. This is not a problem with the content indicators themselves, as Domhoff (2003, Chapter 5) demonstrated empirically by comparing findings for dream reports of varying lengths up to 600 words, finding no significant differences.

The Hall and Van de Castle normative findings are based on 500 dream reports from 100 men and 500 dreams reports from 100 women, which were collected from predominantly middle class Euro-American students at two academic institutions in the late 1940s and early 1950s. These results were replicated with 340 dreams from 69 women and 263 dreams from 53 men collected at another American university in 1979 (Hall, Domhoff, Blick, & Weesner, 1982). The dream content of older Euro-American American adults seems very similar to that of the young adults on whom the norms are based (Hall & Domhoff, 1964; Kramer, Winget, & Whitman, 1971; Krippner & Weinhold, 2002), the one exception being a possible decline, with age, in aggression and negative emotions (Domhoff, 2009).

Hall and Van de Castle (1966) reported a striking difference between men and women's dream reports: men dream about women less often than they dream about men, while women dream about equally for both genders. In addition, men dream less often about clothes and household items while women dream less often about tools and weapons (Schredl, 2007). However, this difference was reversed in Krippner and Weinhold's (2001) study of Brazilian dreams; men dreamed significantly more often about household items than did women.

This is one of several examples where studies of other populations have deviated from Hall and Van de Castle's findings, making generalizations about dream content hazardous.

For Hall and Van de Castle's sample, there were few gender differences in regard to aggression, misfortune, failure, and such negative emotions as anger, apprehension, confusion, and sadness; 80% of men's dreams and 77% of women's have at least one of these negative elements (Domhoff, 2009). Regarding more positive aspects of dream content, such as friendly interactions, good fortune, success, and happiness, about half of the dream reports for both men and women in Hall and Van de Castle's sample had at least one of those elements. Men and women also reported an equal number of dreams in which food or eating was mentioned—about 17% for each gender. An example of an American female's dream report follows:

> An event just ended at which there was a huge buffet. Several men were loading leftover fruit and vegetables on a 4' by 8' plywood tray and putting them on a truck. I asked to help. They said that they did not need me. That was okay! I was pleased we would have an abundance of food left over from the buffet.

Both men and women were more often victims than aggressors in the aggressive interactions in their dreams, and they faced the same attackers, specifically "male strangers" or animals. On a more positive note, both men and women were equally likely to befriend another character in their dreams (Domhoff, 2009). Rubinstein, Hartmann, and Krippner (1996) found more aggression in dream reports of participants living in cities of 40,000 people or more than those living in towns of less than 40,000 people, underlying the possibility that there may be deviations in content data from the same country. This example is illustrative of a female who is attacked by an unknown male, but then befriended:

> I am a knight in a tournament. I feel great, riding a palomino stallion. I am fighting a man, but lose. I am stabbed and start to die. But a Divine Power in the form of a child comes out of nowhere and before I know it, I am completely healed.

The tendency for dreams to feature "negative" events is not atypical and might be adaptive, permitting emotional downloading at night (Levin & Nielsen, 2007). In a wide range of cross-cultural studies, there is more aggression than friendliness and more misfortune than good fortune, and dreamers of both genders are more often the victims than the aggressors in aggressive interactions (Domhoff, 1996, Chapter 6).

American men and women mention about the same number of activities occurring in their dreams, such as talking, walking, looking, listening, and thinking. These activities are very similar except that there are slightly more physical activities in men's dreams than in women's (27% vs. 20%) and slightly more verbal activities in women's dreams (26% vs. 22%). Similarly, American men and women have roughly the same number of objects appearing in their dreams, such as houses, trees, cars, streets, money, and parts of the body. A study of Japanese dreams yielded findings that were almost identical to those for the United States (Yamanaka, Morita, & Matsumoto, 1982).

In the Hall and Van de Castle sample, there was a slight tendency for women to have more characters in their dreams, but this difference has to be tempered by the fact that women's dream reports tended to be about 8% longer than men's on average. There was a gender difference in how often men and women included male and female characters in their dreams: men dreamed twice as often about other men as they do about women (67% vs. 33%), and women dreamed equally about both genders (48% men, 52% women). This was the largest difference found between American men and women. The magnitude of the difference was determined by h, a statistic for effect size that is useful with percentage comparisons (Domhoff, 1996, Appendix D).

The effect size of .38 for this comparison is a large magnitude for studies of dream content. Tartz, Baker, and Krippner (2006–2007) pointed out that computing effect size prevents researchers from regarding small but statistically significant differences as meaningful; it also prevents disregard for statistically nonsignificant results that are in fact meaningful.

This gender difference in the male/female percentage has been found at all ages in many different cultures, including in Argentina, Switzerland, and many small traditional cultures studied in the past by cultural anthropologists (Domhoff, 1996, Chapter 6; Hall, 1984; Schredl, 2007; Tartz & Krippner, 2008). However, it is not a "universal" difference that is invariably found in every group. The dreams of African American male college students at a community college in Chicago in the late 1960s showed a male/female percentage of 53% (males) and 47% (females), which was very similar to the male/female percentage of the African American women in the study (Domhoff, 1996, p. 75). Nor was the difference found in studies of Mexican and Peruvian teenagers and young adults, where the men tended to dream equally of men and women, and the women dreamed more frequently of men (Domhoff, 1996, p. 106). It also was absent in a study of German college students (Schredl, Petra, Bishop, Golitz, & Buschtons, 2003) and studies of Austrian (Stepansky et al., 1998) and English (Tartz, Baker, & Krippner, 2006–2007) participants of various ages. This general finding may be related to the assumption that dreams reflect people's concerns; men in many societies are more concerned about other men than they are about women, whereas women are equally concerned about both men and women (Domhoff, 2009).

For the Hall and Van de Castle sample, another gender difference was that women more often dreamed of characters who were familiar to them than did men—family members, friends, and famous people. This difference is found in most cross-cultural studies (Domhoff, 1996, Chapter 6). An example is a dream reported by a Brazilian woman:

> I had a dream about Professor Cicero from the university. He is meditating with his eyes closed. I can see an aura around his body. Suddenly an amethyst appears in the middle of his head. It is an enormous stone and it represents his "third eye." I think that Professor Cicero must have a great deal of spiritual power.

In the Hall and Van de Castle sample, American men dreamed more often of unfamiliar males than did women (28% vs. 15%), but men and women dreamed equally about familiar males (25% vs. 23%). Conversely, women dreamed more often about familiar females than men did, 29% vs. 16%, but women and men dreamed about equally of unfamiliar females, 11% for women and 10% for men. In short, these comparisons indicate that the difference on familiarity percent is created by the presence of more familiar females in women's dreams and more unfamiliar males in men's dreams. An example is a dream by an Argentine man:

> I dreamed that I was in a deserted place and saw a very big gray statue. Nearby there was an abandoned house made out of wood. In this house, there was a fellow who was hiding like a thief. I came nearer to see the statue. This fellow had a sword and started to move as I came closer, he tried to kill me with the sword. I came into the house and found another sword. I destroyed the house, and the statue fell down, killing the thief.

At a general level, the dreams of the American men and women in Hall and Van de Castle's sample were similar in that about the same percentage of their dreams had at least one aggressive interaction, defined as a deliberate or intentional feeling or act on the part of one character meant to harm or annoy another character (47% for men, 44% for women). This broad definition includes angry thoughts or hostility toward another character as well as threats or physically aggressive acts. An American man reported:

> I am involved in a battle for the independence of Ireland. It is many centuries ago, and the Irish are fighting the English. Lots of people are being killed. Finally, our side wins. I follow the defeated English to the shore to make sure they really get in their boats and leave.

Men and woman in Hall and Van de Castle's group also had about the same percentage of dreams with at least one friendly interaction, defined as a purposeful act involving support, help, kindness, gift giving, or any other type of friendly act toward another character (38% for men, 42% for women). A Brazilian man reported:

> I am in the house of a person who is very nice. He seems to appreciate my presence. He is an Oriental lama. He invites me to stay the night and to sleep in a bed there. Immediately, there emits from my chest a pink light that turns into a brilliant blue. I feel calm and peaceful. We sit on chairs there, in silence.

American men are more often aggressive with other men and are most often friendly with female characters, whereas women have about the same rate of aggressive and friendly interactions with both male and female characters. On the other hand, men and women have the same rate of friendliness per character.

In Hall and Van de Castle's sample, unknown males were the most dangerous human characters in the dreams of both men and women, but the percentage was especially high for men, 72%, suggesting that men's higher male/female percentage may relate to their concern about aggressive interactions with men they do not know. In contrast, men have more friendly than aggressive interactions with women whether they are known or not. Male strangers are their enemies, and women, whether known or not, are their friends. In this dream from an American woman, a known man commits an aggressive interaction:

> I dreamed I got in my car, and the hair on the back of my head stood up. I looked in the rear-view window and saw my father, who had died some time ago. His head popped up from the back seat. He had red eyes and large, snarling vampire fangs, and he was coming for me. I screamed—and I woke up.

English females reported more dreams about physical aggression than English males as well as a larger bodily misfortunes percentage (47% compared to 7% for males). In this dream, from an English female participant, both are represented:

> I had a dream about a man with a gun. He is hunting a group of us. Some members of our group had tackled him and had been killed in the process. But I am not afraid of him. Suddenly, I am at college, carrying a huge folio of art. I am with a classmate. She is a year below me. I am on my own, not knowing what class I am supposed to be in because I have lost my timetable. I feel lost and lonely, so I cut my wrists. I am sitting on a wall. I want people to see me, to understand my pain. But the cuts are only scratches and so nobody takes notice. I decide to look for someplace to die. I go to the toilets, but I feel that I don't want to die there because I might not be found. I realize that I want to be found before I die. Suddenly, the blood starts gushing from my wounds.

To the degree that information is available, these gender differences on aggression are very widespread cross-culturally. For example, the men's dreams from

Mexico, Peru, and Argentina (e.g., Tartz & Krippner, 2008) had more aggression than the women's dreams; men and women in those three countries also had more of their aggressive interactions with male characters than female characters. In some countries, such as the Netherlands and Switzerland, the rates of aggression are much lower than in the United States, but the same gender differences are present. In small traditional societies, the rates of physical aggression are much higher than in the United States or Europe, in good part because of attacks by animals; sometimes the difference between men and women on physical aggression percentage therefore disappears (Domhoff, 1996, Chapter 6).

Contrary to cultural stereotypes about dreams, the dreams reports in Hall and Van de Castle's sample did not often involve sexuality, not even a romantic hug or kiss. Only 12% of American men's dreams and 4% of women's dreams had at least one sexual interaction, and the figures are equally low in the few cross-cultural studies that mention sexuality at all (e.g., Tartz, Baker, & Krippner, 2006–2007).

An example is the Krippner and Weinhold (2001) study of 240 Brazilian dream reports: the number of characters who engage in sexual interactions was 6%; the percentage was the same for both genders. However, the percentage of dreams in which sexual interactions took place were 11% for men and 12% for women. In other words, researchers need to take account of the number of dreams in which an activity occurs as well as the number of characters engaging in that activity. Here is an example of an English woman's dream in which sex is mentioned, even though she does not engage in a sexual activity:

> I am in this unusual pub. I see a sign that says, "There are plenty of beds upstairs." It continues, "Please feel free to use them, as well as the oral sex room downstairs." I sat at an empty seat at a small table and didn't realize that I was sitting directly across from a man. I actually had taken his friend's seat. When his friend came back, they both propositioned me for an act of prostitution. I wasn't too happy about that.

In the Hall and Van de Castle sample, there were more mentions of emotions in women's dream reports, an average of .84 per dream, as compared to an average of .56 for men. However, the percentage of negative emotions (anger, apprehension, sadness, and confusion) was 80% for both men and women. There were some differences in the settings in the dreams of American men and women. The men were more likely to be in outdoor settings than women (52% vs. 39%, h = .26) and more likely to be in unfamiliar settings (39% vs. 22%, h = .38). An American man provided this dream report about an unfamiliar unknown setting:

> I am in a jungle with tribal people and say, "This is not the Berkeley Hills!" People from all nationalities are there, many in loincloths. They tell me that I am in a commune and that they want me to live with them. They drug

me. Four days later I will myself to wake up. I tell them "How dare you keep me here?" I leave the place.

There are related gender differences regarding dreams, at least in those parts of the world where scientific studies have taken place. Women tend to recall dreams, including nightmares, more often than men. Women are more interested in dreams and read more books and articles on the topic than men, and have a more positive attitude toward dreams (Schredl, Kim, Labudek, Schadler, & Goritz, 2013). Most gender differences that were reported for adults were also found in children and adolescents, except that for children between the ages of 3 and 5, no gender differences in dream content were detected (Foulkes, 1982; Strauch, 2004). These data suggest that cultural conditioning and gender roles are an important determinant in the formation of dream content and may explain the differences noted when various samples are compared cross-culturally.

Discussion

From a phenomenological perspective, dreams are experienced as "real" during sleep and are reported in narrative form during wakefulness (Krippner, Bogzaran, & de Carvalho, 2002). A dream report can be conceptualized as a text, hence its content is influenced by the linguistic style of the research participant. Differences in dream content among individuals or groups may reflect their differences in verbal behavior more than any other measure (Winget & Kramer, 1979, p. 14). In a study relevant to this issue, research participants were asked to "make up" a dream while awake and produced narratives that judges could not discriminate from written reports of their nighttime dreams (Cavallero & Natale, 1988–1989).

There are dangers in accepting language as an accurate representation of experience. Instead, language exists in relation to its world; the resulting back-and-forth communication makes it difficult to compare dream reports even within a single culture or group, much less between groups. Even so, the use of dream reports can be an important research tool for cultural psychologists, who have pointed out that there is no group of people (least of all Euro-American males) whose behaviors, activities, and values can become a presumptive universal normative baseline for human development and mental health (Shweder, 1991). Dream reports can provide investigators a window into conceptualizing and appreciating the variety of human worldviews and experiences.

If dream reports were considered to lack meaning, or if they did not reflect daily experience, they could be discounted by social and behavioral scientists. Adler (1938) stressed the match between dreams and the lifestyles of their dreamers, maintaining that the dream does not significantly differ from waking thoughts. Domhoff (2009) has concluded that data emerging from these findings support the idea that there is continuity between the content of dreams and waking life.

Dream reports are in many ways what we might expect based on what is known about the autobiographical memories, interests, and living situations of men and women in waking life. As reflected in their dreams, men and women have many interests, fears and emotional preoccupations in common, such as fear of unknown males and many kinds of animals, and both men and women suffer equally from anger, apprehension, sadness, and confusion.

At the same time, there is ample evidence that differences in dreams relate to differences in waking life (e.g., Krippner & Combs, 2007; Lortie-Lussier, Cote, & Vachon, 2000). There are similarities to findings with reports of autobiographical memories. For example, in a study of 37 men and 37 women ages 45–60 in Poland who were asked to write down their three most vivid memories, the women wrote longer accounts, included more people, used more words about emotions, and provided more descriptive details (Niedzwienska, 2003). All four of these differences have been found in the dream reports of American men and women (Domhoff, 2009).

For Domhoff (2009), it is not surprising that women dream more of indoor settings or household items than do men, due to their greater family responsibilities and greater likelihood of working in an indoor setting. Nor is it surprising that they include more descriptions of clothing. Further, the findings on a higher rate of aggressive interactions in men's dreams, particularly those that involve physical aggression, are consistent with one of the few gender differences found in studies in many different societies. At the same time, the fact that the amount of aggression is lower in some societies and higher in others, and that the gender differences on aggression sometimes decline or disappear, shows that the amount of aggression in dreams is probably closely related to cultural differences.

Future studies of gender similarities and differences in a wider range of countries would be very useful in developing a better theory of dream meaning. Hartmann (2011) suggested that the major function of dreams may be to weave new material into existing memory systems; this is adaptive in that it helps to solve problems and generate new ideas. At the same time, Tedlock (1987) observed that waking consciousness itself is not unitary but is constantly shifting between the internal world and the external world, between arousal and dissociation. This paradox has not kept psychologists from studying waking experience, and it should not keep psychologists from the disciplined inquiry into reported dreams.

Acknowledgments

The general organization of this chapter follows that originated by Domhoff (2009), and readers are advised to read his chapter for a greater elucidation of the topic. Examples of dream reports are taken from the author's personal data base.

The preparation of this chapter was supported by the Saybrook University Chair for the Study of Consciousness.

References

Adler, A. (1938). *Social interest: Challenge to mankind*. London, UK: Faber and Faber.
Cavallero, C., & Natale, V. (1988–1989). Was I dreaming or did it really happen? A comparison between real and artificial dream reports. *Imagination, Cognition, and Personality, 8,* 1924.
Domhoff, G. W. (1996). *Finding meaning in dreams: A quantitative approach*. New York, NY: Plenum.
Domhoff, G. W. (1999). New directions in the study of dream content using the Hall and Van de Castle coding system. *Dreaming, 9,* 115–137.
Domhoff, G. W. (2003). *The scientific study of dreams: Neural networks, cognitive development, and content analysis*. Washington, DC: American Psychological Association.
Domhoff, W. G. (2009). Gender differences in dreams. In S. Krippner & D. J. Ellis (Eds.), *Perchance to dream: The frontiers of dream psychology* (pp. 153–163). New York, NY: Nova Science Publishers.
Foulkes, D. (1982). *Children's dreams: Longitudinal studies*. New York, NY: John Wiley & Sons.
Hall, C. (1984). A ubiquitous sex difference in dreams, revisited. *Journal of Personality and Social Psychology, 46,* 1109–1117.
Hall, C., & Domhoff, G. W. (1964). Friendliness in dreams. *Journal of Social Psychology, 62,* 309–314.
Hall, C., Domhoff, G. W., Blick, K., & Weesner, K. (1982). The dreams of college men and women in 1950 and 1980: A comparison of dream contents and sex differences. *Sleep, 5,* 188–194.
Hall, C., & Van de Castle, R. (1966). *The content analysis of dreams*. New York, NY: Appleton-Century-Crofts.
Hartmann, E. (2011). *The nature and functions of dreaming*. New York, NY: Oxford University Press.
Hyde, J. S. (2014). Gender similarities and differences. *Annual Review of Psychology, 65,* 373–399.
Kramer, M., Winget, C., & Whitman, R. (1971). A city dreams: A survey approach to normative dream content. *American Journal of Psychiatry, 127,* 1350–1356.
Krippner, S., Bogzaran, F., & de Carvalho, A. P. (2002). *Extraordinary dreams and how to work with them*. Albany, NY: State University of New York Press.
Krippner, S., & Combs, A. (2007). Dreams are patterned and have meaning: An argument for continuity between dream life and waking life. *Dream Network, 26*(4), 17–19; 46.
Krippner, S., & Weinhold, J. (2001). Gender differences in the content analysis of 240 dream reports from Brazilian participants in dream seminars. *Dreaming, 11,* 35–42.
Krippner, S., & Weinhold, J. (2002). Gender differences in a content analysis study of 608 dream reports from research participants in the United States. *Social Behavior and Personality, 30,* 388–410.
Levin, R., & Nielsen, T. A. (2007). Disturbed dreaming, posttraumatic stress disorder, and affect distress: A review and neurocognitive model. *Psychological Bulletin, 133,* 482–528.
Lortie-Lussier, M., Cote, L., & Vachon, J. (2000). The consistency and continuity hypotheses revisited through the dreams of women at two periods of their lives. *Dreaming, 10,* 67–76.
Niedzwienska, A. (2003). Gender differences in vivid memories. *Sex Roles, 49,* 321–331.
Rubinstein, K., Hartmann, A., & Krippner, S. (1996, Spring). The geography of dream aggression. *DreamTime: The Association for the Study of Dreams Newsletter,* pp. 15–17.

Schredl, M. (2007). Gender differences in dreaming. In D. Barrett & P. McNamara (Ed.), *The new science of dreaming* (Vol. 2, pp. 29–47). Westport, CT: Praeger.

Schredl, M., Kim, E., Labudek, S., Schadler, A., & Goritz, A. S. (2013). Gender, sex role orientation, and dreaming. *Dreaming, 23,* 277–286.

Schredl, M., Petra, C., Bishop, A., Golitz, E., & Buschtons, D. (2003). Content analysis of German students' dreams: Comparison to American findings. *Dreaming, 13,* 237–243.

Shweder, R. A. (1991). *Thinking through cultures: Expeditions in cultural psychology.* Cambridge, MA: Harvard University Press.

Stepansky, R., Holzinger, B., Schmeiser-Rieder, A., Saletu, B., Kunze, M., & Zeithofer, J. (1998). Austrian dream behavior: Results of a representative population survey. *Dreaming, 8,* 23–30.

Strauch, I. (2004). *Dreams in the transition from childhood to adolescence: A longitudinal study* (in German). Bern, Switzerland: Hans Huber.

Tartz, R. S., Baker, R. C., & Krippner, S. (2006–2007). Cognitive differences in dream content between English males and females attending dream seminars using quantitative content analysis. *Imagination, Cognition and Personality, 26,* 325–344.

Tartz, R. S., & Krippner, S. (2008). Cognitive differences in dream content between Argentine males and females using quantitative content analysis. *Dreaming, 18,* 217–235.

Tedlock B. (1987). Dreaming and dream research. In B. Tedlock (Ed.), *Dreaming: Anthropological and psychological interpretations* (pp. 1–30). New York, NY: Cambridge University Press.

Tonay, V. (1990–1991). California women and their dreams: A historical and sub-cultural comparison of dream content. *Imagination, Cognition, and Personality, 10,* 83–97.

Winget, C., & Kramer, M. (1979). *Dimensions of dreams.* Gainesville: University of Florida Press.

Yamanaka, T., Morita, Y., & Matsumoto, J. (1982). Analysis of the dream contents in college students by REM-awakening technique. *Folia Psychiatrica et Neurologica Japonica, 36,* 33–52.

6

FRIENDS AND FRIENDLINESS

Could They Be the Clue in Psychiatric Patients' Dreams?

G. William Domhoff

UNIVERSITY OF CALIFORNIA, SANTA CRUZ

Introduction

There have been many studies of dream content in various psychiatric populations over the past 55 years, but most of them are anecdotal in nature, use untested coding systems, or include only a small number of dream reports. In addition, there are several possible confounds in past studies, such as variation from hospital to hospital in how patients are diagnosed and classified. Then, too, patients within the same diagnostic categories may have been in different phases of their illnesses. The possible effects of medication and hospitalization on both dream content and the ability to provide full and accurate dream reports usually are not controlled. The best of these studies are summarized by Kramer and one of his colleagues (Kramer, 1970, 2000; Kramer & Roth, 1979) who conclude that there are only a few consistent findings, many of them involving frequency of recall, the degree of emotion present, and the vividness of dreaming. Another review focusing on recent studies, mostly carried out between 2005 and 2013, points to similar findings on the absence or negativity of emotions while noting that studies are often contradictory, but with little assessment of the quality and sample sizes of the specific studies (Skancke, Holsen, & Schredl, 2014). It also may be that there are actually very few differences between patient and nonpatient populations, as shown shortly.

Nor is the closely related literature on the effects of psychotropic medications on dreaming and dream content any more illuminating. In a review of nine studies carried out during the heyday of laboratory dream research, Roth, Kramer, and Salis (1979) note that "few if any of the existing studies were more than pilot studies," and that "there has been a failure to examine even one drug in depth" (pp. 220–221). Moreover, they conclude that "the lack of standardization of methods of assessing quality of dream content has resulted in isolated bits of information that do not yet form a coherent picture" (Roth et al., 1979, p. 221). As a result, the strongest conclusion they can reach is that "some sedative-hypnotic and antidepressant agents may affect the quality of dreams, but the precise nature of the effect is yet to be determined" (Roth et al., 1979, p. 220).

The one rigorous and relatively recent study involving medications and actual dream content adds very little to the earlier picture. It examined dreams as an "add-on" to a major laboratory study comparing the effects of antidepressant medication—either fluoxetine (Prozac) or nefazodone (Serzone)—on the sleep physiology of patients suffering major, nonpsychotic depression (Armitage, Rochlen, Fitch, Trivedi, & Rush, 1995, p. 191). For the dream portion of the study, patients were asked to report any dreams they remembered after they were awakened at a set time in the morning. Only 27 premedication and 32 on-medication dream reports were obtained from 21 of the 89 patients participating in the study. Aside from the low level of recall, which is consistent with earlier studies of depressed patients, the other main findings were that the reports were "short, relatively bland with little emotion" (Armitage, et al., 1995, p. 193). In addition, the dream reports while taking the medication were less vivid and had fewer scenes (Armitage, et al., 1995, p. 196).

Although there are only a few clinically useful or theoretically interesting findings that can be extracted from the literature on the dream content of psychiatric patients, some of the past studies do provide leads as to where future studies might most productively focus their energies, and thereby develop information that could be clinically useful in the future. Generally speaking, social interactions and emotions are the two elements of dream content that are most closely related to waking measures of psychological well-being, and are therefore potentially pathognomonic when greatly different from nonpatients' dreams (Zadra & Domhoff, 2011). In particular, a closer look at friends and friendly interactions in dreams, which can be examined with several different content indicators, might provide a good starting point, especially in conjunction with a consideration of aggressive interactions and/or emotions.

Past studies also provide some good low-budget data-gathering strategies and research designs that could be built upon using new web sites, search programs, and statistical analysis tools that have been developed in the past 15–20 years. The concluding section of the chapter therefore suggests intake questions, dream-collection strategies, and content-analysis methods for future psychiatric studies, any of which could be used without disturbing established clinical procedures in either group-based psychotherapy practices or clinical units.

The Hall and Van de Castle Coding System

The most comprehensive coding system for the quantitative study of dream content, created by Hall and Van de Castle (1966), includes a body of past findings that provide a useful starting point for studying patients' dreams. It has ten general categories and numerous content indicators that cover virtually every element in dream reports. It rests on the nominal level of measurement to avoid the serious reliability problems that plague most ordinal-level (rating) scales for dream content, and uses readily understood percentages and ratios to correct for differences in the length of dream reports. Due to the distortions and mistakes created by skewed distributions and nonrandom samples, both of which are common in dream studies, the system uses the formula for the significance of differences between proportions to determine p values. Proportions also lead seamlessly to the use of an effect size measure called Cohen's h, which is similar in its general logic to Cohen's better-known d statistic for determining effect sizes based on means (Domhoff, 1996, Chapter 4, Appendix D; Domhoff, 2003, Chapter 3; Domhoff & Schneider, 2015).

The Hall and Van de Castle (hereafter HVdC) coding system also includes normative findings for men and women based on samples of 500 dream reports from each gender collected at Case Western Reserve University and Baldwin-Wallace College between 1949 and 1951. These norms were subsequently replicated for men and women at the University of Richmond in 1981, for women at the University of California, Berkeley, in 1985, and for women at Salem College in the late 1980s (Domhoff, 1996, Chapter 4). Several studies of subsamples of varying sizes determined that the normative findings are replicated exactly with 250 dream reports, very well with 125 dream reports, and adequately for some indicators with 100 dream reports (Domhoff, 2003 pp. 92–94, 113–114; Domhoff & Schneider, 2008a, pp. 1262–1264). This large number of dream reports is needed in any quantitative study of dream content for two reasons: first, many dream elements, such as friendly and aggressive interactions, appear in less than half of dream reports; and second, effect sizes are generally small to medium. Very importantly, these studies also show there are only a few differences, primarily on aggressive interactions, between dream reports collected in the sleep laboratory and non-lab settings, which is a big factor in why low-budget dream research could be carried out in psychiatric clinical settings (Domhoff, 2005; Domhoff & Schneider, 1999; Hall, 1966b).

For purposes of this chapter, there are six relevant content indicators that may be indicative of psychopathology when some yet-to-be determined combination of them differs significantly from the norms: (1) friends percent (all known non-family characters divided by the total number of human characters); (2) aggression/friendliness percent (A/F%), which is calculated by dividing all dreamer-involved aggressions by dreamer-involved friendly interactions and aggressions; (3) friendliness per character ratio (F/C index); (4) aggressions per character ratio (A/C index); (5) the percentage of dreams with at least one friendly interaction; and (6) the percentage of dreams with at least one aggressive interaction. The normative figures for these six indicators will be presented in subsequent sections in the context of comparisons with patient populations or individual case studies.

The HVdC content indicators, while individually useful, are best considered together to see if any patterns emerge. In this regard, they are somewhat analogous to a Minnesota Multiphasic Personality Inventory (MMPI) profile. In fact, the content indicators are called an *h-profile* when the differing magnitudes of the effect sizes for each indicator are presented as a bar graph with the male or female normative sample serving as the baseline (Domhoff, 1996, Chapter 4 and Appendix E; Domhoff, 2003, Chapters 3 and 5). Within the context of indicators relating to aggressive and friendly social interactions, the A/F% is valuable because it puts into balance findings concerning the relationship between aggressive and friendly interactions that were reported in many past studies merely as "more aggressions" or without an adequate control group. The A/C and F/C indexes are useful for similar reasons, along with the fact that they normalize comparisons of aggressions and friendliness across samples by using the number of characters as a control. It is often very revealing to consider the A/C and F/C indexes with specific groups of characters (such as men, women, friends, and strangers) or with specific characters (such as mother, father, husband, and wife).

However, as the title of this chapter suggests, it may be that the absence of friends and the lack of friendly interactions (which can occur with family members and strangers as well as friends) is the pair of factors that best indicates the presence of psychopathology. Without the capacity to create friendships and to interact in a friendly way with family, friends, and strangers, a human life is psychologically impoverished.

Studies of Psychiatric Populations

The most systematic study of differences between psychiatric patients and nonpatients employed the HVdC coding system and made comparisons with its male norms (Hall, 1966a). The study was based on 211 dream reports collected from 50 male patients, who were grouped into four diagnostic categories: five patients who were both schizophrenic and alcoholic, 20 patients who were schizophrenic, 15 patients who were alcoholics, and 10 patients with a variety of other diagnoses. The dream reports of the four groups were compared with each other and with the male norms for characters, social interactions, success and failure, misfortune and good fortune, and eating and drinking. Surprisingly, there were very few differences (Hall, 1966a). However, there was one potentially useful difference between the dream reports of the 50 patients as a whole and the male norms: lower percentages and ratios having to do with friends and friendly interactions. Specifically, the patients' friends percent, F/C index, and percentage of dreams with at least one friendly interaction are below the male norms, and the A/F% is above the norms. Since most of these differences are slightly larger for the 105 dreams reports from schizophrenics, Table 6.1 compares the findings from their dreams with the male norms on the six indicators related to aggression and friendliness.

TABLE 6.1 The dreams of male schizophrenics compared to the Hall/Van de Castle male norms on aggression & friendliness indicators.

i	Male Norms	Schizophrenics	h	p
Friends Percent	31%	20%	−.28	.002
A/F%	59%	78%	−.41	.000
A/C Index	.34	.37	+.06	.780
F/C Index	.21	.11	−.29	.000
At Least One Aggressive Interaction	47%	47%	−.01	.316
At Least One Friendly Interaction	38%	17%	−.47	.000

These findings are especially interesting because they are consistent with the findings in several later psychiatric studies in Europe and the United States. For example, low friendliness was a striking finding in a study of female patients in Paris. Fifteen were schizophrenic; 12 were other types of psychotics (Schnetzler & Carbonel, 1976). Although an A/F% was not reported, the figures in Table 3 of the published article can be used to determine that it is 62% in the schizophrenic group and 78% in the other psychotic group, as compared to 47% for the control group of 15 normal female subjects and 52% for the HVdC female norms (Schnetzler & Carbonel, 1976, p. 373). A similar finding is reported in a study of female outpatients in London who suffered from high anxiety states (Gentil & Lader, 1978). Each of 20 patients mailed in five dream reports in stamped envelopes that the researchers provided. These dream narratives were compared with those collected from 25 female volunteers. According to the authors, the lack of friendly interactions is one of the "most significant" findings, but the statistics used do not make it possible to make comparisons with the American normative sample (Gentil & Lader, 1978, p. 301).

Findings in a comparison of dream reports from depressed and schizophrenic patients studied in a laboratory in Cincinnati, Ohio, pointed to a low level of friendliness as well as a lack of friends in patient dreams (Kramer & Roth, 1973). Ten depressed patients, five male and five female, contributed 91 dream reports; 13 schizophrenics, 11 male and two female, contributed 217. There were more strangers in the schizophrenics' dream reports and more family members in the depressed patients' reports, but it is especially notable that both groups had an extremely low friends percent: 18% for the schizophrenics and 22% for the depressives, compared to 31% for the male norms. More recent studies, though mixed in their findings, sometimes report more strangers in the dreams of schizophrenics and more family members in the dreams of depressed patients (see Skancke, et al., 2014, pp. 42–43, for summaries).

The findings on few friends and/or low friendliness in patients' dream reports can be put in a broader context by noting research that focuses on the relationship between dream content and the subjective sense of well-being in nonpatient populations. In particular, a longitudinal study of 28 participants who kept dream journals and completed measures of psychological well-being (PWB) at varying points over a 6–10 year period discovered that "the lower the participants' self-reported levels of PWB, the more their dreams tended to contain aggressive as opposed to friendly interactions, negative emotions as opposed to positive ones, and, to lesser extent, failures and misfortunes as opposed to successes and good fortunes" (Pesant & Zadra, 2006, p. 111). Scores on a neuroticism scale also correlated negatively with the ratio of friendly to aggressive interactions, but not as strongly as did well-being measures.

Evidence From Individual Dream Journals

Dream journals, kept by perhaps 1–2% of people from all walks of life for a month or more for varying reasons, have standing as a form of personal document long recognized in psychology as possessing the potential to provide new insights (Allport, 1942; Webb, Campbell, Schwartz, Sechrest, & Grove, 1981). Dream journals (called *dream series* by quantitative dream researchers) are valued as "nonreactive" measures that have not been influenced by the demand characteristics and expectancy effects that can be a confounding factor in many types of experiments in the psychological and health sciences, including dream research (e.g., Rosenthal & Ambady, 1995). Dream series have their greatest value when several of them, kept for diverse reasons, lead to the same general results. This is because the use of numerous dream series has parallels with drawing a random sample due to the fact that the use of multiple dream series tends to eliminate the effects of irrelevant variables. In addition, studies of dream series go beyond a string of individual case studies because each one of them can be compared very precisely with the male or female normative samples, which is similar to comparing an individual's MMPI scores to the MMPI's norms. Then, too, dream series coded with the HVdC categories can be compared with each other in a very direct way. Statistically, quantitative studies of dream series are on solid ground because the autonomous nature of each dream leads to the empirical finding, based on analyses of subseries from four different dream series, that there is no evidence of autocorrelation (Domhoff & Schneider, 2015).

Quantitative analyses of nearly two dozen individual adult dream series since the late 1940s reveal that dream content is generally consistent for most individuals over months, years, and decades, which is a good example of an important finding that never would have been discovered using standard methods (Domhoff, 1996, Chapter 7). In addition, inferences based on blind analyses of the results of several such studies, which are then corroborated or rejected by the dreamers and their close friends, reveal that most dream content is continuous with waking concerns and interests. This continuity is revealed most clearly in terms of the frequency with which the main people in the dreamer's life appear and the way in which they are portrayed in social interactions (e.g., aggressive, friendly, unresponsive).

There are also clear indications of the dreamer's primary waking interests (e.g., music, sports, traveling). This inference-and-response methodology, which allows the questions to be tailored to the individual case, has proven far superior to the vain attempts from the 1940s through the 1960s to correlate dream findings with the results of personality tests—partly because dreams embody wishes, fears, and abiding preoccupations, and partly because personality tests are blunt instruments (Domhoff, 1996, pp. 154–156).

Unfortunately, there are no studies of psychiatric patients in which the combination of blind analysis and the responses to the inferences that emerged from the blind analysis could be applied. However, there is adequate information for the three cases presented in the remainder of this section to demonstrate that there is continuity between the concerns found in the dream reports and the dreamers' main concerns in waking life. Before turning to that demonstration, though, it is crucial to qualify the general conclusion concerning continuity in three ways so that the presumption of continuity is not overstated and misunderstood. First, the continuity is not with day-to-day events, but with general concerns. Secondly, the continuity usually is with both thought and behavior, but sometimes it is only with thought, particularly in terms of sexual and aggressive fantasies. Third, not all dream elements are continuous with waking concerns and interests. Some of these elements may be metaphoric, but many of them seem to be glitches, perhaps revealing the limits of cognitive capacity during dreaming (Domhoff, 2007).

The Dreams of a Child Molester

An opportunity to study the dream reports of a highly unusual patient unexpectedly arose when "Norman," a child molester in his mid-30s who had been incarcerated for seven years in five different institutions between the ages of 20 and 34, revealed to a clinical psychologist that he had written down 1,368 dream reports for his own personal interest over the previous 3.5 years (Bell & Hall, 1971, pp. 6–9). He was in a mental institution 80% of the time that he was keeping his dream journal, often writing dream reports on paper bags or laundry lists (Bell & Hall, 1971, pp. v, 3). He lived at home with his mother and sister (when he was not institutionalized), had never married, enjoyed reading and swimming, and worked as a helper in printing shops.

A complete HVdC coding of the dream reports revealed that Norman differed from the norms in only a few ways. There were many unusual features in the character patterns in his dream reports, with his mother appearing four times more often than would be expected from the norms, and his sister appearing ten times more often. However, there were no mentions of his father. Norman had a typical number of dream reports with at least one sexual thought or interaction, but his sexual dreams differed from those of other adult males in terms of the variety of characters with whom he was erotically involved and the types of interactions that occurred. Despite his unusual character and sexual patterns, the most striking aspect of his dream reports was the very low percentage of characters in them that were his friends: only 9%, far below the normative figure of 31% for males. There was an especially low incidence of female friends and acquaintances. Beyond his mother and sister, he dreamt primarily of unknown males and unknown females. As for the males who were known to him, they were usually his fellow inmates, not friends of long standing.

Although there were few friends, Norman was not unusually low on friendly interactions; this was largely due to his generally positive interactions with his mother and sister in his dreams, but also because he often befriended or helped children and teenagers. Nor is there anything unusual in his pattern of aggression and friendliness except that he is a little less aggressive than other males. His case is a good example of why it is important to study the percentages and indexes for both interactions and characters in closely examining a set or series of dream reports.

These dream findings fit with the reality of Norman's waking life, in which he was very dependent on his highly controlling mother and his supportive sister, whom he reported were the two most positive influences in his life. Norman's father was often absent in Norman's early years; he was pushed out of the house by Norman's mother when Norman was 12 and died a few years later. Norman had no friends and preferred to be around children. As in his dreams, he had had sex with other males and at least once with an animal. His main sexual outlet, however, was the same compulsive voyeurism present in his dream reports (see Domhoff, 1996, pp. 166–171, for the full case).

The Dreams of a Neurotic Patient

Fifty-eight dream reports recorded by a 28-year-old married man while he was in psychotherapy provided a rare opportunity for dream researchers to quantify the dreams of a neurotic patient. The patient worked as an inventory clerk and came to therapy because of marital tension, general nervousness, and physical symptoms such as stomachaches. The psychotherapist viewed him as psychologically naïve and with little insight into his problems, but he also thought that the patient "appeared genuinely motivated" and "able to interact effectively despite his anxiety" (Moss, 1970, p. 33). The patient improved considerably in the course of 48 sessions. A follow-up inquiry ten months after therapy ended found that he was "reasonably satisfied with his marital and work situations and he had not felt the need for additional psychiatric assistance in the interim" (Moss, 1970, p. 56).

The patient's dream series was striking for its low percentage of friends. In addition, the dreamer was low in friendliness with all classes of characters, including females, and high in aggressive interactions with all classes of characters, again including females. Thus, his A/F% was 81, compared to the normative male percent of 62 ($h = .43$, which is a large effect size). His negative emotions percent was 97, as opposed to the normative percentage of 80 ($h = .58$). There is only one instance of happiness in 58 dream reports (see Domhoff, 1996, pp. 171–176, for the dream findings in this case).

In an autobiographical sketch he wrote before he went into psychotherapy, he said his family upset him because of constant bickering; he felt that nothing he did ever pleased them. He had a younger brother that bullied him and entered into violent quarrels with their father. He was angry with his wife for what he saw as a failure to communicate with him. The patient characterized his general attitude toward people in a way that is consistent with the low levels of both friends and friendly interactions in his dreams: "I try to stay away from them, they make me sick" (Moss, 1970, p. 32).

A College Woman With High Anxiety

The dream reports of a young college woman suffering from a variety of symptoms provided the opportunity to examine the effects of a psychiatric medication on dream content. She had written down 33 dream reports in her first year of college as part of the therapy she was receiving from the campus counseling center for anxiety and mild depression. After abandoning the therapy because she did not feel it was helping her, during her junior year she saw a psychiatrist and was placed on the SSRI sertraline (Zoloft), with her dosage gradually increasing from 25 to 100 milligrams before her light-headedness and panic attacks subsided. A year later, she recorded 40 dreams while still taking Zoloft for possible use in a research project in a psychology course, but without any knowledge of the HVdC system. Kirschner (1999) discovered that the second set of dream reports differed dramatically from the first set on several HVdC content indicators. In particular, she moved further above the norms on the friends percent and the F/C index, and closer to the norms on the A/F%, the A/C index, and the percentage of dreams with at least one aggressive interaction. The full results are displayed in Table 6.2.

TABLE 6.2 Statistical differences between dreams before and after treatment with an SSRI, with the female normative sample included for comparison.

	Unmedicated (33 Dreams)	With Zoloft (40 Dreams)	h	p	Female Norms
Friends Percent	42%	64%	+.44	.003	37%
A/F%	75%	52%	−.82	.000	51%
A/C Index	.78	.39	+.41	.003	.24
F/C Index	.18	.35	−.48	.003	.22
At Least One Aggressive Interaction	65%	50%	−.30	.201	44%
At Least One Friendly Interaction	38%	45%	−.14	.556	42%

Since the study involves only one participant and has fewer than the 125 dream reports for each condition that would be ideal in terms of sample size, it is perhaps best viewed as a pilot study. However, it is one of the few systematic studies of the effects of a medication that detected any changes in dream content, so it might serve as one prototype for the potential pre- and post-studies that are suggested in the concluding section, whether they involve medication or psychotherapy.

Studying Dream Content in Psychiatric Clinics

Based on past research with student populations, the findings from studies of dream series, and the potentially useful findings outlined in this chapter, this section briefly discusses several possibilities for studies that could be done in inpatient and outpatient psychiatric settings that serve a large number of patients. In particular, individual practices and clinics that see long-term patients with specific symptoms, such as anxiety states or obsessive-compulsive disorder, might be especially propitious sites for systematic studies. Clinics that provide medications to patients who visit regularly for check-ups or prescription renewals also might be good settings for well-controlled studies.

Quantitative studies of dream reports in psychiatric settings might begin with one or two simple questions about the patient's personal dream history that were added to a standard intake questionnaire. Most importantly, patients could be asked to write down or tape record their Most Recent Dream when they first arrive to the clinic—and on each return visit. If respondents are primed for recency by asking for the date they recalled the dream, and if reports stating that the dream is a childhood dream or a recurrent nightmare are discarded, then there is good reason to believe—on the basis of past studies—that 125 Most Recent Dreams provide a representative sample of any given population (Avila-White, Schneider, & Domhoff, 1999; Domhoff, 1996 Chapter 4; Domhoff, 2003, Chapter 5).

Using the Most Recent Dream method, it would be possible to do pre- and post-studies that resemble the study of the anxious college woman in the previous section. An even better prototype for such a study was carried out on cancer patients who wrote down Most Recent Dreams before and after their mastectomies. Their dream reports differed from the HVdC normative sample for women. Furthermore, the post-mastectomy dream reports showed a marked concern with bodily disfigurement, as shown by a coding category for body parts (Giordano, et al., 2012).

In addition to requesting a Most Recent Dream, an intake questionnaire could ask if the new patient has ever or is now keeping a dream journal that has 50 or more dream reports—and if so, when and for how long. Although only a small percent of people have kept dream journals, such journals are ideal as baselines for pre- and post-studies with unique patients or with patients who are about to be put on new medication. As explained earlier, the quantitative nature of the HVdC coding system and the existence of replicated normative samples for men and women take such studies beyond a series of separate case studies that are not easily compared.

Space limitations preclude any detailed discussion of how dream reports collected in psychiatric settings could be analyzed. Everything that is needed to do a quantitative study using the HVdC system is available on dreamresearch.net, including a spreadsheet (DreamSAT) for HVdC codings that provides p values and effect sizes, and a correction formula for multiple tests of the same pair of samples (Schneider & Domhoff, 1995). The results provided by DreamSAT are displayed in either tables or the bar graphs called *h-profiles*.

In addition, dream reports can be searched for words, phrases, and word strings, and then analyzed using the programs on DreamBank (www.dreambank.net); the dream reports themselves can be stored in a place that is accessible only to the clinical researchers who collected them (see Domhoff & Schneider, 2008b, for an account of the capabilities built into DreamBank and a summary of the major findings using it; also see Schneider & Domhoff, 1999). Evidence for the value of well-crafted word strings that have been normed using the same dream reports on which the HVdC norms are based can be found in work by Bulkeley (2012, 2014).

Conclusion

The people and social interactions included in the HVdC categories for friends and friendliness reflect the most profound bonds that shape human life—the ability to move outside the family circle to form connections with other human beings, along with the ability to interact in a positive fashion in human groups that include people previously unknown to the person. Without friends and friendly interactions, what's left is a life without emotions—or with only negative emotions and aggressive interactions, which also are features of some psychiatric patients' dreams. Viewed in this light, the findings in this chapter seem all the more relevant if the dreams of psychiatric patients are ever to become more useful in diagnosis and prognosis. However, it would take a program of systematic research, perhaps carried out by several outpatient clinics and in-patient facilities that developed a common data-analysis unit, to determine the usefulness of dream reports in the difficult ongoing effort to help those who suffer from psychopathologies.

Acknowledgements

My thanks to Adam Schneider for his careful editing of the manuscript and for formatting the tables.

References

Allport, G. (1942). *The use of personal documents in psychological science*. New York: Social Science Research Council.

Armitage, R., Rochlen, A., Fitch, T., Trivedi, M., & Rush, A. (1995). Dream recall and major depression: A preliminary report. *Dreaming, 5,* 189–198.

Avila-White, D., Schneider, A., & Domhoff, G. W. (1999). The most recent dreams of 12–13 year-old boys and girls: A methodological contribution to the study of dream content in teenagers. *Dreaming, 9,* 163–171.

Bell, A., & Hall, C. (1971). *The personality of a child molester: An analysis of dreams.* Chicago: Aldine.

Bulkeley, K. (2012). Dreaming in adolescence: A 'blind' word search of a teenage girl's dream series. *Dreaming, 22,* 240–252.

Bulkeley, K. (2014). Digital dream analysis: A revised method. *Consciousness and Cognition, 29,* 159–170.

Domhoff, G. W. (1996). *Finding meaning in dreams: A quantitative approach.* New York: Plenum.

Domhoff, G. W. (2003). *The scientific study of dreams: Neural networks, cognitive development, and content analysis.* Washington, DC: American Psychological Association.

Domhoff, G. W. (2005). The content of dreams: Methodologic and theoretical implications. In M. Kryger, T. Roth, & W. Dement (Eds.), *Principles and practices of sleep medicine* (4th ed., pp. 522–534). Philadelphia: Elsevier Saunders.

Domhoff, G. W. (2007). Realistic simulation and bizarreness in dream content: Past findings and suggestions for future research. In D. Barrett & P. McNamara (Eds.), *The new science of dreaming: Content, recall, and personality correlates* (Vol. 2, pp. 1–27). Westport, CT: Praeger.

Domhoff, G. W., & Schneider, A. (1999). Much ado about very little: The small effect sizes when home and laboratory collected dreams are compared. *Dreaming, 9,* 139–151.

Domhoff, G. W., & Schneider, A. (2008a). Similarities and differences in dream content at the cross-cultural, gender, and individual levels. *Consciousness and Cognition, 17,* 1257–1265.

Domhoff, G. W., & Schneider, A. (2008b). Studying dream content using the archive and search engine on DreamBank.net. *Consciousness and Cognition, 17,* 1238–1247.

Domhoff, G. W., & Schneider, A. (2015). Assessing autocorrelation in studies using the Hall and Van de Castle coding system to study individual dream series. *Dreaming, 25*(1), 69–78.

Gentil, M., & Lader, M. (1978). Dream content and daytime attitudes in anxious and calm women. *Psychological Medicine, 8,* 297–304.

Giordano, A., Francese, V., Peila, E., Tribolo, A., Airoldi, M., Torta, R., et al. (2012). Dream content changes in women after mastectomy: An initial study of body imagery after body-disfiguring surgery. *Dreaming, 22,* 115–123.

Hall, C. (1966a). A comparison of the dreams of four groups of hospitalized mental patients with each other and with a normal population. *Journal of Nervous and Mental Diseases, 143,* 135–139.

Hall, C. (1966b). *Studies of dreams collected in the laboratory and at home.* Santa Cruz, CA: Institute of Dream Research.

Hall, C., & Van de Castle, R. (1966). *The content analysis of dreams.* New York: Appleton-Century-Crofts.

Kirschner, N. (1999). Medication and dreams: Changes in dream content after drug treatment. *Dreaming, 9,* 195–200.

Kramer, M. (1970). Manifest dream content in normal and psychopathologic states. *Archives of General Psychiatry, 22,* 149–159.

Kramer, M. (2000). Dreams and psychopathology. In M. Kryger, T. Roth, & W. Dement (Eds.), *Principles and practices of sleep medicine* (3rd ed., pp. 511–519). Philadelphia: Saunders.

Kramer, M., & Roth, T. (1973). Comparison of dream content in laboratory dream reports of schizophrenic and depressive patient groups. *Comprehensive Psychiatry, 14*, 325–329.

Kramer, M., & Roth, T. (1979). Dreams in psychopathology. In B. Wolman (Ed.), *Handbook of dreams* (pp. 361–367). New York: Van Nostrand Reinhold.

Moss, C. S. (1970). *Dreams, images, and fantasy: A semantic differential casebook*. Urbana: University of Illinois Press.

Pesant, N., & Zadra, A. (2006). Dream content and psychological well-being: A longitudinal study of the continuity hypothesis. *Journal of Clinical Psychology, 62*(1), 111–121.

Rosenthal, R., & Ambady, N. (1995). Experimenter effects. In A. Manstead & M. Hewstone (Eds.), *Encyclopedia of Social Psychology* (pp. 230–235). Oxford: Blackwell.

Roth, T., Kramer, M., & Salis, P. (1979). Drugs, REM sleep, and dreams. In B. Wolman (Ed.), *Handbook of dreams* (pp. 203–225). New York: Van Norstrand Reinhold.

Schneider, A., & Domhoff, G. W. (1995). The quantitative study of dreams. From www.dreamresearch.net.

Schneider, A., & Domhoff, G. W. (1999). DreamBank. www.dreambank.net.

Schnetzler, J., & Carbonel, B. (1976). Etude thématique des recits de rêves de sujets normaux, schizophrènes et autres psychotiques. *Annales Medíco Psychologiques, 3*, 367–380.

Skancke, J., Holsen, I., & Schredl, M. (2014). Continuity between waking life and dreams of psychiatric patients: A review and discussion of the implications for dream research. *International Journal of Dream Research, 7*, 39–53.

Webb, E., Campbell, D., Schwartz, R., Sechrest, L., & Grove, J. (1981). *Nonreactive measures in the social sciences* (2nd ed.). Chicago: Rand McNally.

Zadra, A., & Domhoff, G. W. (2011). The content of dreams: Methods and findings. In M. Kryger, T. Roth, & W. Dement (Eds.), *Principles and practices of sleep medicine* (5th ed., pp. 585–594). Philadelphia: Elsevier Saunders.

7

DREAMS

Thinking in a Different Biochemical State

Deirdre Barrett

I was fascinated by dreams as far back in childhood as I can remember. Magical adventures every night, as vivid as waking events, seemed to be some of the most remarkable and mysterious things in life. Students usually go into psychology and then choose a specialty during graduate school. I did it the other way around: I knew I wanted to study dreams and gradually realized that this meant I should become a psychologist. I suspect this is true of many other authors in this book. Bill Domhoff is the only dream researcher I've ever heard say that his own dreams are not particularly frequent or vivid—in his case Calvin Hall was simply the most compelling researcher at his graduate program. I think most of us get hooked in by the richness of our own dream life.

Over time, I've researched many aspects of dreaming—lucid dreams, nightmares, dreams in particular clinical populations, and the similarities and differences of daydreaming and hypnosis. In this chapter, I'll begin by reviewing my recent studies on dreams and creative problem solving, then summarize other areas, and lastly discuss theoretical conclusions and clinical implications of this work.

Creative Problem Solving

The first stage of my inquiry into problem solving and creative dreams was library research. I was intrigued by dramatic examples repeated in many dream books. Friedrich August Kekulé dreamed the structure of benzene. Mary Shelley dreamed the two main scenes that became *Frankenstein;* Robert Lewis Stevenson also dreamed scenes that inspired *Dr. Jekyll and Mr. Hyde.* Many surrealist masterpieces came directly from dream images.

When I began searching the indexes of history of science books and biographies of prominent inventors and artists, I found many equally striking examples that had been recorded but were less known among dream researchers. Frederick Banting dreamed the first method for concentrating canine insulin so that it could be administered to diabetics and won a Nobel Prize for this work. Otto Loewi dreamed an experiment to demonstrate the role of chemicals in electrical conduction within nerves—another Nobel Prize winner. Biologist Margie Profet had an animated cartoon dream "like those sex education films in elementary school" that showed her the function of menstruation—this one leading to a McArthur Prize. India's greatest mathematician, Srinivasa Ramanujan, said that all his mathematical proofs came to him in dreams. Art generates the most examples, but not all had the overtly "dreamlike" quality of the surrealists. Jasper Johns dreamed of painting a giant American flag—the work that launched his career and now hangs in the New York Museum of Modern Art.

My second area of inquiry into problem-solving dreams was interviewing modern scientists and artists, seeking more detail than is usually in historic accounts. Architects Lucy Davis and museum designer Solange Fabio both described dreams of walking through finished buildings, noting design features—then waking up, sketching these, and eventually building their dreamed structures. Harvard astronomer Paul Horowitz told me that every time he was stuck on some detail of designing telescope controls, he would have a dream in which he watched someone doing the task—arranging a group of lenses or constructing a computer chip—while a voice narrated exactly what to do. Composer Shirish Korde described how music often arrived for him in dreams—sometimes hearing it, but also seeing it as birds at variable heights denoting positions on a music staff or as synesthetic colors denoting tones (1).

A few of these artists and inventors mentioned asking their dreams for help with self-devised techniques similar to the "dream incubation" that Henry Reed (2) and other psychologists developed for solving emotional quandaries and health problems. William Dement (3) and Morton Schatzman (4) had already tried this with objective problems—both asking subjects to try incubation with brainteasers—generating occasional dramatic successes. They concluded the success rate was low because of flagging interest: all of Dement's problem solutions had been dreamed on the very first night that his subjects were assigned the task. Therefore, in my research with college students, I had them select real-life problems that they actually needed to solve. Some chose homework assignments. Then they suggested to themselves for a week at bedtime that they would dream the solution. Whether because of the ease of these problems—all were presumably within the students' abilities—or the relevance to the students' lives, one-half of my students had dreams they felt addressed their problem. One-third dreamed a solution to it. Judges rated only slightly fewer dreams as addressing or solving problems (5).

In all these sets of dreams—historic, interview, and prospective incubation—some occasionally solved objective problems. However, they tended to be much better at two types: problems that require creative thinking, and problems that have solutions that can be visualized. Dreams were particularly good for finding solutions that required thinking outside the box. This makes sense in terms of what we know about physiology of REM sleep: the prefrontal cortex is damped down so that we wouldn't be as quick to censor with "That's not the way to approach it." Dreams are also especially useful when solutions can be visualized. The secondary visual cortex—associated with imagery—is more active during REM than during waking. The most famous of all dream examples illustrates both these characteristics: Kekulé, who when awake was trying to solve benzene as a straight line with right-angle side chains, dreamed of it as a closed ring denoted by a snake made of atoms taking its tail in its mouth.

The Dreams of Clinical and Other Distinctive Populations

I've conducted a number of studies on people who have a particular disorder or who've had some unusual, and potentially traumatizing, life experience, and I've examined how these are reflected in their dreams.

Depression

In 1992, Mike Loeffler and I examined dreams from a group of subjects who scored as depressed on the Beck Depression Inventory but who were not in psychotherapy nor on psychoactive medication (6). They recalled fewer dreams than a nondepressed control group, had shorter dream accounts, had less emotion in their dreams (especially anger), and had fewer characters. There was a nonsignificant trend for them to have less pleasant content, but they were the same as the nondepressed group on unpleasant content. The dreams of the depressed subjects did not contain more fear than the controls. Since our group wasn't on antidepressants, this suggests that the higher rate of nightmares in some other studies may be due to antidepressant medications rather than depression.

Nightmares

Karen Dunn and I conducted a similar study (7) of frequent nightmares sufferers defined as having nightmares at least once a week vs. control subjects with less than one. Subjects completed a questionnaire about characteristics of their nightmares and reactions to them, and also completed seven other psychological questionnaires. Those who experienced frequent nightmares reported a higher rate of other sleep disturbances, more death concerns, and more major life stress than control subjects. Frequent nightmare sufferers did not score higher on general anxiety, emotionality, or minor life stresses. Subjective reports from frequent sufferers indicated that the majority of them believed their nightmares occurred predominantly when facing stresses. These were, in descending order of frequency, school and job pressures, conflicts in relationships, physical illness or exhaustion, and frightening films.

A significant difference between our study and other nightmare research is that we did not define nightmares while other research often used "frightening dreams that wake you up" or similar phrasing. We asked subjects to write out their most recent nightmares so we could check that none used the term for night terrors, apnea, or negative daydreams. They weren't universally frightening. When subjects were asked to rate the order in which different emotions dominated their nightmares, 83% ranked fear first, 13% sadness, and 4% specified other terms such as *helplessness* and *confusion*. No subject ranked anger as the most common nightmare emotion, but it was ranked second by 57%. In their examples, sadness most often dominated in nightmares about the loss of loved ones. In terms of anger, a typical example was:

> My last nightmare was about my sister. She had made me very mad. I was screaming at her. When I woke up I was screaming, "I hate you." When I realized it was a dream, I was still mad at my sister.

A quality of feeling overwhelmed by the events and emotions of a dream seems central to the subjects' criteria for labeling of nightmares, rather than the overwhelming emotion always being fear.

Posttraumatic Stress Disorder (PTSD)

In my 1996 book, *Trauma and Dreams* (8), I gathered a number of authors who'd given talks at either dream conferences or conferences on treating trauma. Their clinical populations varied widely: children who'd been kidnapped, sexually abused, badly burned, or trapped in a war zone; adults who'd been raped, served in war, or survived the Nazi concentration camps. However, there were consistent patterns in the evolution of nightmares in those recovering from trauma. In patients who had not developed full-blown PTSD, posttraumatic nightmares faded over time, interwove with other issues, or evolved into scenarios of mastery. Rape survivors had nightmares repeating the assault over and over for a while. They transitioned to dreams in which they were at work or in a social setting and they'd see the rapist walk by or peer around a corner, but soon he'd be gone. Others had dramatic dreams in which they successfully fought off their attacker, someone else intervened, or the threat was eliminated in a magic, dreamlike manner. Many of the chapter authors wrote about a technique that I'd also experimented with in my practice of coaching people to have mastery dreams. We found this helped reduce nightmares and also reduced waking anxiety and feelings of vulnerability. Barry Krakow had since dubbed this *Dream Rehearsal Therapy* and demonstrated how well it works in systematic research with a wide variety of traumatized populations (9).

In 1991, immediately after the first Gulf War, I was invited to Kuwait to teach a 6-week course on trauma treatment. I collaborated with Kuwaiti psychologist

Jaaffar Behbehani to collect nightmares—retrospectively for ones during the occupation and ongoing for those in the immediate aftermath (10). We found that Kuwaitis were experiencing similar reenactment nightmares to those of trauma survivors in other societies. However, combined with Muslim doctrine and Arabic folk beliefs about dreams foretelling the future, these nightmares provoked even more anxiety than in other cultures that view dreams as reflecting the past. Westernized Kuwaitis with some respect for social science were relieved to hear that people in other traumatized situations consistently have recurring nightmares about those traumas without the events being destined to recur. More fundamentalist, anti-Western dreamers were not particularly interested in such information. Offsetting the cultural beliefs' potential to increase fearfulness, several people we interviewed had dreamed of the invaders being driven out of Kuwait City. They took deep comfort from these dreams throughout the occupation, while a Westerner might have dismissed them as wish-fulfillment.

Trauma and Dreams had its paperback release in mid-September 2011. In the talks and conversations that were already scheduled, I, of course, heard a flood of nightmares about the events of 9/11. While this hardly comprised a formal research project, I was so struck by these dreams that I organized them into a talk at the International Association for the Study of Dreams (IASD) conference the following summer (11). The dreams showed many of the same patterns as in other trauma populations. Some nightmares were straightforward re-enactments: one man who worked across from the World Trade Center described his recurring nightmare as "just an image from waking life—looking back and seeing the building coming down." Another common pattern from other populations repeated here was the nightmares that went a step further than real life, in which the most-feared possibility occurred: a World Trade Center worker repeatedly dreamed of barely escaping, as in real life, but then seeing his wife among the dead in the street. In reality, she worked in the building, but they'd been safely reunited within the hour. Other dreamers showed what has often been termed "survivor guilt" (I'm not sure it's guilt as opposed to close identification with lost colleagues or loved ones). One second-floor World Trade Center worker repeatedly dreamed that he stood frozen at the window on an upper floor with a plane bearing down; he understood this to be the experience of a lost friend. Many recurring nightmares showed the familiar patterns of diminishing or turning into mastery dreams. Two financial-area workers had experienced the doomed World Trade Center occupants jumping out of windows as the most horrifying image they'd personally witnessed. This replayed in their nightmares: sometimes they watch, other times they were forced to jump themselves. After many repetitions, however, they began to equip themselves and other jumpers with parachutes in one case and, more fancifully, umbrellas in the other dream. Danger and anxiety lingered but they no longer overwhelmed the dreamers.

At the time, the media was filled with allusions to the "unprecedented trauma" that "all of the nation" experienced on 9/11. Watching a building explode on television, however, even a hundred times, is a far cry from running from flames and collapsing steel oneself or picking through rubble for body parts while wondering if the remaining structure will hold above you. Among more removed television viewers, people who were more generally anxious or specifically had a high rate of nightmares were likelier to dream about 9/11. I also saw a phenomenon I've noticed in clients: People with a previous personal history of trauma are often triggered by public ones. Some begin to have frequent nightmares combining the events. A childhood sexual abuse survivor dreamed her abuser was part of bin Laden's network and was forcing the dreamer to help them. A rape survivor dreamed she saw the rapist boarding her plane carrying a box cutter and knew he was planning to hijack it.

Dissociative Disorders

Because I ask my clients about dreams, I've observed that those traumatized people who end up with dissociative disorders show not only the kinds of nightmares common in PTSD, but also a wide range of dream phenomena I don't hear from any other group. To get a broader sense of this, I surveyed 16 therapists about the dream characteristics of 48 of their patients with dissociative disorders (12). For most patients, recovery of repressed memories was the most frequent distinctive dream event. Other dream phenomena included a hysterical conversion symptom resolving in a dream and a trauma-related hallucination beginning after a dream of related content. Both of these phenomena occurred in patients with diagnoses of dissociative disorder not-otherwise-specified.

Many other phenomena occurred for patients with dissociative identity disorder (DID), formerly "multiple personality disorder." Sometimes alters' experiences were remembered as dreams. One woman with recurring "nightmares" of catching evil cats by the throat and stuffing them in garbage cans awoke from one of these dreams to find that the velour jogging suit in which she slept had cat fur clinging to it. She didn't own a cat and was so alarmed that she brought in the suit for her therapist to confirm that the fur was present. Another had "dreams" of sitting on the bank of a river at night feeling soothed as she stared at it. Months later, an alter owned up to these being real nocturnal jaunts.

Some patients had dreams that seemed to be depicting their dissociation. One patient, not yet aware of her DID except for losing time and hearing voices that later proved to be her alters', reported a dream that seemed highly symbolic of her multiplicity.

> I was sitting in a photo booth trying to get it to take a picture of me, but all the pictures that came out showed other people—or at least faint outlines of other people. In the mirror, where you see what will come out, the face kept changing, like ghosts.

Alters showed up as dream characters. Two patients who had made suicidal gestures, which they attributed to accidents, had dreams that helped explain them. One dreamed of a woman determined to commit suicide, the other of one vowing to kill the dreamer. These turned out to be alters responsible for cutting and an overdose.

A few patients had dreams that were perceived by several alters from different characters' perspectives. In one, an alter was being abused, another was screaming for help, and yet another came in to club the attacker, while a child alter played obliviously in a corner of the room. Four patients had dreams in which they were their alter. Six had a "dream maker" who could influence the host or other alters' dreams. Sometimes the dream maker had a narrow agenda: one designed "rapist" dreams about any man to whom the dreamer was getting close. Often, however, the dream maker was a helper alter. One told the therapist: "Dreams can test the waters for whether she's ready for a memory" and used the ability to guide the host toward healthy behaviors or to communicate therapeutically. Another patient's alter described dreaming as part of a broader influence campaign: "I show her images a lot, even while she's awake—of memories and things I feel and want to do. But she sees them best if I show them to her while she's dreaming." For two patients, integration took place in dream. One dreamed of a wedding in which only one person stood at the altar by the end of the ceremony and another dreamed of saying goodbye to a character "who faded into me like mist." Parenthetically, Christine Sizemore, the woman written about in *The Three Faces of Eve* (13), in her own account (14) says her final integration happened in a dream.

These results got me to thinking about the similarity of dreaming to the alterations of consciousness in DID, including amnesia. The dream character, as a hallucinated projection of aspects of the self, struck me as a model for the DID alter. Dreaming is the only state in which most of us interact with aspects of ourselves as discrete other people. Dreaming may even be a literal precursor with physiologic mechanisms for amnesia and the manufacture of alternate identities that are recruited in the development of DID. Ross et al. (15) had already suggested that trauma may disregulate sleep stages and suggested that PTSD flashbacks may be physiologically REM imagery intruding into waking. I published a theoretical paper titled "The Dream Character as a Prototype for the Multiple Personality 'Alter'" (16) elaborating on how there are constellations of cognitive and personality processes that operate outside conscious awareness and normally are observable primarily in dreams. Extreme early trauma may mutate or overdevelop these dissociated parts and call upon them to "wake up" and function in the external world. I believe these dream processes parallel what we see in DID much more closely than waking fantasy, which has often been written about as a basis for the disorder.

Bereavement

Another group whose dreams I studied were the recently bereaved (17). The dreams clustered in four categories: back to life, advice, leave taking, and state of death. "Back to life" dreams, making up 39% of the total dreams and typical of early stages of loss, were ones in which the dead sought to change the circumstances of their death, usually futilely, as in the following:

> My grandmother visits me in a hotel. I say, "Oh, you've come back to me," and she says, "Yes, we are going to try it again and see if I live this time." Suddenly she collapses on the bathroom floor. I try to revive her, but I can't. I am panic-stricken and scream, "You can't die. I have to do it right this time."

Another dream involved a friend who had committed suicide winking from her coffin—she hadn't really killed herself yet, but was now going to be buried alive.

"Advice" dreams occurred somewhat later and comprised 23% of the total. In these, the deceased gave counsel about situations in the dreamer's current life, profound or mundane; these were consistently positive dreams. "Leave-taking" dreams, in which the deceased gave loved ones a chance to say good-bye, occurred much later and comprised 29% of the dreams. Eleven percent of these dreams were lucid, as in the following example from the subject who had the "back to life" nightmare about her grandmother quoted earlier:

> I had a lucid dream about my grandmother that was probably the best dream I ever had. In this dream I was little, about five or six years old, and I was in the bathroom at my grandmother's house. She was giving me a bath in this big claw-footed tub. The old steam radiator was turned on, making it very cozy. I knew that I was dreaming and that I was getting to see my grandmother well again. After the bath, she lifted me out onto the spiral cotton rug and dried me with a blue towel. When that was done, she said she had to leave now; this seemed to mean for Heaven. I said, "Good-bye, Grandma. I love you." She said, "I love you too, Mary." I woke up feeling wonderful. She had been delirious in the last months of her life, so I'd never really gotten to say good-bye.

The final category was "state of death" dreams. This category contained 18% of the dreams and had the highest rate of lucidity at 13%. Most surprisingly, in these dreams 53% of the dead telephoned. In one, the dreamer's deceased mother called to tell her that she was pregnant and it was going to be a girl. In another, the dreamer answered the phone and her boyfriend's father's voice began to describe the beauty of the place he was now in. When the dreamer asked, "Is this Pa?" Pa's voice replied, "No, Pa died. How could you talk to him?" but this did not trigger lucidity. State-of-death dreams tended to be positive and seemed to be reassuring the dreamer both about the fate of their loved ones and about issues of their own mortality.

Prisoners

While teaching a summer course in London, I came across a unique set of dreams in the archives of the Wellcome Medical Collection. From 1940 to 1942, Major Kenneth Hopkins had gathered dream accounts every morning from fellow prisoners in the WWII Nazi POW camp Laufen. Hopkins planned to use the data for his dissertation research after the war was over, but he died of a lung ailment in the camp. Its liberators mailed the dream accounts back to his university and they found their way into storage at Wellcome. A group of my students and I applied the Hall–Van de Castle scales and also some ad hoc scales about confinement and escape (18). The POWs' dreams had more content concerning battles, imprisonment, escape, and food than the Hall–Van de Castle normative male dreams from the same era. The POW dreams did not have as much of any type of social interaction. These dreams contained less friendliness, sexuality, and even less aggression than the male norms. However, aggression was unusually extreme when it occurred, and its content was linked to previous battles rather than camp life. The POWs had less good fortune or misfortune in their dreams and also had frequent bland dreams about the tedium of the camp. Their dream characters included higher percentages of males, family members, and the dead; they had fewer friends or animal characters than the male norms. This may simply reflect whom they were in contact with at the camp. Overall, these patterns resembled dreams of other prison populations rather than of other post-combatants, which may be because this particular group was captured early during WWII. One interesting effect lay outside our statistical analyses. Dreams about escaping the camp could be positive or negative: attempts went wrong for many dreamers. However, there was a small subset of dreamers with frequent triumphant escape dreams. After many such dreams, these men disappeared from the data set on the same date. A bit of research revealed that they were a subset of the "Laufen 6" about whom a book, a film, and a board game had been released in England commemorating their daring escape. This was definitely an example of the continuity effect in dreams, though not one we were set up to measure statistically.

Unusual Categories of Dreams

Lucid Dreams

In a study titled "Just How Lucid Are Lucid Dreams?" (19), I examined the lucid dreams of 50 subjects to determine whether they are fully lucid for the following corollaries, which should flow logically from knowing one is dreaming: (1) people in the dreams are dream characters; (2) dream objects are not real (i.e., actions will not carry over concretely upon awakening); (3) the dreamer does not need to obey waking-life physics to achieve a goal; and (4) memory of the waking world is intact rather than amnestic or fictitious. Many lucid dreams were too brief to evaluate on all corollaries. Only about half of the lengthier accounts were lucid for any particular corollary and less than a quarter were lucid on all four. There was trend for more experienced lucid dreamers to be lucid about more corollaries. In the dream journals of these frequent lucid dreamers I examined a related and reciprocal category of dreams that were lucid in terms of some of these four corollaries, but missing the realization that "I'm dreaming." These dreams comprised 4% of the total. Dreamers occasionally realized that events were not real but misattributed the cause to "I'm the director of a play" or "I'm in a deep trance." At other times they simply realized the corollary without ever wondering about its cause, such as in the following two examples:

> This was a special situation and I could just walk through the wall although this would usually be impossible. . . .
> I knew the man wasn't real, that I was making him up, and should be able to make him take it back if I didn't like this. . . .

Flying Dreams

These have anecdotally been suggested to relate to lucid dreams, either by general proximity of occurrence or by flying directly triggering lucidity. I examined 1,910 dreams from 191 subjects (20) and found that flying dreams were likelier to be reported by subjects having lucid dreams or any of three related categories: "prelucid" dreams, dreams about sleep, and false awakenings. When flying and lucidity occurred in the same dream, lucidity preceded flight rather than being triggered by it: "I'm dreaming; I think I'll fly" not "I'm flying, therefore I must be dreaming." Certain characteristics of being close to waking probably cause the dreamer to sense the vestibular system's disequilibrium while also experiencing activation of the prefrontal cortex.

Dreams in Which the Dreamer Dies

People of many cultures traditionally believe that if you are killed in a dream, you will actually die in your sleep at that moment—or similarly, that you *can't* die in a dream. These probably spring from how much more common dreams of impending death are with the dreamer awakening just before it happens. Overt dreams about dying are rare, but not unheard of among healthy young adults. I studied such dreams both by surveying undergrads on whether they'd ever had one and by perusing large collections of dream journals (21). Surprisingly, these dreams were overwhelmingly pleasant. Slightly more than half of these accounts involve a lengthy afterlife sequence and may best be interpreted as symbolizing other psychological processes. The remainder were more focused on the process of dying and seemed to illustrate a struggle to come to terms with mortality. Dreams of almost dying were uniformly terrifying.

Related States

Daydreams and Hypnotic Dreams

In two studies, I examined the relationship of nighttime dreams to daydreams and hypnotic dreams with an eye toward how a person's hypnotizability influences all three categories. In the first study (22), I found that daydreams contained more friends, strangers, and happiness, while nighttime dreams had more family members, more negative emotions, and not surprisingly more "dream-like" distortions and discontinuities. Hypnotic dreams that occur in the trance state tended to fall in between nocturnal and daydreams on all these dimensions. Hypnotizability influenced hypnotic dreams, with subjects who are highly hypnotizable having dreams that resembled nighttime dreams closely. Even the daydreams of subjects who are easily hypnotized had some nocturnal dream characteristics, including bizarreness and discontinuities. These dreams could feel out of control and horrifying; more than one subject coined the term "daymare" to describe them.

In the second study, Neal Zamore and I examined in more detail how hypnotizability influenced dreaming (23). We found a correlation between hypnotizability and dream recall, dream vividness, and dream length, as well as unusual content categories such as lucid dreaming and flying dreams.

Sleep Talking

A group of my Harvard students and I analyzed the content of the somniloquies of Dion McGregor, the most extensive sleep talker ever recorded (24). McGregor, like most longwinded sleep talkers, seems to have spoken from REM periods accompanied by some hybrid waking-like bursts of alpha. We compared the transcripts of his somniloquies to dream accounts from the normative male dreams on the Hall–Van de Castle scales (25) and Allan Hobson's bizarreness scales (26). McGregor's somniloquies contained significantly more female characters relative to males than for the norms, and more familiar characters and friends, but fewer family members. The dreamer-as-character was much more interactive than the male dreamers except that McGregor was much less likely to engage in physical aggression specifically. There were a lower percentage of negative emotions, except that there was more self-negativity. On the Hobson bizarreness scales, McGregor had similar levels of discontinuity of plot, characters, objects, and actions, but had fewer incongruities of plot and many fewer instances of incongruity or uncertainty of thought. The lessened bizarreness of thought probably follows from the waking-hybrid alpha activity, but most of the other differences appeared congruent with McGregor's known quirks. He lived away from family amid a large circle of gay friends, wrote songs for female singers, and authored a book about Greta Garbo.

Clinical Implications

Answers to "What is the function of dreaming?" have ranged from Freud's (27) "wish-fulfillment" to Revonsuo's (28) diametrically opposed "threat simulation." I think there's an inherent problem with the question. We'd never ask the function of waking thought, at least not expecting a simple, limited answer—it's for *everything*. As I've elaborated on elsewhere (29), I believe that dreams are just thinking in a very different biochemical and electrophysiological state. This is how I would interpret the studies I've just reviewed. Prisoners are dreaming about how to escape and what they'll do back home. Bereaved dreamers are struggling to come to terms with the loss—at first obsessing over "He/she can't really be gone" and "What could I have done differently?" but eventually internalizing positive traits from the loved one. Depressed dreamers have the Catch-22 of less energy to fight depression when being depressed, but they nevertheless dream representations of their limited world. DID patients dream hypotheses about why they lose time, while alters plot their sometimes contradictory agendas: gain power through sexuality, gain safety by avoiding men, be cute and sweet so no one would hurt you, be so tough and scary no one could. One patient I treated (30) was violently assaulting his girlfriend in what originally appeared to be sleep episodes but proved to accompanied by a waking EEG. He also had recurring dreams about a violent stranger. In an interpretive dialogue with this dream character, the character told him he was "the man who lived inside your father and took him over sometimes." This led to a flood of memories about his dissociative father's violence and a new understanding of what was going on with himself.

Even types of dreams that don't look adaptive may have been so in ancestral environments. I disagree with Revonsuo about all dreams being threat simulations, but I do think that posttraumatic nightmares probably evolved because they generate anxiety and prompt vigilance: they keep the dreamer ready to fight or flee. This vigilance may have been more useful when a bear or a tribe over the hill who had attacked one night might return the next. In modern times, terrorism may repeat years later, or 1,000 miles away, or never. It likely won't use the same approach the dreams replay. These replays just re-traumatize the modern dreamer. The dreaming mind eventually begins to let go of the instinctual repetitions and generate mastery dreams that reassure and—in a few cases—may provide a model for what to do in a future trauma.

Many people I've seen in therapy have come seeking dream work. In other short-term, symptom-focused therapy, I still always ask, "Have you had any dream related to . . . ?" If a patient offers one, it may be either overtly about the symptom or something subjectively felt to be related to it. At the very least, this offers a concise metaphor for something the patient might not otherwise have been able to articulate. Sometimes it contains the seed of a solution. As I've written about more elsewhere (31), even with physical symptoms presenting in behavioral medicine, I find that dreams can be useful. Inquiring "Have you had any dreams about your pain?" may illuminate whether patients view pain as a shameful stigma, a badge of courage, or a reason for others to nurture them. If they have dreamed of their affliction as a science-fiction monster or a medieval torture device, then they have a more vivid image to use in pain control than most patients would generate awake.

Sometimes dreams simply underline something patients already know enough to make them act on it. One young woman being worked up by her physician for amenorrhea and incubated a dream about what was causing it: She dreamed of exercising and exercising. Her excessive activity did indeed turn out to be the cause of her missed periods, a concept she'd probably had all along, but the dream highlighted it enough for her to report it to her doctor. Another young man (32) came for treatment of insomnia, which he talked about non-psychologically until I suggested he try to dream about the symptom. He had two dreams about little boys at bedtime—one depicted as terribly alone, and the other as dying in his sleep. Working on this dream helped him understand what his fears were about sleep and to devise bedtime rituals to help him sleep easily without anxiety.

Dreams are already inherently therapeutic, problem-solving attempts in which some of our clients will come up with good ideas. However, if we want to maximize the effects of dreams, we, as therapists, can facilitate this by asking questions to help clients see if a dream has handed them a new approach to a waking life concern. Dream incubation can help to harness this power by providing simple steps that encourage our sleeping brain to ruminate on particular concerns.

References

(1) Barrett, D. L. *The Committee of Sleep: How Artists, Scientists, and Athletes Use Their Dreams for Creative Problem Solving—and How You Can Too*. New York: Crown Books/Random House, 2001.

(2) Reed, H. "Dream Incubation: A Reconstruction of a Ritual in Contemporary Form." *Journal of Humanistic Psychology* 16, 1976, p. 53–69.

(3) Dement, W. *Some Must Watch While Some Must Sleep*. San Francisco: W.H. Freeman, 1974, p. 98–102.

(4) Schatzman, M. Sleeping on Problems Can Really Solve Them. *New Scientist*, August 11, 1983, p. 416–417.

(5) Barrett, D. L. The "Committee of Sleep": A Study of Dream Incubation for Problem Solving. *Dreaming: Journal of the Association for the Study of Dreams* 3, 1993, p. 115–123.

(6) Barrett, D. L. and Loeffler, M. The Effect of Depression on the Manifest Content of the Dreams of College Students. *Psychological Reports* 70, 1992, p. 403–406.

(7) Dunn, K. K. and Barrett, D. L. Characteristics of Nightmare Subjects and their Nightmares. *Psychiatric Journal of the University of Ottawa* 13, 1988, p. 91–93.

(8) Barrett, D. L. (Ed.) *Trauma and Dreams*. Cambridge, MA: Harvard University Press, 1996.

(9) Krakow, B., et al. Imagery Rehearsal Therapy for Chronic Nightmares in Sexual Assault Survivors with Posttraumatic Stress Disorder: A Randomized Controlled Trial. *JAMA* 286.5, 2001, p. 537–545.

(10) Barrett, D. and Behbehani, J. Posttraumatic Nightmares in Kuwait Following the Iraqi Invasion, in S. Krippner and T. McIntyre, Eds. *Psychological Effects of War on Civilians: An International Perspective (Psychological Dimensions to War and Peace*. Amityville, NY: Praeger Publishing, 2003, p. 135–144.

(11) Barrett, D. *Night Wars*. Paper presented at the 19th Annual International Conference for the International Association for the Study of Dreams, June 15–19, 2002, Boston, Massachusetts.

(12) Barrett, D. L. Dreams in Dissociative Disorders. *Dreaming: Journal of the Association for the Study of Dreams* 4.3, 1994, p. 165–177.

(13) Thigpen, C. H., and Cleckley, H. M. *The Three Faces of Eve*. New York: Popular Library, 1957.

(14) Sizemore, C. C. *A Mind of My Own*. New York: William Morrow Co., 1989.

(15) Ross, R. J., et al. Rapid eye movement sleep disturbance in posttraumatic stress disorder. *Biological Psychiatry* 35.3, 1994, p. 195–202.

(16) Barrett, D. L. The Dream Character as a Prototype for the Multiple Personality "Alter." *Dissociation* 8, March 1995, p. 61–68.

(17) Barrett, D. L. Through a Glass Darkly: The Dead Appear in Dreams. *OMEGA: The Journal of Death and Dying* 24, 1991, p. 97–108.

(18) Barrett, D. L., Sogolow, Z., Oh, A., Panton, J., Grayson, M., and Justiniano, M. Content of Dreams from WWII POWs. *Imagination, Cognition, and Personality* 33, 2013, p. 293–304.

(19) Barrett, D. L. Just How Lucid Are Lucid Dreams: An Empirical Study of Their Cognitive Characteristics. *Dreaming: The Journal of the Association for the Study of Dreams* 2, 1992, p. 221–228.

(20) Barrett, D. L. An Empirical Study of the Relationship of Lucidity and Flying Dreams. *Dreaming: the Journal of the Association for the Study of Dreams* 1.2, 1991, p. 129–133.

(21) Barrett, D. L. Dreams of Death. *OMEGA: The Journal of Death and Dying* 19, 1988, p. 95–102.

(22) Barrett, D. L. The Hypnotic Dream: Its Content in Comparison to Nocturnal Dreams and Waking Fantasy. *Journal of Abnormal Psychology* 88, 1979, p. 584–591.

(23) Zamore, N. and Barrett, D. L. Hypnotic Susceptibility and Dream Characteristics. *Psychiatric Journal of the University of Ottawa* 14, 1989, p. 572–574.

(24) Barrett, D. L., Grayson, M., Oh, A., and Sogolow, Z. *A Content Analysis of Dion McGregor's Sleep Talking Episodes*. Paper presented at the 30th Conference of the International Association for the Study of Dreams, June 21–25, 2013, Virginia Beach, Virginia.

(25) Hall, C. and Van de Castle, R. *The Content Analysis of Dreams* New York: Appleton-Century-Crofts, 1966.

(26) Hobson, J. A., Hoffman, S. A., Helfand, R., and Kostner, D. Dream Bizarreness and the Activation-Synthesis Hypothesis. *Human Neurobiology* 6.3, 1987, p. 157–164.

(27) Freud, S. *The Interpretation of Dreams*. New York: Macmillan, 1913.

(28) Revonsuo, A. The Reinterpretation of Dreams: An Evolutionary Hypothesis of the Function of Dreaming. *Behavioral and Brain Sciences* 23.6, 2000, p. 877–901.

(29) Barrett, D. L. "An Evolutionary Theory of Dreams and Problem-Solving," in Barrett, D. L. & McNamara, P., Eds. *The New Science of Dreaming, Volume III: Cultural and Theoretical Perspectives on Dreaming*. New York: Praeger/Greenwood, 2007, p. 133–154.

(30) Barrett, D. L. The "Royal Road" Becomes a Shrewd Shortcut: The Use of Dreams in Focused Treatment, *Journal of Cognitive Psychotherapy* 16.1, 2002, p. 56–63.

(31) Barrett, D. L. "The Relation of Dissociative States to Sleep and Dreaming," in Krippner, S., and Powers, S., Eds. *Broken Images, Broken Selves: Dissociative Narratives in Clinical Practice.* New York: Brunner/Mazel, 1999, p. 216–229.

(32) Barrett, D. L. Using Hypnosis to Work with Dreams. *Self and Society: A Journal of Humanistic Psychology* 23, 1996, p. 25–28.

8
THE DIGITAL REVOLUTION IN DREAM RESEARCH

Kelly Bulkeley

Introduction

Starting with Freudian psychoanalysis, most schools of psychotherapy have treated dreams as a valuable resource in their clinical work. Dreams help therapists better understand the concerns and preoccupations of their clients by revealing memories of formative moments from their past, reflecting their current conflicts and struggles, and illuminating their personality strengths and capacities for growth. Dreams have been likened to an emotional thermostat (1), and the comparison is certainly apt. The patterns in people's dreams offer a surprisingly accurate gauge of their feelings, thoughts, and meaningful experiences in waking life.

The challenge is how to make the most of this resource in clinical practice. Some of the best insights only emerge from carefully studying a long series of the client's dreams—not an easy task, even for those with great expertise. Few psychotherapists receive any education in working with dreams, and the time pressures of short-term therapy leave little room for a deep, systematic exploration of the client's dream experiences.

This chapter argues that new digital tools of dream analysis, if well designed and appropriately deployed, have the potential to overcome these obstacles and make it easier for therapists to understand and benefit from their clients' dreams. The word *potential* must be emphasized, because the technologies in this field are still at a very early stage of development. But as I will argue, the research foundations are being built to support an empirically grounded, data-driven approach to identifying clinically significant patterns in dream content.

First I describe a system of digital analysis that uses word searches to study large collections of dreams. Then I show how this method can be applied to the dreams of people who are going through some kind of psychological crisis or emotional difficulty. I will discuss three brief case studies: a depressed young man (Will), a middle-aged woman with relationship problems (Smith), and a young woman with bouts of severe anxiety (Bea). I conclude the chapter with thoughts about future developments in these technologies and their most promising applications in clinical practice.

A Word Search Approach

My interest in new technologies of dream analysis has grown over the course of several experiments, each of which has yielded encouraging results (2, 3, 4). These projects have used simple word searching tools to analyze large collections of dreams. Each project has successfully identified a number of meaningful connections between people's dreams and their waking-life concerns and activities. Compared to traditional methods of hand-coding dreams, the word search method has enormous advantages in speed, simplicity, flexibility, and reliability. To be clear, word searches are not perfect or infallible, and they are not meant to remove humans from the analytic process. A word search approach is best conceived as a means of enhancing human-centered dream interpretation, providing a quick and objective overview of a data set. This digitally generated overview is the beginning of the interpretive process, not the end. It's a way of letting computers do what they do best—sorting through huge quantities of data—so we humans can do what we do best, using our intuitive skills of pattern recognition to find meaningful connections between the dreams and waking life.

I initially learned how to use the word search functions of DreamBank (www.dreambank.net), Bill Domhoff and Adam Schneider's highly useful online archive of systematically gathered dream reports. Then, starting in 2009, with the help of software engineer Kurt Bollacker, I began developing my own online archive and search engine called the Sleep and Dream Database, or SDDb. Although it is still a work in progress, I have been using the SDDb to explore various collections of dreams—big sets of dreams from demographically diverse populations, long series of dreams from individuals over many years, and classic collections of dreams used by other researchers, past and present. The SDDb has a word search function with a built-in template of 40 categories of content, divided into eight classes. The 40 categories are rooted in the content analysis system of Calvin Hall and Robert Van de Castle, with additional influence from G. William Domhoff, Tracey Kahan, Milton Kramer, Ernest Hartmann, and many others. The template, now in its 2.0 version, makes it easy to compare the results of word search studies on different collections of dreams.

The Hall and Van de Castle norm dreams, with approximately 500 male and 500 female dream reports, have long served the field as a measuring stick of average, ordinary patterns in dream content. For word searches on the SDDb I have created a new measuring stick that combines the HVDC norm dreams with several other sources of high-quality, systematically gathered data to provide a bigger and more diverse representation of what counts as "normal" dreaming. The SDDb baseline dreams include a total of 5,245 reports of "most recent dreams" (female

N = 3,110, male N = 2,135). These baselines are not a perfect map of human dream content, but they do offer a useful standard for measuring and comparing the patterns of word usage in a given collection of dreams.

Example 1: Will

Will was a 26-year old man who participated in a research project I initiated in 2006 (5). He kept a year-long sleep and dream journal, and I interviewed him at several points during the year to ask about various aspects of his life. The focus of the project was political and religious beliefs, so I did not ask detailed questions about his mental health history. But Will volunteered that he had struggled with depression, mood disorders, and poor sleep for many years. At least a couple of times his problems became severe enough that he sought out professional help, and he had been prescribed a variety of medications to control the worst of it. He lived at home with his parents, had trouble keeping a job, and did not enjoy much of a social life.

Despite these difficulties, Will was an extremely intelligent and charming young man. Literate, intellectually curious, and artistically creative, he had a gentle and generous spirit that had prompted him a couple of years earlier to care full-time for his grandmother during the final weeks of her life.

During the year-long research project, Will recorded 96 dreams. Table 8.1 shows the results of applying the 40 categories of the SDDb 2.0 word search template to this series of dreams, comparing Will's results to the corresponding frequencies in the SDDb male baseline dreams. The percentages show how many dreams in the set contain at least one reference to a word in the given category.

If you knew nothing else about Will but his patterns of dream content compared to the baselines, you would likely be able to tell that he was an unusual and troubled person. Looking at the categories for emotions, Will's low frequencies of fear and anger and his higher references to sadness were accurate reflections of his depressive, melancholic temperament. The high proportions of references to falling and death corresponded to his waking concerns about the fragility of his personal relationships (for example, with his deceased grandmother, who appeared frequently in his dreams). The low frequency of references to sexuality mirrored his limited romantic experience in waking life.

Will's dreams also had unusually high frequencies of words referring to sensory perception, thinking, and reading and writing. These mirrored his intellectual strengths and the well-developed cognitive skills he brought to his interactions with the waking world.

The most unusual aspect of Will's dream series regarded his use of words relating to the four classical elements of fire, air, water, and earth. His frequencies for all four elements were dramatically higher than the male baselines, the highest I have ever seen, in fact. Looking at these dreams in more detail revealed that many of them involved transcendental experiences of merger and union, with

TABLE 8.1 Word Search Analysis of Will's Dream Series

	Will's Journal N = 96 Average word length: 128		SDDb Male Baselines N = 2135 Average word length: 105
	Percent	*Four Most-Used Words*	*Percent*
Perception			
Vision	51	see, watching, eyes, watch	29
Hearing	27	hear, listen, sound, ears	9
Touch	25	hand, holding, touches, hands	12
Smell & Taste	6	smells, smell	1
Color	33	blue, white, red, black	13
Emotion			
Fear	4	upset, fear, anxiety	15
Anger	2	angry, furious	5
Sadness	8	sad, depressed, depressing, sadness	3
Wonder	16	suddenly, wondering, puzzled	18
Happiness	8	happy, relaxed, relieved, contented	6
Characters			
Family	51	family, brother, grandmother, father	27
Animals	11	hamster, birds, bear, fish	12
Fantastic beings	1	demons	2
Male references	34	his, he, him, father	40
Female references	53	her, she, grandmother, woman	35
Social Interactions			
Friendliness	39	friend, friends, goodbye, save	34
Physical aggression	20	fight, hit, shot, rob	21
Sexuality	1	kisses	6
Movement			
Walking & Running	26	walk, walking, run, runs	27
Flying	8	floating, float, flying, flies	6
Falling	28	fall, falling, falls, drop	8
Death	25	died, dying, death, dead	7
Cognition			
Thinking	59	think, sense, thinking, notice	38
Speaking	39	talking, say, says, talk	32
Reading & Writing	17	reading, reads, writing, written	5
Culture			
Architecture	45	room, house, door, home	41
Food & Drink	21	eating, soup, drink, milk	12

(Continued)

TABLE 8.1 (Continued)

	Percent	Four Most-Used Words	Percent
Clothing	11	dress, wearing, dressed, vest	11
School	15	school, teacher, university, professors	13
Transportation	29	street, car, path, boat	28
Technology & Science	17	video, engineering, email, phone	8
Money & Work	19	work, office, dollars, money	22
Weapons	4	guns, knife, gun	5
Sports	4	soccer, basketball, football	4
Art	19	singing, song, poem, songs	7
Religion	19	Christmas, Christian, heaven, temple	6
Elements			
Fire	26	sun, fire, burned, burn	4
Air	14	wind, air, breath, breathe	5
Water	41	water, lake, river, ocean	12
Earth	17	earth, rocks, rock, dirt	10

extraordinary shifts in awareness and perceptual sensitivity. Will associated these mystically tinged dreams with his waking belief in a non-theistic spirituality of nature, which conflicted with the strict religious beliefs of his Catholic family. A therapist might also look at these unusual dreams for clues to his family relations, his typical defense strategies, his long-term ideals, and perhaps a tendency toward dissociation.

This kind of analysis is intended to give an initial orientation towards the major features of a new set of dreams, highlighting unusual themes and making it easier to pursue deeper explorations. In Will's case, the word usage patterns in his dreams accurately reflected the distinctive contours of his emotional life, personal relationships, psychological strengths, spiritual beliefs, and ongoing vulnerabilities.

Example 2: Smith

Smith was a woman in her late 40s who agreed with her therapist to contact me, via another researcher, for assistance in understanding her dreams. They shared her diary of 67 dream reports, which she had recorded over a period of several months during the therapy process. In this case, I was almost entirely "blind" at the start of the analysis. I knew Smith's age and gender and the fact she was in therapy, which I had to assume indicated some kind of mental health issue. Other than that, I knew nothing about her. When I applied the word search template to her dreams, I looked at the results (shown in Table 8.2, with a comparison to the

TABLE 8.2 Word Search Analysis of Smith's Dream Series

	Smith's Journal N = 67 Average word length: 304		SDDb Female Baselines N = 3110 Average word length: 100
	Percent	*Four Most-Used Words*	*Percent*
Perception			
Vision	49	see, saw, eyes, watch	37
Hearing	25	heard, noise, ear, hear	10
Touch	46	hand, fingers, holding, finger	12
Smell & Taste	10	tasted, nose, taste, delicious	2
Color	48	white, blue, red, green	18
Emotion			
Fear	27	worried, scared, embarrassed, worry	23
Anger	9	furious, irritated, angry, disgusting	8
Sadness	3	sad, disappointed	5
Wonder	28	suddenly, wondered, shocked, wondering	18
Happiness	9	happy, relaxed	9
Characters			
Family	40	married, dad, mother, family	40
Animals	39	dog, cat, fish, animals	13
Fantastic beings	4	aliens, spirits, dragon	2
Male references	70	he, his, him, man	47
Female references	58	she, her, girl, lady	44
Social Interactions			
Friendliness	57	help, friend, offered, wedding	46
Physical aggression	25	hit, struggled, fight, killed	14
Sexuality	9	sex, kissed, had sex, having sex	4
Movement			
Walking/Running	57	walked, ran, running, walking	27
Flying	10	flying, flew, fly, floating	4
Falling	21	dropped, fell, drop, collapsed	7
Death	7	death, dead, die, died	9
Cognition			
Thinking	54	decided, thought, thinking, think	39
Speaking	70	said, call, talking, called	35
Reading/Writing	16	book, read, letter, books	6
Culture			
Architecture	82	door, room, house, home	47
Food & Drink	48	drink, wine, food, lunch	14

(Continued)

TABLE 8.2 (Continued)

	Percent	Four Most-Used Words	Percent
Clothing	40	dress, wearing, clothes, wear	14
School	9	school, students, university, test	17
Transportation	52	car, stairs, train, road	24
Technology	27	phone, phones, computer, DVD	7
Money and Work	55	work, office, bought, buy	18
Weapons	3	swords, weapon	3
Sports	4	basketball, gymnastic, tennis	4
Art	25	movies, song, music, dance	10
Religion	15	hell, god, spirits, Easter	7
Elements			
Fire	9	fire, sun, burn	4
Air	12	air, breath, breathed	4
Water	21	water, ice, snow, pond	13
Earth	27	hill, stone, dirt, dirty	10

SDDb female baselines) and made inferences about her waking-life concerns and preoccupations. I sent the inferences to Smith and her therapist, both of whom sent responses confirming or disconfirming my predictions.

Most of the inferences turned out to be correct. Smith was a sociable and talkative woman who was close to both parents, had no children of her own, and had several cats and dogs as pets. She was very concerned about money and finances, but was not otherwise an emotionally expressive individual. She was preoccupied about getting married and having a wedding. She was not highly educated, nor was she religiously or spiritually active. She spent a great deal of time reading books and watching movies and television. All of this information emerged from a study of nothing more than the patterns of word usage in Smith's dreams, before knowing almost anything else about her.

After sharing these results with Smith and her therapist, our ensuing conversation filled in the general picture of her situation. Smith had begun therapy for help with two principal concerns: feeling stuck in job she didn't like, and feeling stuck in a long-term relationship with a man who did not want to get married. She wanted to quit the job with its long commute (reflected in her high transportation frequency) and try something new, but the turbulent economy and dangers of unemployment made her hesitant. Her decision was complicated by the fact that she financially supported her boyfriend, meaning any change in her job would impact their relationship. It turned out Smith was not only an avid reader but also an energetic writer of fantasy fiction, reflecting the literary creativity she developed over the years despite a very modest educational background.

I do not know what Smith and her therapist ultimately did with her dream series beyond their discussions with me. I encouraged them to view the word search analysis as an invitation to a more detailed and probing interpretive process. Having an overview of the patterns in her dreams would give them a common frame of reference for looking at particular areas of concern, conflict, or possible growth.

It might also give both client and therapist an opportunity to reflect on aspects of her situation they might be overlooking or exaggerating. For Smith, she said she accepted her boyfriend's unwillingness to get married, but her dreams contained numerous references to weddings and marriage, suggesting this theme preoccupied her more than she was acknowledging (a point her therapist strongly agreed with). However, the therapist blamed some of Smith's problems on the dehumanizing effects of modern technological society, but in Smith's dreams and waking comments she seemed fairly comfortable with technology, suggesting the therapist may have been more concerned about this issue than she was.

Example 3: Bea

Bea initially contacted G. William Domhoff with two series of dreams, which he forwarded to me for a blind word search analysis. I knew nothing about Bea beyond the facts that she was a young woman and the first series of dreams (N = 183) came before the second series (N = 40). Using an earlier version of the word search template, I calculated Bea's word usage frequencies in the two series, compared them to the HVDC female norms, and made a number of blind inferences about her waking life in the two time periods. (The detailed statistical results do not need to be repeated here, since they were published in a 2010 article in the journal *Dreaming* (4).)

With Domhoff serving as intermediary, Bea confirmed most of the inferences (11 of 15) as correct. She was a student who had moved from high school (series 1) to college (series 2), and I could tell she had become more academically challenged, was playing more field hockey and less soccer, had a boyfriend, was more sexually active, felt more concerned about her family (mother, father, and one brother), and had experienced a negative emotional downturn between the times of series 1 to series 2.

In a follow-up conversation Bea said that during her first year of college she sought counseling for recurrent bouts of anxiety, with persistent fantasies about threats to her family. She said my inference about the negative emotional shift from the first to second series of dreams was "spot on." Even though she was living on her college campus during her second series, she was dreaming more about her parents (and the family dog) during that time than during the first series when she was living at home. This underscores an important point about dreaming-waking continuities identified by word searches: we tend to dream about people we are concerned about, not necessarily people who are physically around us in our daily lives.

For Bea, leaving home and going to college elicited a host of fears about her family's safety, which her dreams accurately reflected. These anxieties grew so intense that she finally sought help at the campus mental health center. The counseling went well, and after a few months the anxiety dissipated and she could finally settle into the routines of school.

Bea contacted us a couple of years after the time of her counseling, so the word search analysis could have no part in her treatment. But the experiment Domhoff and I performed showed that this kind of analysis could play a valuable role in a therapeutic process by providing a quick, objective, and accurate measure of an individual's emotional state over time.

Future Challenges

The method of word search analysis outlined here offers many benefits for psychotherapeutic practice. The three examples of Will, Smith, and Bea suggest that word searching, even at this very early stage of development, is an effective means of gauging a dreamer's emotional welfare, daily activities, personal relationships, and cultural beliefs. Therapists from any background could benefit from timely access to this kind of information about their clients.

However, many obstacles must be overcome before the full potential of such technologies can be realized:

- Any digital tool that works with personal material like dreams will have to ensure the security and confidentiality of people's data, otherwise nobody will want to try these methods of studying their dreams.
- Better, more user-friendly systems will have to be developed to make it easier for people to record their dreams, archive them, and explore them for their own interests.
- To work in a clinical context, systems of digital dream journaling will have to be integrated with analytic tools that therapists can use to track the dream patterns of their clients.
- Above all, much more research (using word searches and other methods of study) will be needed to create an evidence-based map of recurrent patterns of dream content across various groups of people. This map will serve as a necessary guide for the new technologies and the people who use them, making sure they stay connected to the best scientific knowledge about the realities of human dream experience.

These are not insurmountable challenges. In coming years we are likely to see a proliferation of sophisticated new digital tools for dream analysis. The most successful of these tools will develop technologies to enhance, rather than overwhelm, people's understandings of their dreams. The key is integrating the quantitative and qualitative dimensions of the analysis. In the studies presented here, blind word searching was the quantitative method, and personal interviews and questionnaires were the qualitative methods. A great deal can be learned from either method alone, but my experiences with the SDDb have convinced me that much more can be gained from using them in tandem.

Recently I read a newly published book that makes essentially the same point in a larger social context. Clive Thompson, an editor at *Wired* magazine, wrote *Smarter Than You Think*, in which he argues that new digital technologies are transforming the world into a (mostly) better place (6). A key passage comes in the first chapter, when he describes the evolution of chess-playing computers. In the 1990s the world chess champion Garry Kasparov had several public matches with IBM's Deep Blue supercomputer. Thompson says that Kasparov's experiences led to "an audacious idea":

"What would happen if, instead of competing against one another, humans and computers *collaborated*? What if they played on teams together—one computer and a human facing off against another human and a computer? That way, [Kasparov] theorized, each might benefit from the other's peculiar powers. The computer would bring the lightning-fast—if uncreative—ability to analyze zillions of moves, while the human would bring intuition and insight, the ability to read opponents and psych them out. Together, they would form what chess players later called a centaur: a hybrid beast endowed with the strengths of each . . . In essence, a new form of chess intelligence was emerging. You could rank the teams like this: (1) a chess grand master was good; (2) a chess grand master playing with a laptop was better. But even that laptop-equipped grand master could be beaten by (3) relative newbies, if the amateurs were extremely skilled at integrating machine assistance. [Kasparov concluded,] 'Human strategic guidance combined with the tactical acuity of a computer . . . was overwhelming." (pp. 3, 5, emphasis in original)

With a couple of tweaks to Thompson's chess example, we can easily foresee the emergence in the not-too-distant future of *centaurs of dream interpretation*, integrated systems that smoothly and harmoniously combine the strengths of human intelligence and computer data analysis. To get there, we have to experiment, tinker, and innovate; we have to gather as much high-quality data as possible, put every hypothesis to the empirical test, and be prepared for some false starts and dead ends. But the technology already exists to create really amazing dream interpretation centaurs. All that is lacking is the input of highly skilled and richly experienced people like the contributors to this book, and many of its readers, too. They, and you, are the "grand masters" of the dream game, people who are uniquely well-qualified to teach the machines how to work better.

Conclusion

This chapter has shown how a simple word search method can generate clinically useful information about a series of dreams quickly, reliably, and accurately. The results are encouraging for efforts to develop new centaurs of dream interpretation that can give therapists, counselors, and others in the helping professions new resources for gaining insights into the most meaningful concerns and preoccupations of their clients' lives.

I will leave you with this jet-pack and robot-car kind of image of what therapists may see some day in the future: Your clients keep a regular dream journal in a safe, private digital space. Before each session together you get an automatically generated report summarizing the significant patterns and changes in the client's dreams, just like a medical doctor gets a chart with current temperature and blood pressure before seeing a patient. This report would not tell you what to do, but it would prime your empathetic sensitivities and deepen your familiarity with the most important concerns and activities in your client's life. Perhaps it might signal an impending problem or hidden danger. It might also illuminate the emergence of potentials for growth and healing that you might not otherwise have noticed.

References

1. Bulkeley K. 2009. Seeking patterns in dream content: A systematic approach to word searches. Consciousness and Cognition. 2009;18: 905–16.
2. Bulkeley K, Domhoff GW. 2010. Detecting meaning in dream reports: An extension of a word search approach. Dreaming. 2010;20(2): 77–95.
3. Bulkeley K. Dreaming in adolescence: A "blind" word search of a teenage girl's dream series. Dreaming. 2012;22(4): 240–52.
4. Bulkeley K. American dreamers. Boston: Beacon Press; 2008.
5. Kramer M. The dream experience: A systematic exploration. New York: Routledge; 2007.
6. Thompson C. Smarter than you think. New York: Penguin; 2014.

9

THE MANIFEST DREAM REPORT AND CLINICAL CHANGE

Myron L. Glucksman

CLINICAL PROFESSOR OF PSYCHIATRY
NEW YORK MEDICAL COLLEGE, VALHALLA, N.Y.

Milton Kramer

EMERITUS PROFESSOR OF PSYCHIATRY
UNIVERSITY OF CINCINNATI
COLLEGE OF MEDICINE, CINCINNATI, OHIO

Traditionally, psychoanalysts have considered the manifest dream report (MDR) less significant than the latent dream content. Freud (1900/1958) focused on what he considered to be the hidden wishes or impulses in the latent content. In his "Introductory Lectures on Psychoanalysis," he stated: "We will describe what the dream actually tells us as the manifest dream content, and the concealed material, which we hope to reach by pursuing the ideas that occur to the dreamer, as the latent dream-thoughts" (Freud, 1916/1963, p. 120). Nevertheless, a number of clinicians have emphasized the manifest dream content as an important source of clinical information. Warner (1983) observed certain changes in the manifest content of successive dreams that corresponded with clinical improvement. These included increased self-esteem, greater self-soothing capability, and less masochism. More specifically, he described "turning point dreams" that reflected the achievement of a therapeutic milestone or a significant change in the patient's psychodynamics (Warner, 1987). Glucksman (1988, 2001) pointed out the importance of manifest content as a metaphorical presentation of the dreamer's conflicts, problems, feelings, and relationships. In addition, he described how both manifest and latent content can be used to document and facilitate clinical change during treatment. Other investigators have also emphasized the importance of understanding or "translating" manifest content (Kramer and Roth, 1977; Palombo, 1984; Mendelsohn, 1990; Greenberg and Pearlman, 1993). Kramer and colleagues (Kramer, Whitman, Baldridge, and Lansky, 1964; Kramer, 1993) described how multiple MDRs during the night are linked together to achieve emotional problem solving. Specifically, the change in mood from night to morning relates primarily to the individuals who appear in the manifest content.

Numerous studies have identified specific variables relevant to clinical change and outcome in psychotherapy and psychoanalysis (Luborsky, Chandler, Auerbach, Cohen, and Bachrach, 1971; Kernberg, Coyne, Horwitz, Appelbaum, and Burstein, 1972; Bachrach, Weber, and Soloman, 1985; Karasu, 1986; Kantrowitz, Katz, and Paolitto, 1990). Of interest is that many of these variables are similar or identical to the known functions of dreaming. These include: problem solving and conflict resolution (Cartwright, 1986; Greenberg, Katz, Schwartz, and Pearlman, 1992; Domhoff, 1993; Koulack, 1993; Hobson, 1999), mood or affect regulation (Lowy, 1942; Kramer et al., 1964; Kramer, 1993), learning and mastery (Koulack, 1993; Smith, 1993; Fiss, 1993; Hobson, 1999), and self-awareness (Dewald, 1972; Purcell, Moffitt, and Hoffman, 1993). In view of the similarity between certain dream functions and some of the key variables involved in clinical change, it seems likely that a linkage between them exists. In fact, there have been reports of a relationship between MDRs and clinical change, but these have been anecdotal and lack experimental validation (Bonime, 1962; French and Fromm, 1964; Hall and Van de Castle, 1966; Saul, 1972; Warner, 1983; Warner, 1987). In order to explore this topic in a more systematic way, we chose to examine MDRs during the course of psychiatric treatment. We selected MDRs because they can be reliably rated according to specific variables by independent observers. Hall and Van de Castle (1966) developed a reliable, valid system for quantifying MDR content. Their system, as well as the observations of others (Winget, Kramer, and Whitman, 1972), revealed that manifest content differences corresponded to demographic variables as well as mental illnesses, including schizophrenia and depression (Kramer and Roth, 1973). However, their protocol was developed for dreams of 100 words or more, and excluded those consisting of fragments or briefer MDRs.

We began our investigation of the relationship between MDRs and clinical change by examining dreams during the early and later stages of treatment (Glucksman and Kramer, 2004). Our hypothesis was that there would be significant differences between the MDRs of those patients who either showed signs of improvement or did not. One of us (MG) selected 12 patients from his private practice who had completed either psychoanalysis or psychodynamically oriented therapy. They were divided into two groups: (1) six patients who demonstrated significant clinical improvement, and (2) six patients who demonstrated limited or no clinical improvement. The manifest content of an early as well as a later MDR for each patient was selected verbatim from MG's therapy notes. The 12 MDR pairs were presented randomly to MK without any other identifying data (MK was an independent observer who had no clinical knowledge of the patients). His task was to place six MDR pairs into the clinically improved group, and six MDR pairs into the clinically unimproved group. MK placed each of the MDR pairs correctly into the improved and unimproved groups. This was a highly significant statistical result ($p < .001$).

The following are examples of MDR pairs from one of the six most clinically improved and one of the six least clinically improved patients:

Most Improved Patient

Dream From Initial Phase of Treatment

> "I returned to teaching after a nervous breakdown. Another female teacher said: "You just made it back in time or you would have been fired." A choir director was trying to get me to sing alone. We were in an old Victorian house, and I saw a panther. I was frightened."

Dream From Later Phase of Treatment

> "I was at a beach resort where I won a beauty contest. I looked for my husband to tell him. I felt no urgency in finding him, and savored the experience."

Least Improved Patient

Dream From Initial Phase of Treatment

> "I was with a group of college friends talking about having kids. I stayed out of the conversation, and someone asked why I was staying out of the discussion. I told them about the conflict between my husband and myself. I felt badly about telling them."

Dream From Later Phase of Treatment

> "I was on a sailboat with a man. He fell asleep. I tried to wake him up, but he wouldn't get up. I was totally on my own to sail the boat."

The most improved patient entered treatment with anxiety symptoms, phobias, feelings of inadequacy, and dependency on others. Her mother was extremely controlling and devalued her. Her symptoms significantly diminished during therapy, and she became more self-reliant. The least-improved patient entered treatment with depressive symptoms; she wanted to have a baby, but her passive-aggressive husband was opposed to it. She continued to be depressed, and the conflict with her husband over becoming pregnant remained unresolved.

The encouraging results of the previous study led to a second one in which we attempted to correlate changes in MDRs with the degree of clinical improvement in the same group of 12 patients (Glucksman and Kramer, 2004). MG (the treating clinician) rank ordered the patients according to clinical improvement based on the following criteria: (1) symptom reduction, (2) resolution of central conflict(s), (3) level of functioning, (4) ego strength, (5) interpersonal relationships, (6) transference resolution, (7) affect resolution, and (8) self-analytic capacity. MG selected the first and last dreams of treatment and provided MK with 12 randomized MDR pairs. MK evaluated and rank ordered the 12 MDR pairs according to the following criteria: (1) negative to positive, or positive to negative, changes in mood; (2) negative to positive, or positive to negative, changes in behavior; (3) negative to positive, or positive to negative, changes in self-image; and (4) effective or ineffective problem/conflict solving. The correlation between MG's clinical rankings and MK's 12 MDR pair rankings was significant: almost the .05 level of probability ($r = .45, p = .069$).

The following are examples of the first and last MDR pairs from one of the most improved and one of the least improved patients:

Most Improved Patient

First Dream of Treatment

"I was put into a mental hospital."

Last Dream of Treatment

"I'm at an airport boarding a plane with a man. We climb up the stairs to the plane until there are no more rungs or stairs. I'm terrified. A little girl jumps off and is killed. But I climb to safety with the man and am glad that I survived. However, I'm angst-ridden over the little girl."

Least Improved Patient

First Dream of Treatment

"I was trying to escape from a foreign country. It was a very repressive regime."

Last Dream of Treatment

"I was on a ship. It was fired on and I was hit by bullets in my back. I knew I was dying."

The most improved patient entered treatment depressed and suicidal. Following a brief hospitalization, she was less symptomatic, and became more satisfied with her job and marriage. The least improved patient entered treatment feeling depressed about her job and marriage. She failed to improve, and left treatment still symptomatic and despondent about her future.

Among the variables we used for rating MDRs was affect. The central role of affect in understanding the motivation and meaning of dreams has been emphasized by a number of investigators (Freud, 1900; Bonime, 1962; Hall and Van de Castle, 1966; Kramer, Winget, and Whitman, 1971; Stairs and Blick, 1979; Foulkes, Sullivan, Kerr, and Brown, 1988; Kramer, 1993). However, affect is not always present in spontaneous and sleep laboratory dream reports (Bonime, 1962; Strauch and Meier, 1996; Kramer and Birk, 2002; Kramer and Glucksman, 2006). We decided to further explore the role of affect in dreams and whether or not its presence changes over the course of treatment (Kramer and Glucksman, 2006). MG selected the first and last MDRs of 24 patients who had either completed treatment or were well along. According to MG, each of these patients had made significant clinical improvement. MK did not know the clinical history or gender of any of the 24 patients. Both MG and MK rated the 24 MDR pairs for the presence or absence of reported affect, and whether the valence of reported affect was positive or negative. There was 94% agreement between MG and MK regarding the presence or absence of affect in the MDRs. Moreover, there was 100% agreement between them on the positive or negative valence of affect in the 24 MDR pairs. In view of the high level of agreement between MG and MK on the presence, absence, and valence of affect, we chose to report MK's ratings since he was the less-biased observer (having no clinical knowledge about the patients). MK found that affect was present in 58% of MDRs. On one hand, initial MDRs had a great deal more negative (77%) than positive affect (19%). On the other, last MDRs had more positive (53%) than negative affect (47%). In essence, there was a shift from negative to positive affect in MDRs over the course of treatment.

The following is an illustration of the shift in affect valence from the first to last MDRs of treatment:

First MDR of Treatment

"I was back in college as a freshman. I was going to classes where I didn't know anybody. It was an unpleasant feeling. Someone asked me if I was Bob's brother."

Last MDR of Treatment

"I was teaching at a medical school and interacting with medical students. I was enjoying it."

The patient was a physician who entered treatment with depressive symptoms, low self-esteem, and doubts about his professional competency. He had been unhappy as a freshman in college, and felt overshadowed by his more popular brother. Toward the end of treatment, he was no longer depressed and felt more self-confident. In addition, he felt a great deal of satisfaction from his position as a professor in a medical school.

Although the change in affect valence of MDRs from the beginning to the end of treatment may have been partially due to the passage of time as well as the effect of medication, it was most likely a result of the beneficial influence of psychotherapy. Of interest is that MG found affect in 98% of MDRs and patients' associations to them. The latter observation, along with MK's finding that 58% of MDRs contain affect, reinforced the hypothesis that affect is an intrinsic part of the dream experience.

Our next study of the role of MDRs in treatment focused on the clinical and predictive value of the initial MDR in therapy (Glucksman and Kramer, 2011). Historically, the initial dream of analysis was considered to be of special significance. Saul (1940) concluded that early dreams reveal the patient's core psychodynamics. Stekel (1943) proposed that the first reported dream revealed the patient's entire life history. Beratis (1984) observed that the initial dream communicates the patient's salient psychodynamic themes. Kradin (2006) termed the initial dream of treatment the *herald dream,* because it presents the major psychodynamic issues that concern the patient and anticipates the trajectory of the ensuing treatment. Unfortunately, all of these studies were based on anecdotal clinical reports. Therefore, we decided to study the initial dream of treatment in a more systematic, unbiased fashion.

We collected the initial MDRs from 63 patients in MG's practice who had either terminated treatment or were still engaged. The sample included 33 females and 30 males, ranging in age from 18 to 76 years. Each MDR was assigned a number randomly and printed without any other identifiers, such as the name of the patient, age, gender, or associations. Initial MDRs were rated according to the following variables: (1) affect and affect valence, (2) affect in associations, (3) psychodynamic theme, (4) psychodynamic theme as predictor of core psychodynamic issues, (5) transference, (6) gender, and (7) dream theme category. Both MG and MK independently rated MDRs for each variable, except where familiarity with the patient precluded them from doing so (e.g., gender), or where the therapist's clinical knowledge of the patient was necessary (e.g., associations, transference).

MG and MK had a high level of agreement (89%) on their independent ratings of affect and affect valence of the 63 initial MDRs. In view of this, MK's ratings were used in this study because of his lack of clinical knowledge about the patients. He found affect in 44% of initial MDRs, which was consistent with our previous study (Kramer and Glucksman, 2006) where 58% of MDRs contained affect. Negative affect occurred in 32% of initial MDRs, and positive affect was found in only 11% of initial MDRs, similar to our previous study (Kramer and Glucksman, 2006). When associations were included with MDRs, affect was observed in 86% of MDRs, also consistent with our previous study (Kramer and Glucksman, 2006).

An example of an initial MDR with negative affect is the following:

"I went to a building where I used to work. I drove a Subaru coupe there. But nobody was there; I felt alone and sad."

The patient entered treatment with depressive symptoms following the loss of his job, as well as a myocardial infarction. Perhaps the major reason for the preponderance of negative affect in initial MDRs is because most patients are in a dysphoric state at the beginning of treatment. As in this case, major depressive disorder is a common reason for patients to seek treatment.

The psychodynamic theme of an initial MDR was defined as a phenomenological, dynamic description of the dream imagery. It was not based on any particular psychoanalytic model or orientation. MG and MK agreed on 90% of psychodynamic themes of initial MDRs. Because of this high level of agreement, MK's conceptualizations of psychodynamic themes were chosen because of his lack of familiarity with the patients. Each initial MDR's psychodynamic theme was then compared to MG's description of the core psychodynamic issues that emerged during that particular patient's treatment. Psychodynamic themes of 94% of initial MDRs were judged to be consistent with the core psychodynamic issues that arose during subsequent treatment.

The following is an initial MDR, the psychodynamic theme, and the salient psychodynamic issues that were identified during the ensuing treatment:

> "I was playing bridge with my wife and we were in a bidding sequence. I knew I was in a bad situation and was afraid I'd make a mistake with a bad result. I would be a failure and everyone would see it."

Both MG and MK agreed that the psychodynamic theme of this initial MDR involved a sense of inadequacy, fear of being exposed, failing, and experiencing humiliation or shame. The following psychodynamic issues emerged during treatment: The patient was extremely controlling and compulsive. He was afraid of being criticized for making mistakes, especially by male authority figures. His mother has been very critical of him while he was growing up, and often did not speak to him for days when she was angry with him. His father was emotionally distant, and his occasional temper outbursts were frightening for the patient. The latter was highly competitive, as well as a perfectionist at his job, socially, and even in his leisure activities. His feelings were strongly controlled, and he was afraid of revealing any vulnerabilities. Over the course of therapy, it became evident that he was terrified of abandonment by his mother and wife as well as physical injury or humiliation by his father or other men. Clearly, the major or core psychodynamic issues that emerged during therapy were embedded in the psychodynamic theme of his initial MDR.

Transference in the initial MDR was defined as the presence of the therapist (MG), a person, object, or situation serving as a projection and displacement of the therapist. According to these criteria, transference was observed by MG in 44% of initial MDRs. When present, it was negative in 61% of initial MDRs and positive in 32% of initial MDRs. The therapist was not present as himself in any initial MDRs, which was consistent with other observations (Harris, 1962; Yazmajian, 1964; Rosenbaum, 1965; Bradlow and Coen, 1975). More women than men manifested transference in the initial MDRs.

An example of negative transference in an initial MDR is the following:

> "A man was attacking me and trying to cut my back with a knife. The cops couldn't catch him and he got away with it."

The patient had been sexually and physically abused by her father from childhood until adolescence. Her ex-husband had also abused her physically and verbally. She was extremely distrustful of men, including the therapist, and avoided any heterosexual relationships following her divorce. Self-mutilation (cutting) was a major presenting symptom.

An example of positive transference in an initial MDR was the following:

> "I went to the doctor and he did an MRI on my neck. He found something that explained all my symptoms. I felt relieved and happy."

The patient entered treatment with somatic symptoms associated with anxiety, including neck and back pain. A complete medical workup failed to reveal an organic cause for her pain. She was initially hopeful that the therapist would diagnose and treat her symptoms successfully. These clinical examples were illustrative of the fact that transference in the initial MDR can be informative regarding the patients' expectations, attitudes, and perceptions of the therapist.

Previous studies have demonstrated male/female differences in manifest dream content (Hall and Van de Castle, 1966; Winget et al., 1972; Winget and Kramer, 1979). Women are more likely to have dreams containing friendly social interactions, emotions, and home and family references. Men have dreams with more aggression, competitiveness, hostility, and sexuality. MK, who had no knowledge of the gender or other identifying clinical information connected to the patients in this study, correctly predicted the gender of 62% of the patients from the initial MDR. His observations supported the previous reports of systematic differences in the dreams of males and females.

The initial MDRs in this study were grouped into one of seven dream theme categories. These included: (1) relational (interpersonal relationships involving attachment, rejection, abandonment, reunion, separation, intimacy), (2) injury (actual or feared physical and emotional injury, harm, abuse, mutilation, humiliation), (3) control (loss of control, helplessness, mastery, power, domination, submission), (4) self (physical or emotional aspect of self, including traits, qualities, characteristics), (5) problem solving (resolving problems, issues, conflicts, decision making), (6) sexual (actual or wished-for sexual activity, lust, orgasm), and (7) loss (actual or feared loss, death, disappearance, absence of spouse, friend, job, status, money, possessions). Although these dream theme categories were arbitrary, and clearly overlapped one another, we were curious regarding their frequency. MG rated the dream theme categories because he was intimately aware of the patients' psychodynamic issues and their clinical progress. However, his observations lacked interrater reliability, and therefore could not be statistically validated. Of interest, he found that relational and injury dream themes occurred more frequently in initial MDRs than any of the others. The most likely explanation for this finding is that interpersonal and attachment issues, as well as threats of actual or potential harm, are part of developmental experience and ubiquitous throughout life. Dream themes of loss, although infrequent, occurred in older patients (as might be expected). In summary, our observations suggested that the initial MDR was a useful predictor of the core psychodynamic issues and themes that emerged during treatment.

Our most recent study (Glucksman and Kramer, 2012) was a further investigation of the initial and last MDRs of treatment. This was an attempt to replicate our previous findings using a larger patient population (Glucksman and Kramer, 2004; Kramer and Glucksman, 2006; Glucksman and Kramer, 2011). In addition, we expanded the MDR variables to include other measurements of clinical change. MG selected 30 of the 63 patients from our study of the initial MDR of treatment. Five patients in that study had already terminated treatment, while 25 remained at an advanced stage of treatment and were making satisfactory progress. The other 33 patients had either terminated treatment prematurely or failed to make satisfactory progress. The 30 patients selected were judged by the treating clinician (MG) to have made significant clinical progress according to criteria that others have employed to evaluate therapeutic outcome (Luborsky et al., 1971; Kernberg et al., 1972; Bachrach et al., 1985; Karasu, 1986; Kantrowitz et al., 1990). These criteria included: (1) symptom reduction, (2) resolution of central conflicts or problems, (3) affective regulation, (4) interpersonal relationships, (5) self-image, (6) transference resolution, (7) level of functioning, and (8) self-analytic capacity. Ages of the patients ranged from 35 to 76 years, and the mean length of treatment was 11.5 years. The relatively long duration of treatment for many patients was due to the fact that they believed that ongoing self-exploration and contact with the therapist was helpful. Diagnoses included Axis I and Axis II disorders, but excluded psychotic conditions. Psychotropic medication was taken by 90% of the patients at some point during treatment. The initial and last MDR of each patient (30 pairs) were retrospectively collected from MG's therapy notes and printed without reference to name, age, or gender. The initial MDR was the first dream reported in treatment, while the last MDR was a dream reported just prior to termination, or the last dream reported during successful ongoing treatment. The following MDR variables were rated: (1) affect and affect valence of MDR, (2) affect and affect valence of associations to MDR, (3) direction of association themes to MDR, (4) narrative of MDR, (5) psychodynamic formulation of MDR, and (6) transference in MDR. The 30 pairs of MDRs were presented to the rater(s) in a randomized fashion without any identifying information.

There was a high level of agreement (88%) between MG and MK, who independently rated the 30 MDR pairs for affect and affect valence. In view of the high interrater reliability, MK's ratings were used because he had no clinical knowledge of the patients and was therefore less biased. MK noted affect in 47% of initial MDRs, which was similar to our previous studies (Kramer and Glucksman, 2006; Glucksman and Kramer, 2011). Affect was present in 63% of last MDRs, which was almost identical to a previous study (Kramer and Glucksman, 2006). Negative affect occurred in 43% of initial MDRs, and 37% of last MDRs. Positive affect occurred in 3% of initial MDRs, and in 23% of last MDRs. There was a definite trend suggesting a difference in affect valence between the initial and last MDRs ($p = .065$). This finding was consistent with an earlier study (Glucksman and Kramer, 2004).

The following is an example of a change in affect valence from the initial to last MDR:

Initial MDR

"I was walking through the woods in a wool tweed suit. There were spots of blood all over it. I was sweating blood and felt tired, weak, and had a headache. My clothes were all soaked in blood."

Last MDR

"You asked me to have a cup of coffee with you after our session. You were dressed in khakis, a t-shirt, and jacket. I declined, but then you suggested supper together. I was thrilled and jumped at the chance. However, I tamped down my feelings of attraction to you."

The patient was a young woman in her second marriage to an older man. She wanted to have children with him, but he was reluctant because he already had children from his first marriage. Feeling rejected and devalued by him, she became very depressed. After several years of treatment, she persuaded him to have another child and subsequently became pregnant. The last MDR was a transference dream reflecting her positive feelings for the therapist.

Affect and affect valence of associations in the 30 MDR pairs was rated by MG, who had direct knowledge from therapy notes of each patient's associations to MDRs. Affect occurred in 83% of initial and last MDR associations. On one hand, negative affect occurred in 67% of initial MDR associations and 40% of last MDR associations. On the other, positive affect was present in only 3% of initial MDR associations and 30% of last MDR associations. There was a significant difference between the affect valence of initial and last MDR associations ($p = .007$). The changes of affect valence in associations mirrored the changes of affect between initial and last MDRs.

The direction of association themes was rated by MG, who had access to this material from therapy notes. MG defined the direction of association themes as either positive or negative memories, feelings, events, relationships, or behavior in the content of associations. There was a highly significant change in the direction of association themes from the initial to last MDRs of treatment ($p < .001$). This shift more than likely represented an overall improvement in clinical status and life circumstances.

The following is an illustration of the positive or negative change in direction of association themes from initial to last MDRs:

Initial MDR

"I was at work and was flooded with emails. I threw up my hands and walked away. I felt like had done all I could do."

Associations to Initial MDR (Negative)

"My job is very stressful. I just had a review with my boss and it was a lower rating than I expected. I'm frustrated with the work, and I'm looking at other job possibilities."

Last MDR

"I'm driving my car and see a tornado coming. It hits me and the car is tossed around. Somehow, I get around it and everything is OK."

Associations to Last MDR (Positive)

"I just saw a tornado on a TV show—they're very dangerous and destructive. If you're in a car, you can get seriously hurt or killed. I was involved in a difficult situation at work that didn't seem proper. I told my boss to stop the transaction, and he did. I felt relieved, and that it was a vote of confidence in me. Actually, it made me feel more confident."

The patient was a corporate executive who had entered treatment because of extreme anxiety and insomnia. He felt overwhelmed by his job and unappreciated by his boss. In addition, he often found himself in questionably unethical situations. During the course of treatment, he found a position with another firm where he felt more effective and validated.

The shift in affect valence of associations from negative to positive, as well as the change in direction of association themes from negative to positive, was another indication of clinical improvement during treatment.

The *dream narrative* is a phenomenological, non-psychodynamic description of MDR imagery. MG and MK rated the dream narratives of the 30 MDR pairs as either positive or negative, depending on the nature of the imagery. They agreed on 93% of initial and last MDR narratives. In view of their high level of agreement, MK's ratings were used because of less likelihood of his being biased. On one hand, he found that initial MDRs had 77% negative narratives, and 13% positive narratives. On the other, last MDRs had 60% negative narratives, and 40% positive narratives. There was a statistically significant difference between initial and last MDR narratives ($p = .016$). The change from negative to positive dream narratives in initial and last MDRs strongly indicated a beneficial response to treatment.

The following is an illustration of the difference between initial and last dream narratives:

Initial MDR

"I'm in Iraq and the Iraqis are trying to kill me. I'm frightened and hiding."

Dream Narrative (Negative)

"The dreamer is in a combat setting and feels mortally threatened. She is frightened, and tries to hide in order to avoid being killed."

Last MDR

"I'm back at work and saving a co-worker, Dave. He was in trouble and I helped him. I made him look good."

Dream Narrative (Positive)

"The dreamer is in a work setting and helps a co-worker who is having difficulty. In doing so, she helps him improve his image."

The patient began treatment because of difficulty in her marriage and problems at work. She was depressed, felt extremely vulnerable, and had a poor self-image. During the course of treatment she addressed her marital and job issues. As a result, she felt less depressed, resolved her marital problems, and felt more effective at her job.

The psychodynamic formulation of MDRs was a generic, psychodynamic interpretation or translation of the manifest dream content. It was rated according to its positive or negative quality. MG and MK agreed on the psychodynamic formulation of 92% of the 30 MDR pairs. Because of this high level of agreement, MK's ratings of psychodynamic formulation were used because he was less biased. He found 80% negative and 10% positive psychodynamic formulations in initial MDRs. Conversely, he observed 53% negative and 33% positive psychodynamic formulations in last MDRs. There was a statistically significant difference between the psychodynamic formulations of initial and last MDRs ($p = .054$).

The following is an illustration of the difference between psychodynamic formulations of initial and last MDRs:

Initial MDR

"An evil force enveloped me and followed me around. It stalked the family I lived with and it looked like a person. It killed one of the children in the family."

Psychodynamic Formulation (Negative)

"The dreamer is frightened of some kind of injury or death. It may be part of the external surround, or an externalization of an inner feeling. The evil may be within or a destructive force coming from others."

Last MDR

> "Some friends invited me to go ice skating. A very nice Asian man was also invited to meet me. We hit it off and skated around the pond together. I felt good."

Psychodynamic Formulation (Positive)

> "The dreamer wishes to be accepted by others and to begin a romantic relationship with a man. The Asian man may represent her therapist with whom she feels secure and trusting."

The patient entered treatment with depressive and paranoid symptoms. She was alienated from both parents because they had abused her physically and emotionally during childhood. At times, she believed her mother might kill her, and she identified with the child in the initial dream. She was suspicious and distrustful of people, including the therapist. As treatment progressed, she became more trusting and eventually began a romantic relationship with a man she met at work. The shift from negative to positive psychodynamic formulations between the initial and last MDRs suggested that meaningful intrapsychic and interpersonal changes occurred during her treatment.

Transference in the MDR was defined as the actual therapist, persons, or objects in the manifest dream imagery that represented projections or displacements of the therapist. MG rated the 30 MDR pairs for evidence of transference because he was clinically informed about each therapeutic relationship. He observed the presence of transference in 53% of initial and 40% of last MDRs. This finding was similar to our previous study (Glucksman and Kramer, 2011). On one hand, negative transference appeared in 43% of initial and 17% of last MDRs. On the other, positive transference occurred in 7% of initial and 23% of last MDRs. There was a statistically significant difference in the type of transference exhibited between initial and last MDRs ($p = .037$).

The following is an illustration of the presence and change in type of transference between initial and last MDRs:

Initial MDR

> "My father kissed me on the cheek. I wanted him to kiss me on the other one, but he didn't. It was a weak kiss."

Transference (Mixed or Ambivalent)

> "The patient wishes to be loved and affirmed by the therapist. Instead, he feels disappointed by the tepid show of affection. His father was unaffectionate and seldom praised him. The dream reflects the patient's ambivalent feeling toward the therapist, as well as his father."

Last MDR

"I'm doing research at the maritime museum in Hyannis. The curator is surprised to see me, and greets me enthusiastically."

Transference (Positive)

"The patient wants to be recognized and praised for his work. He feels affirmed and accepted by the therapist. His feelings toward his father may have also changed."

The patient entered treatment because he felt inadequate socially and professionally. He was afraid of being criticized and humiliated, particularly by male authority figures. His father was unaffectionate and distant, while his mother was coercive and manipulative. He was initially ambivalent and guarded with the therapist, but gradually became more trusting and comfortable as treatment progressed.

Although transference was rated by only one rater (MG) who is subject to bias, his clinical knowledge of the patients was useful in identifying transference in MDRs. Despite the lack of interrater reliability regarding the identification of transference in MDRs, the shift from negative to positive transference between initial and last MDRs was informative. It suggested that transference in MDRs may change from negative to positive during the course of successful therapy. This variable, though not independently rated by more than one observer, deserves further evaluation.

In summary, this study duplicated the findings in our earlier studies (Glucksman and Kramer, 2004; Kramer and Glucksman, 2006) regarding changes in MDRs from the beginning to the end of treatment. Of note is that a large number of patients in this study received medication, and their clinical improvement was most likely due to the synergistic action of medication and psychotherapy. Regardless of the factors that facilitated clinical improvement, the findings of this study once again indicated that manifest dream content may change during treatment in a manner consistent with improvement in other areas of psychological and behavioral functioning. With the exception of our initial study (Glucksman and Kramer, 2004), we have not examined the relationship between MDRs and lack of progress in treatment.

In conclusion, we believe that our studies have systematically demonstrated the clinical usefulness of MDRs in treatment. Nevertheless, we recognize that latent dream content may also be helpful in order to fully understand and confirm the meaning of manifest dream content. Our studies have repeatedly emphasized the centrality of affect in the formation and content of dreams. In addition, affect and the valence of affect in MDRs, as well as associations to MDRs, were reliable guides to clinical improvement during treatment. The dream narrative was also an important element of dreams, and changes in MDR narratives from negative to positive over the course of treatment reflected clinical improvement (Foulkes et al., 1988). Likewise, changes in psychodynamic formulations of MDRs from negative to positive during treatment indicated clinical progress. The psychodynamic theme of the initial dream of treatment was a strong indicator of the types of psychodynamic issues and conflicts that emerged during therapy. Relational and injury dream themes occurred most frequently in the initial MDRs of treatment. Transference was a recognizable feature of certain dreams, and it changed from negative to positive during successful treatment.

In summary, our studies have demonstrated that a number of relevant MDR variables can be systematically rated with high interrater reliability. These MDR variables were found to have significant predictive and clinical value during therapy. On the basis of our studies, we believe that the MDR can be used as a reliable instrument for measuring clinical progress over the course of treatment.

References

Bachrach, H., Weber, J., and Soloman, M. (1985): Factors associated with the outcome of psychoanalysis (clinical and methodological considerations) of the Columbia Psychoanalytic Center research project (IV). International Review of Psychoanalysis, 43, 161–174.

Beratis, S. (1984): The first analytic dream: mirror of the patient's neurotic conflicts and subsequent analytic process. The International Journal of Psychoanalysis, 65, 461–469.

Bonime, W. (1962): The Clinical Use of Dreams. New York, Basic Books.

Bradlow, P. A., and Coen, S. J. (1975): The analyst undisguised in the initial dream of psychoanalysis. The International Journal of Psychoanalysis, 56, 415–425.

Cartwright, R. (1986): Affect and dream work from an information processing point of view. Journal of Mind and Behavior, 7, 411–428.

Dewald, P. (1972): Assessment of structural change. Journal of the American Psychoanalytic Association, 20, 119–132.

Domhoff, G. W. (1993): The repetition of dreams and dream elements: a possible clue to a function of dreams, in A. Moffitt, M. Kramer, and R. Hoffman (eds.), The Functions of Dreaming. Albany, State University of New York Press, 293–320.

Fiss, H. (1993): The "royal road" to the unconscious revisited: a signal detection model of dream function, in A. Moffitt, M. Kramer, and R. Hoffman (eds.), The Functions of Dreaming, Albany, State University of New York Press, 381–418.

Foulkes, D., Sullivan, B., Kerr, N., and Brown, L. (1988): Appropriateness of dream feeling to dreamed situations. Cognition and Emotion, 2, 29–39.

French, T. and Fromm, E. (1964): Dream Interpretation: A New Approach, New York: Basic Books, Inc.

Freud, S. (1900/1958): The Interpretation of Dreams, in J. Stratchey (trans. and ed.), The Standard Edition of the Complete Psychological Works of Sigmund Freud. Vols. 4 and 5, London, The Hogarth Press.

Freud, S. (1916/1963): Introductory Lectures on Psychoanalysis, in J. Stratchey (trans. and ed.), The Standard Edition of the Complete Psychological Works of Sigmund Freud. Vol. 15, London, The Hogarth Press, 120.

Glucksman, M. L. (1988): The use of successive dreams to facilitate and document change during treatment. Journal of the American Academy of Psychoanalysis, 16, 47–70.

Glucksman, M. L. (2001): The dream: a psychodynamically informative instrument. Journal of Psychotherapy Practice and Research, 10:4, 223–230.
Glucksman, M. L., and Kramer, M. (2004): Using dreams to assess clinical change during treatment. Journal of the American Academy of Psychoanalysis and Dynamic Psychiatry, 32 (2), 345–358.
Glucksman, M. L., and Kramer, M. (2011): The clinical and predictive value of the initial dream of treatment. Journal of the American Academy of Psychoanalysis and Dynamic Psychiatry, 39 (2), 263–283.
Glucksman, M. L., and Kramer, M. (2012): Initial and last manifest dream reports of patients in psychodynamic psychotherapy and combined psychotherapy/pharmacotherapy. Psychodynamic Psychiatry, 40 (4), 617–634.
Greenberg, R., Katz, H., Schwartz, W., and Pearlman, C. (1992): A research based reconsideration of psychoanalytic dream theory. Journal of the American Psychoanalytic Association, 40, 531–550.
Greenberg, R., and Pearlman, C. (1993): An integrated approach to dream theory: contributions from sleep research and clinical practice, in A. Moffitt, M. Kramer, and R. Hoffman (eds.), The Functions of Dreaming. Albany, State University of New York Press, 363–380.
Hall, C., and Van de Castle, R. (1966): The content analysis of dreams. New York, Appleton-Century-Crofts.
Harris, I. (1962): Dreams about the analyst. International Journal of Psychoanalysis, 43, 151–158.
Hobson, J. A. (1999): The new neuropsychology of sleep: implications for psychoanalysis. Neuro-Psychoanalysis, 1 (2), 157–183.
Kantrowitz, J., Katz, A. L., and Paolitto, F. (1990): Follow-up of psychoanalysis five to ten years after termination: II. Development of the self-analytic function. Journal of the American Psychoanalytic Association, 38 (3), 637–654.
Karasu, T. B. (1986): The specificity versus nonspecificity dilemma: toward identifying therapeutic change agents. American Journal of Psychiatry, 143 (6), 687–695.
Kernberg, O., Coyne, L., Horwitz, L., Appelbaum, A., and Burstein, E. (1972): Psychotherapy and psychoanalysis: final report of the Menninger Foundation psychotherapy research project. Bulletin of the Menninger Clinic, 36, 3–275.
Koulach, D. (1993): Dreams and adaptation to contemporary stress, in A. Moffitt, M. Kramer, and R. Hoffman (eds.), The Functions of Dreaming. Albany, State University of New York Press, 321–340.
Kradin, R. (2006): The herald dream: an approach to the initial dream in psychotherapy. London, Karnac Books.
Kramer, M. (1993): The selective mood regulatory function of dreaming: an update and revision, in A. Moffitt, M. Kramer, and R. Hoffman (eds.), The Functions of Dreaming. Albany, State University of New York Press, 139–195.
Kramer, M., and Birk, I. (2002): Affective processing by dreams across the night. Sleep, 25 (suppl. A), 180–181.
Kramer, M., and Glucksman, M. L. (2006): Changes in manifest dream affect during psychoanalytic treatment. Journal of the American Academy of Psychoanalysis and Dynamic Psychiatry, 34 (2), 249–260.
Kramer, M., and Roth, T. A. (1973): A comparison of dream content in laboratory reports of schizophrenic and depressive patient groups. Comprehensive Psychiatry, 14, 325–329.
Kramer, M. and Roth T. (1977): Dream translation. Israel Annals of Psychiatry and Related Disciplines, 15, 336–351.

Kramer, M., Whitman, R., Baldridge, B., and Lansky, L. (1964): Patterns of dreaming: the interrelationship of the dreams of the night. Journal of Nervous and Mental Disorders, 139, 426–439.

Kramer, M., Winget, C., and Whitman, R. (1971): A city dreams: a survey approach to normative dream content. American Journal of Psychiatry, 127, 1350–1356.

Lowy, S. (1942): Psychological and Biological Foundation of Dream Interpretation. London, Butler and Tanner Ltd.

Luborsky, L., Chandler, M., Auerbach, A., Cohen, J., and Bachrach, H. M. (1971): Factors influencing the outcome of psychotherapy. Psychological Bulletin, 75 (3), 145–185.

Mendelsohn, R. M. (1990): The Manifest Dream and Its Use in Therapy. New York, Jason Aronson.

Palombo, S. R. (1984): Deconstructing the manifest dream. Journal of the American Psychoanalytic Association, 32 (2), 405–420.

Purcell, S., Moffitt, A., and Hoffman, R. (1993): Waking, dreaming, and self-regulation, in A. Moffitt, M. Kramer, and R. Hoffman (eds.), The Functions of Dreaming. Albany, State University of New York Press, 197–260.

Rosenbaum, M. (1965): Dreams in which the analyst appears undisguised—a clinical and statistical study. The International Journal of Psychoanalysis, 46, 429–437.

Saul, L. (1940): Utilization of early current dreams in formulating psychoanalytic cases. Psychoanalytic Quarterly, 9 (4), 453–469.

Saul, L. (1972): Psychodynamically Based Psychotherapy. New York, Science House.

Smith, C. (1993): REM sleep and learning: some recent findings, in A. Moffitt, M. Kramer, and R. Hoffman (eds.), The Functions of Dreaming. Albany, State University of New York, 341–362.

Stairs, P., and Blick, K. (1979): A survey of emotional content of dreams of college students. Psychological Reports, 45, 839–842.

Stekel, W. (1943): The Interpretation of Dreams. Vol. 1, New York, Liveright Publishing.

Strauch, I., and Meier, B. (1996): In Search of Dreams. Albany, State University of New York Press.

Warner, S. L. (1983): Can psychoanalytic treatment change dreams? Journal of the American Academy of Psychoanalysis, 11 (2), 299–316.

Warner, S. L. (1987): Manifest dream analysis in contemporary practice, in M. L. Glucksman and S. L. Warner (eds.), Dreams in New Perspective: The Royal Road Revisited. New York, Human Sciences Press, 97–117.

Winget, C., Kramer, M., and Whitman, R. (1972): Dreams and demography. Canadian Psychiatric Association Journal, 17 (suppl. 2), ss203-ss208.

Winget, C., and Kramer, M. (1979): Dimensions of Dreams. Gainesville, University Press of Florida.

Yazmajian, R. V. (1964): First dreams directly representing the analyst. Psychoanalytic Quarterly, 33, 536–551.

10
THE HILL COGNITIVE–EXPERIENTIAL MODEL

An Integrative Approach to Working With Dreams

Patricia T. Spangler
UNIFORMED SERVICES UNIVERSITY OF THE HEALTH SCIENCES

Clara E. Hill
UNIVERSITY OF MARYLAND

The cognitive–experiential dream model, or CEDM (Hill, 1996, 2004), was developed as a means for studying the effects of working with dreams in therapy. Many existing approaches to dream work in therapy were valid and useful, but no single approach included aspects that facilitated exploring dream material, gaining insight into the meaning of the dream, and developing a plan of action based on the dreamer's newfound insights. In addition, most approaches did not have the clarity and structure that would allow for training, replicability, and adherence check in a research setting. The CEDM was developed to address these issues.

Assumptions underlying the model are that dreams are a continuation of waking thought without input from the external world; the meaning of dreams is personal (standard symbols or dream dictionaries are not useful or applicable); working with dreams requires a collaborative process between the therapist and client; dreams are a useful tool for helping people understand themselves; dreams involve cognitive, emotional, and behavioral components; and therapists must have expertise in basic helping skills before they can be effective in using the dream model.

Structure of the Model

The CEDM comprises three stages: exploration, insight, and action. The model is based on client-centered theory in that the therapist serves as a guide in helping the client explore her or his dreams rather than serving as an expert who has *the* interpretation.

The goal of the exploration stage is to activate the cognitive schema related to the dream by exploring dream images. Therapist and client collaborate on selecting three to five key images to explore in the order in which they appeared in the dream. The therapist then guides the client sequentially through a thorough exploration of the image using the DRAW steps:

- **D**escribe the image in intricate detail, including people, places, actions, colors, shapes, smells, and sounds.
- **R**e-experience the feelings experienced during the image.
- **A**ssociate the image and the thoughts and feelings related to it to past experiences.
- **W**aking-life events that may have triggered the image.

This stage requires in-depth exploration of each image and takes about 45 minutes.

In the insight stage, the goal is for the therapist to work with the client to co-construct a personally relevant meaning of the dream. This stage is informed by psychodynamic theory and technique. The therapist begins by asking the client what the dream means to him or her. The level of insight shown by the client gives the therapist some idea as to the level of interpretation that is the most likely to fit for the client. If the client understands only part of the dream and is still puzzled by or has left out some key images, the therapist can help the client integrate those puzzling or missing components into a new meaning that brings greater insight.

The meaning made of the dream may be at one of three levels. On one level, the dream itself may be considered an experience (rather than as symbolic or metaphorical) with the therapist guiding the client toward a deeper understanding self through examining the thoughts and feelings related to the experience in the dream. On another level, the dream can be considered a reflection of waking-life concerns. Given that dreams often are triggered by immediate concerns, thinking about the dream at this level often seems fitting.

At a deeper level, the dream can be interpreted as relating in three ways to inner personality dynamics:

- Parts of self—The client can consider key images in the dream as parts of himself or herself that represent unresolved internal conflicts being projected onto people or other objects. The therapist might ask, for example, "What part of you is a coyote?" and "What part is a shepherd?" To resolve conflicted parts of self, the therapist can use the two-chair technique, directing the client to play each part and have the parts talk to each other.
- Early childhood conflicts—The dream can be interpreted as reflecting the client's unresolved childhood conflicts that are causing current relational or other problems. For example, the therapist might ask about the jealousy the client experienced in the dream and how that might reflect competition for attention from a parent.

- Existential/meaning-of-life/spiritual concerns—The dream might be interpreted as relating to meaning-of-life issues or to the client's relationship with a higher power. If, for example, a male client who dreamed about being on an unfamiliar road without his GPS is struggling with leaving the church in which he was raised, the therapist might help the client examine his anxiety about the changes in his beliefs.

Clients' initial interpretations often relate to waking life. For example, a female client may interpret her dream about taking an exam for a class she had not enrolled in as being about upcoming finals (waking life). Further work with her dream, however, may reveal the student's anxiety about her parents' expectations that she major in engineering rather than pursue a career as a social worker (childhood conflict and meaning of life). An important point in constructing a meaning of the dream is let the client know that there is no one correct meaning of the dream, but the interpretation should seem to the client like a good "fit." Finally, the therapist can ask the client to summarize her or his new understanding to help the client integrate what she or he has learned. Depending on the client's level of understanding, this stage takes 20 to 30 minutes and may require circling back to exploration.

In the action stage, the goal is to help the client use the new understanding of the dream to begin thinking about making changes in waking life. Some clients readily see changes they would like to make from the work they have done in previous stages, whereas other clients may need more preparation and direction. To begin the process of thinking about change, the therapist asks the client how he or she would change the dream. The therapist then bridges the change to waking life (e.g., "You said you would change the dream so that you were more aware of your feelings when you were feeling them. How might that translate to waking life?"). The therapist might then use behavioral strategies to help the client strategize how to implement changes in waking life, or might help the client develop a ritual to honor the dream.

Research on the Model

CEDM has been investigated in more than 25 studies to date. In this section, unless otherwise noted, we rely on the reviews by Hill and Goates (2004) and Hill and Knox (2010) rather than citing individual studies. We present here results on process, outcome, predicting who benefits from the model, cultural factors as they relate to the model, and training.

Process of Dream Work

Components of CEDM

Components of the model have been experimentally manipulated such that some components were delivered or not and then the effects on outcome were tested.

In a study of the exploration stage, results indicated that both description and association were helpful, although exploration and insight gains were significantly greater in the association-only condition. In tests of components of the insight stage, no differences were found in outcomes for waking life versus parts-of-self interpretations, and no differences were found in nonspiritual outcomes for waking-life versus spiritual interpretations. In investigating the action stage, clients who completed the exploration, insight, and action stages had better action ideas and rated sessions higher on problem solving than did clients who did not receive the action stage. In addition, clients' perception of how much the therapist used action skills predicted their intention to carry out the action plan, the degree of client involvement, and the difficulty of the action plan.

Furthermore, four qualitative studies revealed that clients indicated that gaining insight, making links to waking life, experiencing cathartic feelings, and hearing new ideas for change were helpful components of CEDM. In addition, Tien, Chen, and Lin (2009) found that clients perceived waking-life association, parts-of-self exploration, gaining insight, and developing action ideas as helpful components of the model. Finally, Pesant and Zadra (2006) investigated the most helpful events in dream sessions using the Hill model and found that insight was the most frequently reported of all helpful events.

Client Factors

Four studies found evidence that client involvement is related to the outcome of individual dream work, although one study did not find that client involvement was related to outcome in group dream work. In addition, Kline and Hill (2014) examined the DRAW steps of the exploration stage and found that client involvement in each of the steps was positively related to client involvement in all other steps, clients were more involved in the description step than other steps, and client involvement during the description step predicted session outcome.

A series of three case studies shed further light on insight development in dream sessions. Two clients who acquired insight were consistently motivated and involved, nonresistant, trusting, and affectively engaged but not overwhelmed during the sessions. Their therapists used probes for insight and were able to manage their countertransference reactions. By contrast, the client who did not gain insight was resistant, untrusting, and emotionally overwhelmed in the session, and the therapist was not as skillful or as able to manage her negative countertransference as in the other cases.

Therapist Factors

Therapist adherence to the model and competence in applying CEDM related to session outcome. In addition, volunteer clients gained more from working with therapists than they did from using the model on their own, although a small subgroup of clients preferred the self-help modality. In addition, clients in three studies indicated that liking the therapist and the therapist's input were helpful components of the process.

Summary of Process Findings

All components of CEDM appear to be helpful, although therapists need to tailor their work to the individual client. In addition, clients thought that the most valuable components of the model were cathartic release, new insights, and links to waking life. Therapist and client involvement and motivation are key to working with the model. Specifically, helpful tools for therapists are probes for insight and monitoring countertransference; clients need to not feel overwhelmed by reexperiencing emotions, and they need to be open to and trust the therapist.

Outcomes of Dream Work

Session Quality

The quality of sessions involving CEDM has been assessed by post-session ratings of depth, working alliance, and satisfaction. In 12 studies, clients consistently rated the quality of CEDM significantly higher than regular therapy sessions. Clients seemed to feel better about the quality of the sessions focused on dreams than on other topics.

Goals of Dream Work

A number of studies using various approaches to investigating CEDM have yielded convincing evidence that clients gained insight into their dreams. Interestingly, in one study, clients had a moderate level of insight into their dreams prior to sessions and gained insight after both the exploration and insight stages of dream work, and also reported gaining additional insight at a 2-week follow-up. These findings reflect that clients might be stuck prior to sessions in terms of understanding their dreams, but they can rapidly improve their ability to gain a deeper understanding of their dreams through using the model.

In terms of action ideas, studies have shown that clients clarified and focused their thinking about what they could do differently in their waking lives based on what they learned about themselves in CEDM. Interestingly, the quality of action ideas was lower than insight both before and after sessions, suggesting that action lags behind insight. In addition, clients changed in functioning on the target problem reflected in the dream, and clients reported changes in terms of the impact of divorce and loss.

Yet another dream-related outcome is change in attitudes toward dreams. Tien et al. (2006) applied the Hill model in Taiwan and found that volunteer clients presenting dreams reported better attitudes toward dreams after two to three dream sessions than did controls who did not receive a dream session.

Outcomes Not Related to Dreams

Some research on CEDM has found decreases in general symptoms and in depression, as well as increases in existential well-being when spiritual insight was the focus of the dream work. Mixed results have been reported for changes in interpersonal functioning. Furthermore, clients in dream groups scored higher in self-esteem and insight than did those in the wait-list control. Finally, there have been increases in other dyadic perspective-taking but no changes in dyadic adjustment, primary communications, and self-dyadic perspective with couples' dream work.

Summary of Outcome Findings

Positive changes have been reported in session quality and in outcomes specifically related to dream work (e.g., insight, action ideas, target problems, and attitudes toward dreams). Less clear evidence has been reported on outcomes not specifically targeted in dream work (e.g., depression, anxiety, and self-esteem). Given that dreams may not necessarily reflect these broader outcomes, it is not surprising that fewer changes have been found in broader outcomes than in outcomes specific to dream work.

Who Benefits From Dream Work

Client Characteristics

Not surprisingly, clients with positive attitudes toward dreams had positive outcomes. Taken together with the finding that the people who volunteered for dreams sessions had more positive attitudes toward dreams than those who did not volunteer, valuing dreams seems to be an important precondition for dream work. In addition, clients who profited most from dream work presented dreams that seemed potent or powerful to them. Self-efficacy for working with dreams also seems important, in that clients needed to feel that working with dreams would help them accomplish their goals. Furthermore, clients who profited most from dream sessions had poor initial functioning on the problem reflected in the dream, low initial insight into the dream, and poor initial action ideas related to the dream.

Dream Characteristics

Research on the valence of dreams has garnered less consistent results. In one study, the best session outcomes were found when dreams were moderately unpleasant or extremely pleasant, and the worst outcomes when dreams were moderately pleasant or extremely unpleasant. In another study, however, session outcomes were best when dreams were pleasant. In yet another study, no relationship emerged between dream valence and session outcome. Similarly, recency of the dream had little impact in a recent study (Gupta & Hill, 2014). Perhaps, rather than looking at valence or recency, dreams should be categorized into several types: positive interpersonal, negative interpersonal, interpersonal agency, interpersonal nightmares, noninterpersonal dreams, and all others. Indeed, there is some evidence for positive process and outcome for clients with dreams with positive, agency, and noninterpersonal themes than for clients with negative dreams and nightmares.

Summary of Predictors

CEDM seems to be most effective with clients who have positive attitudes toward dreams and are willing to discuss them in therapy, have high self-efficacy or confidence in their ability to work with their dreams, have salient dreams that are puzzling or reflect underlying concerns, and have low initial insight and action ideas related to the dreams. Minimal evidence exists for the importance of other client characteristics (e.g., sex/gender, race/ethnicity, psychological mindedness) and other dream-related characteristics (e.g., recency, vividness, arousal, distortion) in terms of outcome of dream sessions.

Cultural Factors

Dream Work With Men

Men who reported higher gender-role conflict discussed themes related to their conflict (e.g., work-family conflicts, restricted emotionality, and preoccupation with achievement and competition) during dream sessions. Men with both high and low gender-role conflict rated the dream sessions as equally helpful, indicating that once the men agreed to work on their dreams, they found it helpful regardless of their level of gender-role conflict.

Dream Work With East Asian Clients

One study testing the widely held belief that East Asian clients prefer a directive approach found no overall differences in outcome between clients in an empathy-only condition (probes and reflections) versus those in an empathy-with-directive-input-condition (probes and reflections plus interpretations and suggestions for action). Client individual differences did, however, moderate the outcomes such that those who were more anxiously attached and lower on Asian values had better outcomes in the empathy-only condition, whereas those who were less anxiously attached and higher on Asian values did better in the empathy-plus-input condition. In a follow-up study of first- and second-generation female Asian students, interpersonal and academic/career issues were typical themes for both groups, but first-generation Asian women more often disclosed issues related to immigration, cultural issues, adjustment, and physical well-being than did second-generation Asian women. Both subgroups talked about interpersonal behavioral changes, with first-generation Asian women focusing more on changing thoughts and feelings than did second-generation Asian women. Hence, not only might race/ethnicity be a factor in outcome, but immigration status also may play a role in what clients talk about during dream sessions.

Spirituality and Dream Work

We examined how spiritually centered dream work relates to outcome for clients who are spiritually oriented. Clients in a spiritual interpretation condition gained more spiritual insight and had greater increases in existential well-being than did clients whose therapists offered waking-life interpretations.

Training Therapists to Use CEDM

Although many therapists have been trained to use CEDM, only one small-sample study has been conducted on such training. In this study, therapists felt more self-efficacy for working with dreams, had more positive attitudes toward dreams, and had higher self-reported competence for working with dreams following a didactic-experiential workshop, individual feedback, and practice. Furthermore, supervisor feedback led to higher levels of self-efficacy, more positive attitudes toward dreams, and increased ability to conduct dream sessions.

Adapting the Hill Model for Trauma-Related Nightmares: Nightmare Deconstruction and Reprocessing

Despite evidence (Boe, Holgersen, & Holen, 2010; Mellman, David, Bustamante, Torres, & Fins, 2001) of the role that nightmares have in the development and chronicity of posttraumatic stress disorder (PTSD), these dreams are not targeted by and often are resistant to evidence-based treatments. Imagery rehearsal therapy (IRT) is one evidence-based treatment that does target trauma-related nightmares, but its focus is on rescripting the nightmare (Krakow & Zadra, 2010). In IRT, processing nightmare content is avoided, which misses the opportunity to reconsolidate the trauma memory.

Schiller, Monfils, Raio, Johnson, LeDoux, and Phelps (2010) found that trauma memories could be updated with less fear-inducing information during the reconsolidation window when fear memories are labile. Given that dreams and nightmares are thought to have an essential role in consolidating waking-life events into long-term memory, developing a method for reconsolidating nightmare content so that it less distressing also may facilitate reconsolidation of waking-life intrusive memories. Given the increased prevalence of PTSD among veterans and military personnel over the past decade, and consequent interest in PTSD treatment development, we adapted CEDM to work specifically with trauma-related nightmares.

The new treatment, called *Nightmare Deconstruction and Reprocessing* (NDR), was adapted with the goals of decreasing the intensity and frequency of nightmares, and of understanding and reprocessing their content to facilitate reconsolidation of trauma memories. Case study evidence with an Iraq War veteran indicated that both waking-life and sleeping PTSD symptoms decreased post-NDR (Spangler, 2014). In a case example of NDR in group modality, U.S. sailors and Marines with PTSD reported decreased nightmare frequency post-treatment (A. Hummel, LT MSC USN, personal communication 12/12/12).

Designed as a brief therapy, NDR typically comprises six to eight sessions. The first session includes assessment of the client's nightmare pattern; psychoeducation about PTSD, nightmares, and sleep; an overview of NDR; assessment of client motivation for using the model; and practice of stress reduction techniques such as diaphragmatic breathing or progressive muscle relaxation for use in session and for returning to sleep after waking from a nightmare. Because deconstructing nightmare images can be very distressing, describing NDR in the first session and assessing the client's motivation for engaging in the treatment are essential to treatment effectiveness. If the client has a recurrent intense nightmare that is too intense for the client to reexperience, the therapist can ask for a less-disturbing dream, help the client become comfortable with deconstruction, build confidence in her or his ability to gain mastery over the dream, and then work with a more-disturbing nightmare in subsequent sessions.

In subsequent sessions, therapist and client work collaboratively through three stages: (1) deconstruction of and exposure to nightmare images; (2) reprocessing distressing material through meaning making and challenging maladaptive beliefs to reconsolidate nightmare images and traumatic memories; and (3) rescripting nightmare content to facilitate mastery over the nightmares and making waking-life changes.

During Stage 1, the client describes the distressing dream or nightmare in the first person, present tense, to facilitate reexperiencing. Three to five key images are chosen and deconstructed using the DRAW steps described earlier. Deconstruction serves an exposure function, triggers fear-memory retrieval, and provides a basis for gaining a deeper understanding in the next stage.

An important aspect of the deconstruction stage is the client's level of emotional arousal. The client must be engaged enough to activate the distressing memory and achieve the memory lability necessary for reconsolidation. If reexperiencing is too intense, however, it may be counter to the goal of reconsolidating the nightmare material and actually reinforce the traumatic memory. The therapist should assess the client's distress level during the exploration of each image using the Subjective Units of Distress Scale (SUDS), which uses a scale of 1 to 100, where 100 is unbearable (Wolpe, 1969). Optimally, the SUDS should be somewhere between 50 and 90, depending on what the client is able to tolerate. If the distress level is too high, the therapist can use the stress-reduction techniques practiced during the first session. If the SUDS level is too low, the therapist may focus more on the "R" (reexperiencing) of the DRAW steps to engage the client more deeply. Summarizing the deconstructed images prepares the client for the next stage.

At the beginning of Stage 2, the therapist asks the client what he or she believes the meaning of the nightmare is. Meaning making and reprocessing in Stage 2 then facilitate deeper understanding of the nightmare content and trauma memory through processing grief and loss, evaluating fear and anxiety, and challenging negative self-image related to guilt or moral injury. This is a two-step process: (1) collaborating with the client in constructing a meaning of the nightmare and (2) guiding the client through reprocessing his or her thoughts and feelings and, if necessary, challenging maladaptive beliefs and assumptions (e.g., "Why did I get to live when my buddy was killed? It should have been me."). The meaning may relate to current waking-life issues, early life experiences, and/or existential issues as described in CEDM. Meaning making and reprocessing often center on the image causing the most distress (i.e., the image with the highest SUDS level). Reprocessing the images sets the stage for changing the nightmare.

In Stage 3, the goal is to help the client gain mastery over the nightmare and begin to change nightmare content so that less distressing emotions related to the trauma are reconsolidated into long-term memory. There are three key components to this stage: (1) detailed description of new dream images based on the work done in the first two stages, (2) emotional engagement with the new images through behavioral rehearsal of changes to the nightmare both in session and before going to bed, and (3) making changes in waking life based on the meaning made in Stage 2 and changes to the nightmare made in Stage 3.

In subsequent sessions, the client presents the dream again, complete with any images that have been successfully changed. The new dream images are deconstructed as before. During meaning making and reprocessing, the focus is on the new images and what the client believes the changes in these images mean. New changes to the dream in the third stage are made based on the client's understanding the new images.

It may take several sessions for the client to gain enough mastery to transition to making changes to waking life. These changes should be based on the meaning making, reprocessing, and changes made to the nightmare, and can include (1) specific behaviors, such as more interaction with a spouse/partner or activities that help the client feel less isolated; (2) conducting a ritual to honor the new dream, such as listening to a lost buddy's favorite song; and (3) continuing to work on the dream through journaling. NDR is designed to progress through all three stages in each 75- to 90-minute session; however, it can be adapted so that deconstruction and exposure occur in a 45- to 50-minute session, then progressing to meaning making, reprocessing, and changing the nightmare in later sessions.

Conclusion

We have compelling evidence for the effectiveness of CEDM in a variety of settings. Research results to date have indicated that CEDM facilitates investigating dream work in therapy; that clients like and benefit from sessions using the model; that its components are useful for helping clients explore and understand their dreams, and to begin to make changes in waking life; that it helps to decrease symptoms such as depression and to increase well-being; and that the model has multicultural applicability. CEDM's clinical utility and integrative structure facilitate training and use in both clinical and research settings.

References

Boe, H. J., Holgersen, K. H., & Holen, A. (2010). Reactivation of posttraumatic stress in male disaster survivors: The role of residual symptoms. *Journal of Anxiety Disorders, 24*, 397–402.

Gupta, S., & Hill, C. E. (2014). The outcome of dream sessions: The influence of dream recency, emotional intensity, and salience. *Dreaming, 24*, 89–103.

Hill, C. E. (1996). *Working with dreams in psychotherapy*. New York: Guilford Press.

Hill, C. E. (Ed.) (2004). *Dream work in therapy: Facilitating exploration, insight, and action*. Washington, DC: American Psychological Association.

Hill, C. E., & Goates, M. K. (2004). Research on the Hill cognitive–experiential dream model. In C. E. Hill (Ed.), *Dream work in therapy: Facilitating exploration, insight, and action* (pp. 245–288). Washington, DC: American Psychological Association.

Hill, C. E., & Knox, S. (2010). The use of dreams in modern psychotherapy. In A. Clow & P. Mcnamara (Eds.), *International Review of Neurobiology: Vol. 9, Dreams and dreaming* (pp. 291–317). Waltham, MA: Academic Press.

Kline, K. V., & Hill, C. E. (2014). Client involvement in the exploration stage of the Hill cognitive–experiential dream model. *Dreaming, 24*(2), 104–111.

Krakow, B., & Zadra, A. (2010). Imagery rehearsal therapy: Principles and practice. *Sleep Medicine Clinics, 5*(2), 289–298.

Mellman, T. A., David, D., Bustamante, V., Torres, J., & Fins, A. (2001). Dreams in the acute aftermath of trauma and their relationship to PTSD. *Journal of Traumatic Stress, 14*(1), 241–247.

Pesant, N., & Zadra, A. (2006). Évaluation de l'utilité clinique de séances d'interprétation du rêve basées sur un modèle cognitif-expérientiel. [Assessment of the clinical usefulness of dream interpretation session based on a cognitive–experiential model.] *Revue Quebeoise de Psychologie, 27*(10), 153–170.

Schiller, D., Monfils, M. J., Raio, C. M., Johnson, D.C., LeDoux, J. E., & Phelps, E. A. (2010). Preventing the return of fear in humans using reconsolidation update mechanisms. *Nature, 463* (7277), 49–53.

Spangler, P. T. (2014). Nightmare deconstruction and reprocessing for trauma-related nightmares: An integrative approach. *Psychotherapy Bulletin, 49*(1), 31–35.

Tien, H. S., Chen, S, Lin, C. (2009). Helpful components involved in the cognitive–experiential model of dream work. *Asia Pacific Education Review, 10*(4), 547–559.

Tien, H. S., Lin, C. H. Chen, S. C. (2006). Dream interpretation sessions for college students in Taiwan: Who benefits and what volunteer clients view as most and least helpful. *Dreaming, 16*(4), 246–257.

Wolpe, J. (1969). *The practice of behavior therapy*, New York: Pergamon Press.

11
POSTTRAUMATIC NIGHTMARES

From Scientific Evidence to Clinical Significance

Lutz Wittmann
INTERNATIONAL PSYCHOANALYTIC UNIVERSITY, BERLIN, GERMANY

Thérèse de Dassel
INTERNATIONAL PSYCHOANALYTIC UNIVERSITY, BERLIN, GERMANY
THE ROYAL BRISBANE AND WOMEN'S HOSPITAL, BRISBANE, AUSTRALIA

Incidence and Persistence of Posttraumatic Nightmares

The incidence of nightmares in the general population according to representative samples is around 5% (e.g., Stepansky et al., 1998). It is, however, necessary to take into account that the lifetime prevalence of posttraumatic stress disorder (PTSD) in the general population can be roughly estimated to be 10% (Kessler, Sonnega, Bromet, Hughes, & Nelson, 1995). Thus, a representative nontraumatized sample from the general population would probably result in even lower nightmare incidences. In a large but nonrepresentative sample of 498 psychiatric outpatients with a broad range of psychiatric diagnoses (Swart, van Schagen, Lancee, & van den Bout, 2013), 27.7% of patients without PTSD were reported to suffer from nightmares. In patients with a diagnosis of PTSD, this number was elevated to 66.7%. The incidences of nightmares in traumatized individuals from representative samples are strongly elevated by factors between 4.5 (Ohayon & Shapiro, 2000) and 10.9 (Neylan et al., 1998), and they range from 39.8% (Kilpatrick et al., 1998) to 71% (Leskin, Woodward, Young, & Sheikh, 2002; 96% for subjects with PTSD and comorbid panic disorder).

Resembling the time course of PTSD (Kessler et al., 1995), nightmares after trauma appear to follow a bimodal distribution. About two-thirds of the disaster survivors in Holen's study (1990) reported remission of nightmares within 12 months. The remaining individuals suffered from nightmares for at least 3 years. The potential chronicity of posttraumatic nightmares is impressively demonstrated by a recent study on World War II (WWII) prisoner-of-war (POW) veterans

(Rintamaki, Weaver, Elbaum, Klama, & Miskevics, 2009). More than 65 years after the war, 47% of this sample reported dreaming of their POW experiences. Ethnological research tells us that posttraumatic nightmares are an ubiquitous phenomenon rather than being restricted to Western societies only (Hinton, Hinton, Pich, Loeum, & Pollack, 2009).

Sleep

Undoubtedly, posttraumatic nightmares negatively impact sleep quality. Blank, Kelly, Bootzin, and Haynes (2009) report strong correlations of nightmare frequency and intensity with sleep efficiency ($r = -.51$) and total sleep time ($r = -.62$) as measured by actigraphy. Hinton et al. (2009) found 52% of their sample not falling asleep again for 1–2 hours after awakening from a nightmare, while 31% were unable to sleep again all night.

To answer the question concerning how altered sleep parameters may explain quantitative or qualitative aspects of posttraumatic dreaming is much more challenging. Given the growing number of reviews on sleep in PTSD (e.g., Germain, 2013) we emphasize only a few findings of interest in relation to nightmares.

The meta-analysis by Kobayashi, Boarts, and Delahanty (2007) found more stage 1 sleep and less slow-wave sleep in PTSD patients compared with controls. These authors also report elevated REM density in PTSD patients, possibly accounted for by the high comorbidity of PTSD with depressive disorders (Riemann, Berger, & Voderholzer, 2001). As for REM sleep parameters, Germain (2013, p. 375) arrives at the conclusion that "findings on the nature and magnitude of [. . .] REM sleep disturbances in PTSD are equivocal."

Polysomnographic studies have described posttraumatic nightmares as appearing out of REM as well as NREM sleep (Wittmann, Schredl, & Kramer, 2006). Given the lack of polysomnographic studies on the occurrence of nontraumatic (idiopathic) nightmares throughout the sleep cycle, it is difficult to decide on the significance of this finding beyond its implications for the REM-NREM controversy (e.g., Solms, 2000). In conclusion, the mechanisms by which dimensions of sleep physiology relate to posttraumatic dream experiences remains an exciting research field.

Content of Posttraumatic Nightmares

Schreuder, Igreja, van Dijk, and Kleijn (2001) have devised a classification system in which a dream is considered to be posttraumatic when the subject associates its content with a traumatic event. Posttraumatic dreams are subcategorized with respect to the degree of similarity to the original event by denoting whether dreams are replicative (posttraumatic reenactments, used interchangeably throughout with the term replicative nightmare), mixed (similar to the traumatic event), or nonreplicative (symbolically related to the trauma).

Unfortunately, application of different categories as well as further methodological differences impedes valid conclusions when integrating findings. Most studies, however, describe substantial proportions—often around 50%—of replicative posttraumatic nightmares (Davis, Byrd, & Rhudy, 2007; Harb, Thompson, Ross, & Cook, 2012; Hinton et al., 2009; Wittmann et al., 2006). Traumatic replication is associated with traumatic repetition of a dream (Schreuder, van Egmond, Kleijn, & Visser, 1998; Wittmann, Zehnder, Schredl, Jenni, & Landolt, 2010).

In our previous review (Wittmann et al., 2006) we arrived at the conclusion that "an adequate characterization of the phenomenology of the disturbing dream in PTSD remains to be done" (p. 33). Since that time, only a few—but very noteworthy—contributions add to our knowledge. In an exemplary study, Harb et al. (2012) present a detailed description of target nightmares selected in the treatment of 48 Vietnam veterans. Beyond a depiction of sensory details, death scenes, life threat, perpetration and related emotions in the nightmares, they list dominant nightmare themes. The five most frequently dominant themes were fear of death, being under attack, lack of self-efficacy, lack of control, and perception of war as disgusting and horrible. Pigeon, Martinez, and Mellman (2004) recorded dreams of recently hospitalized trauma patients and compared them with a normative sample. Dreams of trauma patients had significantly less aggression, friendliness, sexuality, and good fortune, and more physical aggression, bodily misfortune, and self-negativity than the normative sample. Duval and Zadra (2010) provide a literature review considering the association between specific aspects of dream content and different trauma types, whereas Hinton, Field, Nickerson, Bryant, and Simon (2013) observe potentially culture specific aspects of dream reports of Cambodian refugees engaged in treatment. Two promising psychoanalytic approaches to the study of posttraumatic dreams by Varvin, Fischmann, Jovic, Rosenbaum, and Hau (2012) urgently require replication based on a larger dream sample. As for the change of posttraumatic nightmare content over time (Nader, Pynoos, Fairbanks, & Frederick, 1990; Rasmussen, 2007; Terr, 1983), the absence of longitudinal studies is to be regretted.

Posttraumatic Dreams and Their Relationship to Psychopathology

Posttraumatic nightmares have been consistently shown to be associated with other symptoms of PTSD, including reexperiencing (Schreuder et al., 1998) and hyperarousal (Gerhart, Russ, Hall, & Canetti, 2014) as well as PTSD severity (Blank et al., 2009; Gerhart et al., 2014). Neylan et al. (1998) found that frequent or very frequent nightmares perfectly differentiated between subjects with and without PTSD.

Beyond their close relation with posttraumatic stress, posttraumatic nightmares have been found to be associated with a number of non–trauma-specific mental health outcomes. Blank et al. (2009) found significant correlations between nightmare frequency and depression scores (r = .51). Posttraumatic nightmare frequency was a significant predictor of psychiatric symptoms, psychosomatic reactivity, and time off work in disaster survivors (Holen, 1990). Gerhart et al. (2014) examined the predictiveness of sleep disturbances and nightmares on PTSD, depression, and sense of intrapersonal resource loss (sense of self-efficacy and hope) in a sample of 779 Palestinians. Controlling for initial PTSD, nightmares predicted later PTSD, depression, and sense of intrapersonal resource loss but not vice versa.

Evidence is accumulating for a specific association linking replicative posttraumatic nightmares with the development of PTSD. Subjects describing initial dreams similar to the traumatic incident scored higher on concurrent PTSD severity than those reporting other categories of dreams or no dreams (Mellman, David, Bustamante, Torres, & Fins, 2001). Those subjects also had higher PTSD severity at 6 weeks follow-up than subjects without dream recall. Wittmann et al. (2010) conducted detailed nightmare interviews with children 10 days post-accident and demonstrated that the presence of early replicative nightmares significantly predicted PTSD total scores both at 2 and 6 months follow-up, but not depression scores. Similarly, in a trauma-exposed treatment-seeking sample, Davis et al. (2007) showed that PTSD diagnosed subjects had more replicative nightmares than those without. Other studies (e.g., Schreuder, Kleijn, & Rooijmans, 2000) provide further supporting evidence. Finally, Fosse, Fosse, Hobson, and Stickgold (2003) showed that the repetition of complete episodic memory traces are virtually nonexistent in nontraumatized subjects.

Treatment of Posttraumatic Nightmares

The specific treatment of posttraumatic nightmares is a topic that has received much attention during the last decade. Suggested treatments include a broad range of behavioral and pharmacological interventions (for an overview, see Nappi, Drummond, & Hall, 2012). The treatment approach that has been most extensively studied is imagery rehearsal therapy, or IRT (Krakow, Kellner, Pathak, & Lambert, 1995). Essentially, patients write down a nightmare, change its content in any way they wish, and then record the new dream plot. Applying imagery techniques, this new dream is then rehearsed. An increased sense of mastery over the nightmare is considered to be a central therapeutic factor (Krakow, Hollifield et al., 2001). As a growing number of clinical trials demonstrate, this short-term cognitive-behavioral treatment can reduce nightmare frequency and intensity as well as reduce further symptoms of posttraumatic stress. Given the large number of available reviews on this topic (e.g., Casement & Swanson, 2012) we restrict ourselves to a few comments only. Based on their review of 16 clinical trials, Harb et al. (2013) critically remark that "greater scrutiny of the characteristics and the quality of these trials and reports, as well as of fundamental differences among imagery rehearsal protocols, calls into question the strength of the current evidence base" (p. 576). For instance, mean inclusion rate is reported to be

54.9% and drop-out rates from randomized controlled trials (RCT) amount to 33.4%. Additional concerns arise from the results of a RCT applying exemplary methodological rigor as well as a credible active comparison condition (Cook et al., 2010). Intention to treat analyses of the primary outcome measures showed no improvement of the IRT group as compared to the sleep and nightmare management group. Number of nightmares improved in 21% of the overall sample and worsened in 15%. In summary, although IRT appears to be an extremely economical and helpful tool for many traumatized nightmare sufferers, several questions remain to be answered by further research: Is it possible to identify specific predictors (e.g., patient and dream characteristics, process variables) for treatment outcome? What preventative measures can reduce the drop-out rate from this short-term treatment? How could IRT be integrated into broader approaches of trauma specific psychotherapy? How does IRT compare to other active treatment conditions (Hansen, Hofling, Kroner-Borowik, Stangier, & Steil, 2013)?

Posttraumatic Nightmares in Children

Child development research notes that nightmares peak during early childhood and incidence diminishes with age (Schredl & Pallmer, 1997). The incidence of nightmares in a representative sample of 10-year-old children was 2.5% (N = 4,826; parent report) to 3.5% (N = 4,507; self-report of children; Schredl, Fricke-Oerkermann, Mitschke, Wiater, & Lehmkuhl, 2009).

With incidences of up to 61% (Mertin & Mohr, 2002), the frequencies of posttraumatic nightmares in children are akin to those found in adults. However, no representative samples are available and methodological shortcomings have to be noted with respect to many studies on children's posttraumatic nightmares.

A wealth of research using dream diaries with children living in conditions of war and military violence sheds light on the content of children's posttrauma nightmares. Valli et al. (2005) found that threat content in dreams was highest in trauma-exposed children, when compared with less-exposed and nontraumatized children. Helminen and Punamäki (2008) reported heightened intensity and a higher degree of negative emotions in dreams of traumatized children compared with controls. Punamäki, Ali, Ismahil, and Nuutinen (2005) demonstrated that traumatic events were associated with dreams typical of earlier developmental stages, emphasizing the putative role of regressive effects of trauma and its impact on posttraumatic nightmares.

Langston, Davis, and Swopes (2010) investigated nightmares in 47 traumatized children attending outpatient therapy, with nightmare categorization based on the temporal start point of nightmares. Seven (54%) of 13 children who also reported pretrauma nightmares described their current nightmare content as the same as the trauma, while three (24%) described it as similar. Of 11 children whose nightmares had started posttrauma, eight (73%) described the content as the same as the trauma, while an additional two (18%) described it as similar. Over the course of a 6-month longitudinal investigation of 32 children hospitalized after motor vehicle accidents (12.6% diagnosed with full or subsyndromal PTSD 2 months postaccident), six (18.8%) reported nontraumatic nightmares, five (15.6%) reported mixed replicative nightmares, and 10 (31.3%) reported replicative nightmares (Wittmann et al., 2010).

Comparing the children with posttraumatic nightmares (but not pretrauma ones) to those in the sample with no nightmares, Langston et al. (2010) found that the posttraumatic nightmare group fared more poorly on measures of fear of sleep, feeling sad when waking, depression, PTSD severity, and global sleep quality.

A treatment study conducted with a small sample of teenaged girls experiencing chronic nightmares provides preliminary evidence for the use of IRT for the reduction of posttraumatic nightmares in children (Krakow, Sandoval et al., 2001). Encel and Dohnt (2007) focused efforts on developmentally appropriate modifications to IRT for child populations; however, the effectiveness of these remains unknown.

Explaining Replicative Posttraumatic Nightmares

The occurrence of nightmares in traumatized individuals is hardly surprising based on the continuity hypothesis (Schredl, 2003a). As noted before, the study by Fosse et al. (2003) shows, however, that the replicative dream appears to be unique for the posttraumatic condition. If the exact replication of complete episodic memory traces is indeed limited to dreaming after trauma, explanations for this striking phenomenon are imperative. In this section, we review a selection of hypotheses on the etiology of posttraumatic reenactments as well as related empirical evidence.

Hypothesis I: Posttraumatic Reenactments as Especially Intensive Nightmares

Levin and Nielsen (2007) assume a continuum of dream experiences reflecting increasing intensity. Thus, these authors do not perceive a fundamental difference between replicative and other forms of dreams. Rather, they consider reenactments to be the most intense form of dreaming. They specify several factors which are assumed to determine an individual's position in this continuum: affect load, affect distress, and trauma severity. Posttraumatic reenactments thus result from the joint effect of severe traumatization, strong current stress load and low stress tolerance.

Schredl (2003b) demonstrated that current stress and especially emotional reactivity (neuroticism) contribute to the variance explanation for the frequency of nontraumatic nightmares. Whether this association may be of relevance for the differentiation of replicative vs. nonreplicative posttraumatic nightmares is, however, an open research question. As discussed previously, an increasing number of studies indicate a relationship between replicative nightmares and posttraumatic psychopathology. Again, this finding does not allow for conclusions on the relation of traumatic and nontraumatic nightmares. In summary, available evidence remains equivocal on the question if there is a quantitative or rather a categorical difference between replicative and other forms of dreaming.

Hypothesis II: Posttraumatic Reenactments as Flashbacks During Sleep

Another striking item from the PTSD-reexperiencing symptom cluster are intrusions known as flashbacks (Hackmann, Ehlers, Speckens, & Clark, 2004). Flashbacks are characterized by intense sensory contents and fragmented memories with limited if any capacity for being organized into a narrative. They are also typically associated with a limited awareness of time and the impression that the respective event is being experienced anew. As these characteristics can—at least partially—be attributed to posttraumatic reenactments as well, reenactments could be interpreted as flashbacks triggered by cognitive activity or body sensations during sleep.

Frequency of flashbacks and nightmares was significantly correlated ($r = .31$) in a study by Duke, Allen, Rozee, and Bommaritto, (2008). Van der Kolk and Fisler (1995) report results from a sample of 46 participants diagnosed with PTSD. Participants with replicative nightmares reported that their reenactments were identical to their flashbacks. In a study of Dutch survivors of Asiatic WWII concentration camps, Merckelbach, Dekkers, Wessel, and Roefs (2003) did not find differences between nightmares and flashbacks with respect to frequency distribution or sensory qualities. However, similarity to the trauma was reported to be higher for flashbacks as compared to nightmares. Associations between the occurrence of nightmares and flashbacks have also been observed for two samples by Burstein (1984, 1985). While empirical research appears to support the association of flashbacks and nightmares, it needs to be considered that all reported studies suffer from methodological shortcomings. Especially, a lack of detailed assessment of flashbacks and nightmares as well as of longitudinal designs should be noted.

Hypothesis III: Posttraumatic Reenactments as Ironic Processes of Mental Control

Typical PTSD symptoms comprise the active avoidance of trauma-related mental activity. The cognitive theory of ironic processes of mental control (Wegner, 1994) describes two processes involved in the suppression of mental content. The first process is a monitoring process screening for contents to be suppressed, which is assumed to require only limited cognitive resources. The second process is responsible for the suppression of the identified content. This process is assumed to require greater use of cognitive resources. An ironic effect appears when the suppression process fails due to lacking cognitive resources. The thought to be suppressed is then activated by the monitoring process. At the same time, the process responsible for suppression fails due to limited cognitive resources available during sleep (Harsh & Badia, 1990). It can be concluded that replicative nightmares are a paradoxical effect of posttraumatic cognitive avoidance during waking.

Wegner, Wenzlaff, and Kozak (2004) showed that the frequency of suppressed thoughts in dreams is elevated. This finding has been replicated and extended (Bryant, Wyzenbeek, & Weinstein, 2011; Taylor & Bryant, 2007). None of these studies, however, recruited traumatized individuals. When controlling for reexperiencing and hyperarousal symptom severity, Babson et al. (2011) found that avoidance symptoms did not predict nightmares in a large representative sample with a history of at least one traumatic event. In summary, the cognitive model of Wegner (1994) needs to be specifically tested in a sample of individuals diagnosed with PTSD, including a detailed comparison of suppressed waking mentation and frequency of different types of posttraumatic nightmares.

Hypothesis IV: Posttraumatic Nightmares as Screen Memories

Lansky (1995) has presented a different perspective on reports of replicative posttraumatic nightmares, based on observations of 15 severely traumatized inpatients suffering from chronic nightmares. Lansky noticed that all nightmares the patients considered to be replicative revealed deviations from the original traumatic event when closely examined. In consequence, Lansky doubts the existence of truly replicative nightmares. The basic assumption of his model is the mechanism of wish fulfillment by alteration of a current affect (shame) into a traumatic one (anxiety). By means of the retrospective evaluation "it was only a dream about the past," this allows for the defense of the current conflict. His model comprises the following processes: Childhood trauma predisposes to experiences of dissociation, lack of coherence, or shame. In this chronic posttraumatic condition, the individual is vulnerable for anxiety, dissociation, etc., which are experienced as a narcissistic injury and shame inducing. When narcissistic injuries or interpersonal problems of the day preceding the dream induce shame, the following dream repeats a traumatic scene unrelated to the experience of shame. The dream work is thus assumed to transform shame into anxiety using the traumatic event in the sense of a screen memory— using one (possibly not correct) memory from the past in order to mask another.

Lansky derives his conclusions from impressive clinical material. His doubts referring to the replicative nature of one group of posttraumatic dreams remind us that none of the dream content studies cited so far have applied a methodology allowing for a sound validation of the actual existence of posttraumatic reenactments. However, because it is based solely on clinical observations from a limited sample, Lansky's theory needs to be tested applying sound methodological standards.

Clinical Application

From the previous sections, it is obvious that nightmares and sleep complaints will be the rule rather than the exception when working with trauma survivors. The summarized scientific evidence may be used for clinical decisions in several ways. For instance, the specific characteristics of posttraumatic nightmares may be helpful as screening tools for posttraumatic stress severity and an individual's capacity to symbolize the posttraumatic event (Varvin et al., 2012). A growing number of empirical findings relate posttraumatic reenactments closely and specifically to posttraumatic stress. The few studies on the time course of posttraumatic nightmares (e.g., Terr, 1983; compare p. 137) putatively indicate that remission of PTSD may be associated with more symbolic dreams. Thus, the occurrence of certain nightmare types can be considered to have diagnostic and prognostic values. Accordingly, changes in content of nightmares should be carefully noticed. In this section we will give clinical case vignettes illustrating the integration of posttraumatic nightmares in psychotherapy.

Case Report 1

In his work for a private security company, Mr. R. had been responsible for the nighttime protection of a rather large industrial complex. One night, he noticed the presence of an intruder whom he hunted for some time through several buildings. Eventually, Mr. R. was confronted with a group of several armed criminals who appeared ready to kill him, so he ran off and was pursued by the intruders. With his excellent knowledge of the area, he found somewhere to hide, remaining concealed there overnight due to his fear of being discovered and killed. Several times a year, Mr. R. would have an apparently replicative and repetitive nightmare of his flight with the persecutors on his heels. Some years later, Mr. R. commenced psychotherapy for PTSD and several related comorbid conditions. One day he noticed that his psychotherapist was suffering from an acute, obvious impairment of health. He spent the first minutes of the session focusing on the therapist and feeling sorry for him. When it became evident that he may spend the entire session being worried about the therapist, the therapist replied that it may be very difficult to use the therapeutic space for his own—at that time rather pressing—issues when he needed to be concerned with the therapist's well-being. Later in the session, Mr. R. mentioned that he had experienced the dream again, with a slight modification for the first time. When running away from the criminals, this time he was not alone in the dream but in the company of his younger sister. She impeded his flight, and in addition, burdened him with a heavy feeling of responsibility.

According to the previous section, the development from a replicative towards a mixed-replicative posttraumatic nightmare may be considered as prognostically favourable. Confirming this perspective, many of Mr. R.'s severe posttraumatic and comorbid symptoms would decline over the course of the treatment, the trauma-focus of which would shift more and more towards a focus on personality development. Furthermore, the dream illustrates another change, which is mirrored by the manifestation of the transference at the beginning of the session under discussion. In both situations, positively connotated objects (here the sister, there the therapist) appear. Simultaneously, the full ambivalence of social relations in Mr. R.'s life becomes apparent. In both instances, the presence of the object hinders him from caring for himself. The new element of the dream may even reflect a motive explaining the reasons why Mr. R. mostly avoids social bonds: a deep need to protect himself and his conviction that social bonds make him vulnerable. Thus, together with information from a client's interactions within and outside of psychotherapy, the content of posttraumatic nightmares can be used to derive hypotheses on important psychic material a patient may currently be processing. Elaborating this information in a joint manner may provide an important source of insight for both patient and therapist.

Case Report 2

Unfortunately, not all posttraumatic nightmares give us reason to be optimistic. As a child survivor of a genocide, Mr. F. suffered from severe structural impairments (Doering et al., 2014) and posttraumatic stress symptoms. He reported having reexperienced his most extreme traumatic memory at least once every single night for more than 30 years. When approaching this memory during waking, Mr. F. would switch into a completely dissociative state full of frightening behaviors for which he would have no memory afterwards. A joint session together with his partner provided the therapist with the knowledge that Mr. F. would not awaken out of his nightmares but rather engage in the same frightening behaviors as in therapy (reminding us of the study by Hinton et al. [2009] reporting that 72% of Cambodian refugee participants experienced flashbacks upon wakening out of a nightmare).

As Mr. F. had no memory of these states, he had not been able to mention them in therapy. An effort to approach the dreams by IRT turned out to be unsuccessful. Although Mr. F. was very creative in changing the content of his nightmare, rehearsing the new version would trigger dissociative episodes. Therefore, the traumatic memory was worked through many times in therapy, whenever the spontaneous course of the sessions stimulated its reexperiencing or related signs of avoidance. This work was supported by antidissociative techniques which were first applied under the instruction of the therapist and later applied by the patient without further need of support. With increasing control of his daytime intrusions, Mr. F. learned to waken himself when having the nightmare—which was not only a huge relief to himself but also to his partner. Although the patient gratefully welcomed his increasing control over day- and nighttime intrusions, this case vignette reminds us also of our limits when working with the consequences of traumatic events. Although Mr. F. developed a better functional level regarding everyday demands, the replicative and repetitive dream—as Mr. F. characterized his nightmare—may remain a part of his life.

Nevertheless, not every replicative posttraumatic nightmare is replayed night by night. When reexperienced less frequently, even the occurrence of strictly replicative dreams may contain psychologically important information. Gardner and Ørner (2009) illustrate possibilities of working with repetitions in dreams that are very much in line with the mentioned approach by Lansky (1995). "This perspective emerges from a construction of repetitions, not as symptoms of underlying pathology (DSM-IV, APA, 1994), memory dysfunction (van der Kolk, 2006) or incorrect cognitions (Ehlers & Clark, 2000), but as potentially helpful signals to be explored for their guiding role in identifying concurrent problems and adversities the resolution of which might promote improved adjustment (Ørner, 2008). Occasional recurrence of trauma-related dreams may be adaptive as indicators of a continuing presence of important life problems" (Gardner and Ørner, 2009, p. 31). The publications by Lansky as well as Gardner and Ørner remind us that trauma survivors must never be reduced to their traumas. The overwhelming power of the trauma reenactment may easily attract all of our attention. However, if it is not related to pretrauma as well as current experiences in and outside the context of psychotherapy, the posttraumatic replication remains meaningless and an important means to facilitate understanding and mastery may be missed.

References

Babson, K., Feldner, M., Badour, C., Trainor, C., Blumenthal, H., Sachs-Ericsson, N., & Schmidt, N. (2011). Posttraumatic stress and sleep: differential relations across types of symptoms and sleep problems. *J Anxiety Disord, 25*(5), 706–713.

Blank, Y., Kelly, M., Bootzin, R. R., & Haynes, P. L. (2009). Does sleep mediate the relationship between nightmares and symptom severity in patients with PTSD and depression? *Sleep, 32*(Abstract Supplement), A358.

Bryant, R. A., Wyzenbeek, M., & Weinstein, J. (2011). Dream rebound of suppressed emotional thoughts: the influence of cognitive load. *Conscious Cogn, 20*(3), 515–522.

Burstein, A. (1984). Dream disturbance and flashbacks. *J Clin Psychiatry, 45*, 46.

Burstein, A. (1985). Posttraumatic flashbacks, dream disturbances, and mental imagery. *J Clin Psychiatry, 46*(9), 374–378.

Casement, M. D., & Swanson, L. M. (2012). A meta-analysis of imagery rehearsal for post-trauma nightmares: effects on nightmare frequency, sleep quality, and posttraumatic stress. *Clin Psychol Rev, 32*(6), 566–574.

Cook, J. M., Harb, G. C., Gehrman, P. R., Cary, M. S., Gamble, G. M., Forbes, D., & Ross, R. J. (2010). Imagery rehearsal for posttraumatic nightmares: a randomized controlled trial. *J Trauma Stress, 23*(5), 553–563.

Davis, J. L., Byrd, P., & Rhudy, J. L. (2007). Characteristics of chronic nightmares in a trauma-exposed treatment-seeking sample. *Dreaming, 17*(4), 187–198.

Doering, S., Burgmer, M., Heuft, G., Menke, D., Baumer, B., Lubking, M., . . . Schneider, G. (2014). Assessment of personality functioning: validity of the operationalized psychodynamic diagnosis axis IV (structure). *Psychopathology, 47*(3), 185–193.

Duke, L. A., Allen, D. N., Rozee, P. D., & Bommaritto, M. (2008). The sensitivity and specificity of flashbacks and nightmares to trauma. *J Anxiety Disord, 22*(2), 319–327.

Duval, M., & Zadra, A. (2010). Frequency and content of dreams associated with trauma. *Sleep Medicine Clinic 5*, 249–260.

Encel, J. S., & Dohnt, H. K. (2007). Cognitive-behavioural treatment of trauma-related nightmares in children: a developmental adaptation of imagery rehearsal therapy. In D. A. Einstein (Ed.), *Innovations and advances in cognitive-behaviour therapy* (pp. 57–68). Bowen Hills: Australian Academic Press.

Fosse, M. J., Fosse, R., Hobson, J. A., & Stickgold, R. J. (2003). Dreaming and episodic memory: a functional dissociation? *J Cogn Neurosci, 15*(1), 1–9.

Gardner, S. E., & Ørner, R. J. (2009). Searching for a new evidence base about repetitions. An exploratory survey of patients' experiences of traumatic dreams before, during and after therapy. *Counselling and Psychotherapy Research, 9*(1), 27–32.

Gerhart, J. I., Russ, E. U., Hall, B. J., & Canetti, D. (2014). Sleep disturbances predict later trauma-related distress: Cross-panel investigation amidst violent turmoil. *Health Psychol, 33*(4), 365–372.

Germain, A. (2013). Sleep disturbances as the hallmark of PTSD: where are we now? *Am J Psychiatry, 170*(4), 372–382.

Hackmann, A., Ehlers, A., Speckens, A., & Clark, D. M. (2004). Characteristics and content of intrusive memories in PTSD and their changes with treatment. *J Trauma Stress, 17*(3), 231–240.

Hansen, K., Hofling, V., Kroner-Borowik, T., Stangier, U., & Steil, R. (2013). Efficacy of psychological interventions aiming to reduce chronic nightmares: a meta-analysis. *Clin Psychol Rev, 33*(1), 146–155.

Harb, G. C., Phelps, A. J., Forbes, D., Ross, R. J., Gehrman, P. R., & Cook, J. M. (2013). A critical review of the evidence base of imagery rehearsal for posttraumatic nightmares: pointing the way for future research. *J Trauma Stress, 26*(5), 570–579.

Harb, G. C., Thompson, R., Ross, R. J., & Cook, J. M. (2012). Combat-related PTSD nightmares and imagery rehearsal: nightmare characteristics and relation to treatment outcome. *J Trauma Stress, 25*(5), 511–518.

Harsh, J., & Badia, P. (1990). Stimulus control and sleep. In R. R. Bootzin, J. F. Kihlstrom & D. Schacter (Eds.), *Sleep and cognition* (pp. 58–66). Washington, DC: American Psychological Association.

Helminen, E., & Punamäki, R.-L. (2008). Contextualised emotional images in children's dreams: Psychological adjustment in conditions of military trauma. *Int J Behav Dev, 32*(3), 177–187.

Hinton, D. E., Field, N. P., Nickerson, A., Bryant, R. A., & Simon, N. (2013). Dreams of the dead among Cambodian refugees: frequency, phenomenology, and relationship to complicated grief and posttraumatic stress disorder. *Death Studies, 37*(8), 750–767.

Hinton, D. E., Hinton, A. L., Pich, V., Loeum, J. R., & Pollack, M. H. (2009). Nightmares among Cambodian refugees: the breaching of concentric ontological security. *Culture, Medicine and Psychiatry, 33*(2), 219–265.

Holen, A. (1990). *A long-term outcome study of survivors from a disaster. The Alexander L. Kielland disaster in perspective*. PhD thesis, University of Oslo, Oslo.

Kessler, R. C., Sonnega, A., Bromet, E., Hughes, M., & Nelson, C. B. (1995). Posttraumatic stress disorder in the National Comorbidity Survey. *Arch Gen Psychiatry, 52*(12), 1048–1060.

Kilpatrick, D. G., Resnick, H. S., Freedy, J. R., Pelcovitz, D., Resick, P., Roth, S., & van der Kolk, B. (1998). Posttraumatic stress disorder field trial: evaluation of the PTSD construct—criteria A through E. In T. A. Widiger & A. J. Frances (Eds.), *DSM-IV sourcebook* (Vol. 4, pp. 803–844). Washington, DC: American Psychiatric Press.

Kobayashi, I., Boarts, J. M., & Delahanty, D. L. (2007). Polysomnographically measured sleep abnormalities in PTSD: a meta-analytic review. *Psychophysiology, 44*(4), 660–669.

Krakow, B., Hollifield, M., Johnston, L., Koss, M., Schrader, R., Warner, T. D., . . . Prince, H. (2001). Imagery rehearsal therapy for chronic nightmares in sexual assault survivors with posttraumatic stress disorder: a randomized controlled trial. *JAMA, 286*(5), 537–545.

Krakow, B., Kellner, R., Pathak, D., & Lambert, L. (1995). Imagery rehearsal treatment for chronic nightmares. *Behav Res Ther, 33*(7), 837–843.

Krakow, B., Sandoval, D., Schrader, R., Keuhne, B., McBride, L., Yau, C. L., & Tandberg, D. (2001). Treatment of chronic nightmares in adjudicated adolescent girls in a residential facility. *J Adolescent Health, 29*(2), 94–100.

Langston, T. J., Davis, J. L., & Swopes, R. M. (2010). Idiopathic and posttrauma nightmares in a clinical sample of children and adolescents: Characteristics and related pathology. *Journal of Child and Adolescent Trauma, 3*(4), 344–356.

Lansky, M. R. (1995). *Posttraumatic nightmares: psychodynamic explorations.* Hillsdale, NJ: Analytic Press.

Leskin, G. A., Woodward, S. H., Young, H. E., & Sheikh, J. I. (2002). Effects of comorbid diagnoses on sleep disturbance in PTSD. *J Psychiatr Res, 36*(6), 449–452.

Levin, R., & Nielsen, T. A. (2007). Disturbed dreaming, posttraumatic stress disorder, and affect distress: a review and neurocognitive model. *Psychol Bull, 133*(3), 482–528.

Mellman, T., David, D., Bustamante, V., Torres, R., & Fins, A. (2001). Dreams in the acute aftermath of trauma and their relationship to PTSD. *J Trauma Stress, 14*(1), 241–247.

Merckelbach, H., Dekkers, T., Wessel, I., & Roefs, A. (2003). Amnesia, flashbacks, nightmares, and dissociation in aging concentration camp survivors. *Behav Res Ther, 41*(3), 351–360.

Mertin, P., & Mohr, P. B. (2002). Incidence and correlates of posttrauma symptoms in children from backgrounds of domestic violence. *Violence and Victims, 17*(5), 555–567.

Nader, K., Pynoos, R., Fairbanks, L., & Frederick, C. (1990). Children's PTSD reactions one year after a sniper attack at their school. *Am J Psychiatry, 147*(11), 1526–1530.

Nappi, C. M., Drummond, S. P., & Hall, J. M. (2012). Treating nightmares and insomnia in posttraumatic stress disorder: a review of current evidence. *Neuropharmacology, 62*(2), 576–585.

Neylan, T. C., Marmar, C. R., Metzler, T. J., Weiss, D. S., Zatzick, D. F., Delucchi, K. L., . . . Schoenfeld, F. B. (1998). Sleep disturbances in the Vietnam generation: findings from a nationally representative sample of male Vietnam veterans. *Am J Psychiatry, 155*(7), 929–933.

Ohayon, M. M., & Shapiro, C. M. (2000). Sleep disturbances and psychiatric disorders associated with posttraumatic stress disorder in the general population. *Compr Psychiatry, 41*(6), 469–478.

Pigeon, W. R., Martinez, J., & Mellman, T. A. (2004). Dreams of recently hospitalized trauma patients and their relationship to PTSD. *Sleep, 27*(Abstract Supplment), A63.

Punamäki, R.-L., Ali, K. J., Ismahil, K. H., & Nuutinen, J. (2005). Trauma, dreaming, and psychological distress among Kurdish children. *Dreaming, 15*(3), 178–194.

Rasmussen, B. (2007). No refuge: an exploratory survey of nightmares, dreams, and sleep patterns in women dealing with relationship violence. *Violence Against Women, 13*(3), 314–322.

Riemann, D., Berger, M., & Voderholzer, U. (2001). Sleep and depression-results from psychobiological studies: an overview. *Biol Psychol, 57*(1–3), 67–103.

Rintamaki, L. S., Weaver, F. M., Elbaum, P. L., Klama, E. N., & Miskevics, S. A. (2009). Persistence of traumatic memories in World War II prisoners of war. *J Am Geriatr Soc, 57*(12), 2257–2262. doi: 10.1111/j.1532-5415.2009.02608.x

Schredl, M. (2003a). Continuity between waking and dreaming: A proposal for a mathematical model. *Sleep and Hypnosis, 5*, 38–52.

Schredl, M. (2003b). Effects of state and trait factors on nightmare frequency. *Eur Arch Psy Clin N, 253*(5), 241–247.

Schredl, M., Fricke-Oerkermann, L., Mitschke, A., Wiater, A., & Lehmkuhl, G. (2009). Longitudinal study of nightmares in children: stability and effect of emotional symptoms. *Child Psychiatry Hum Dev, 40*(3), 439–449.

Schredl, M., & Pallmer, R. (1997). Nightmares in children. *Prax Kinderpsychol Kinderpsychiatr, 46*(1), 36–56.

Schreuder, B., Igreja, V., van Dijk, J., & Kleijn, W. (2001). Intrusive reexperiencing of chronic strife or war. *Advances in Psychiatric Treatment, 7*, 102–108.

Schreuder, B. J., Kleijn, W. C., & Rooijmans, H. G. (2000). Nocturnal reexperiencing more than forty years after war trauma. *J Trauma Stress, 13*(3), 453–463.

Schreuder, B. J., van Egmond, M., Kleijn, W. C., & Visser, A. T. (1998). Daily reports of posttraumatic nightmares and anxiety dreams in Dutch war victims. *J Anxiety Disord, 12*(6), 511–524.

Solms, M. (2000). Dreaming and REM sleep are controlled by different brain mechanisms. *Behav Brain Sci, 23*(6), 843–850.

Stepansky, R., Holzinger, B., Schmeiser-Rieder, A., Saletu, B., Kunze, M., & Zeitlhofer, J. (1998). Austrian dream behavior: results of a representative population survey. *Dreaming, 8*, 23–30.

Swart, M. L., van Schagen, A. M., Lancee, J., & van den Bout, J. (2013). Prevalence of nightmare disorder in psychiatric outpatients. *Psychother Psychosom, 82*(4), 267–268.

Taylor, F., & Bryant, R. A. (2007). The tendency to suppress, inhibiting thoughts, and dream rebound. *Behav Res Ther, 45*(1), 163–168.

Terr, L. C. (1983). Chowchilla revisited: the effects of psychic trauma four years after a school-bus kidnapping. *Am J Psychiatry, 140*(12), 1543–1550.

Valli, K., Revonsuo, A., Palkas, O., Ismail, K. H., Ali, K. J., & Punamaki, R. L. (2005). The threat simulation theory of the evolutionary function of dreaming: Evidence from dreams of traumatized children. *Conscious Cogn, 14*(1), 188–218.

Van der Kolk, B. A., & Fisler, R. (1995). Dissociation and the fragmentary nature of traumatic memories: overview and exploratory study. *J Trauma Stress, 8*(4), 505–526.

Varvin, S., Fischmann, T., Jovic, V., Rosenbaum, B., & Hau, S. (2012). Traumatic dreams: symbolisation gone astray. In P. Fonagy, H. Kächele, M. Leuzinger-Bohleber & D. Taylor (Eds.), *The significance of dreams. Bridging clinical and extraclinical research in psychoanalysis*. London: Karnac.

Wegner, D. M. (1994). Ironic processes of mental control. *Psychol Rev, 101*(1), 34–52.

Wegner, D. M., Wenzlaff, R. M., & Kozak, M. (2004). Dream rebound: the return of suppressed thoughts in dreams. *Psychology Science, 15*(4), 232–236.

Wittmann, L., Schredl, M., & Kramer, M. (2006). Dreaming in PTSD: a critical review of phenomenology, psychophysiology, and treatment. *Psychother Psychosom, 76*, 25–39.

Wittmann, L., Zehnder, D., Schredl, M., Jenni, O. G., & Landolt, M. A. (2010). Posttraumatic nightmares and psychopathology in children after road traffic accidents. *J Trauma Stress, 23*(2), 232–239.

12

NIGHTMARE THERAPY

Emerging Concepts From Sleep Medicine

Barry Krakow

SLEEP AND HUMAN HEALTH INSTITUTE

Introduction

Sleep medicine specialists view the problem of chronic nightmare disorder as an independent sleep disorder. When patients seek treatment for chronic nightmares, a direct intervention may be offered regardless of the putative causes. This approach derives from the assumption that nightmares may persist because they "take on a life of their own" (Krakow & Zadra, 2006a) despite the fact that nightmares are generally triggered by clear-cut life stressors such as traumatic exposure or a protracted course of psychiatric illness. In contrast, sleep medicine does not view nightmares exclusively as a symptomatic feature of a primary disorder, whereas the psychiatric community and its nosology have long maintained that nightmares are best understood as a secondary phenomenon for which treatment need only be directed at the inciting disorder (Brewin, Lanius, Novac, Schnyder, & Galea, 2009). In this standard model, the nightmares may provide additional value in so far as working with bad dreams uncovers critical emotional conflicts and meaningful insights to help treat the primary disorder, but the nightmares themselves do not—and some would say should not—receive primary attention for fear that essential psychodynamic processes may be masked, undermined, or lost (Parker-Pope, 2010).

The depth and breadth of this chasm between the fields of psychiatry or psychology and sleep medicine is further predicated upon the current and longstanding qualifier in the nosology that states "does not occur exclusively during another mental disorder," which by definition makes nightmare disorder a rarity, because nightmares almost invariably occur in the presence of another mental disorder, most commonly the anxiety condition, posttraumatic stress disorder (PTSD), and not infrequently in depressive disorders (Diagnostic and Statistical Manual of Mental Disorders, 2000). This approach reiterates that treatment must focus on the PTSD diagnosis in a trauma survivor or in the depressed patient with nightmares, because nightmares allegedly improve when the disorder improves.

Imagery Rehearsal Therapy

Notwithstanding this well-entrenched mental health perspective, several randomized controlled trials, some dating back 20 years, offer an alternative explanation that implies a bidirectional relationship between nightmares and psychiatric distress (Kellner, Neidhardt, Krakow, & Pathak, 1992; Miller & DiPilato, 1983). That is, direct nightmare treatment with either desensitization techniques or imagery rehearsal therapy (IRT) markedly decreases chronic nightmare frequency as well as distress-symptom severity, notably anxiety and posttraumatic stress symptoms. IRT is a cognitive-imagery technique through which the awake patient changes the content of the nightmare and rehearses the images of the "new dream" a few minutes each day. (See Figure 12.1 for a summary of the IRT protocol.)

The most remarkable of these studies was a randomized controlled trial of nightmare treatment using IRT for sexual assault survivors with PTSD (Krakow et al., 2001a). In the study, a total of 114 sexual assault survivors, who were randomized to treatment or wait-list control groups, completed follow-up at 3 or 6 months. Comparing baseline to follow-up, IRT significantly decreased nights per week with nightmares (Cohen $d = 1.24$; $P = .001$) and number of nightmares per week (Cohen $d = 0.85$; $P = .001$) as well as PTSD symptoms (Cohen $d = 1.00$; $P = .001$). Controls showed small, nonsignificant improvements (mean Cohen $d = 0.21$). An intent-to-treat analysis ($n = 168$) confirmed significant differences between treatment and control groups for nightmares and PTSD (all $P = .02$) with moderate effect sizes for treatment (mean Cohen $d = 0.60$) and small effects for controls (mean Cohen $d = 0.14$). Posttraumatic stress symptoms decreased by at least one level of clinical severity in 65% of the treatment group compared with symptoms worsening or not changing in 69% of controls (Chi-square(1) = 12.80; $P = .001$) (Krakow et al., 2001a).

Several review articles in the past few years, written largely from a behavioral sleep-medicine perspective, coupled with recent practice parameters from the American Academy of Sleep Medicine (AASM), now designate IRT as the only first-line (Grade A), nonpharmacalogic therapy for chronic nightmares (Aurora et al., 2010). Prazosin is the only medication attaining a similar Grade A status for nightmare treatment, albeit the general view is that when the drug is withdrawn, nightmares return in most patients (Dierks, Jordan, & Sheehan, 2007). However, long-term follow-up studies indicate IRT yields sustained results (measured in years) after just a few weeks of implementation (Krakow, Kellner, Neidhardt, Pathak, & Lambert, 1993; Krakow, Kellner, Pathak, & Lambert, 1996).

To my knowledge, there are no comparable practice parameters for the treatment of nightmares in either the fields of psychiatry or psychology. In fact, the AASM practice parameters list "no rating" for the use of psychotherapeutic

Session 1
- Deemphasizing discussion of past traumatic events or traumatic content of nightmares
- Describing past research to address treatment credibility
- Linking nightmares to insomnia
- Discussing how nightmares pass from an acute phase to a chronic disorder
- Showing how nightmares originally may benefit the patient

Session 2
- Discuss how nightmares might persist as a learned behavior long after traumatic exposure
- Report research findings demonstrating decreased distress with direct nightmare treatment
- Review the concept of symptom substitution and why it may not arise
- Engage the patient to discuss nightmare triggers as trauma-induced vs "habit"-sustained
- Explain principles and practice of general imagery and pleasant imagery
- Offer solutions for overcoming obstacles to waking imagery practice

Session 3
- Broader discussion of waking imagery and possible relationship to dream imagery
- Imagery as a vehicle for change in behavior
- Recognizing the development of the nightmare sufferer identity
- Preparing to change the nightmare identity to a "good dreamer"

Session 4
- Provide the general framework of IRT for nightmares
  - Selecting a nightmare
  - Changing the nightmare any way you wish
  - Rehearsing the new dream with imagery session
- Review patient's first attempt at changing and rehearsing the "new dream"
  - Discuss obstacles and plans for continued home practice

*Extracted from Krakow, B. & Krakow, J. (2002). *Turning Nightmares into Dreams*. Albuquerque, NM: The New Sleepy Times.

FIGURE 12.1 Main therapeutic principles in four weekly IRT sessions delivered to individuals or groups.*

treatments for chronic nightmares due to the absence of controlled treatment studies, but nevertheless include this statement: "The literature describes high-level effectiveness of this treatment modality [therapeutic alliance, psychoanalysis, etc.] in case reports and descriptive treatment protocols. RCTs and comparative studies are unavailable" (Aurora et al., 2010, p. 397). Last, Grade C is the only level attained for the multiple medications currently in use for the treatment of PTSD, which are purportedly prescribed with the expectation these drugs will also diminish PTSD nightmares, yet high-level evidence for such effects is rare to nonexistent (Aurora et al., 2010).

On a personal note, I feel compelled to point out that despite all the successes we have achieved with IRT, I remain a firm proponent of dream interpretation and related psychodynamic techniques for the treatment of chronic nightmares. The most well-known form of IRT in fact was developed by two psychiatrists, one of whom (Dr. Joseph Neidhardt) possessed an exceptionally rich background in dream interpretation work; we coauthored the first book on comprehensive treatments for chronic nightmares, of which one-third of the content is devoted to a traditional approach to disturbing dreams (Krakow & Neidhardt, 1992). Despite the lack of rigorous scientific evidence for traditional dream therapy techniques, I am strongly persuaded that IRT is not the right treatment for every patient, and the role of dream interpretation and related psychodynamic work is highly relevant in many situations.

Emerging Trends & Perspectives

The divergence in perspectives described here is problematic because it engenders too much of an "either-or" decision point. Right now, the behavioral sleep medicine field is ascending in the treatment of chronic nightmares with techniques such as IRT that are not only efficacious but also cost effective. For mild to moderate individual cases of nightmares, treatment might comprise a single session or a few brief sessions, while for more severe cases involving moderate to severe PTSD patients, we have seen successful outcomes with a range of treatment time as short as one 3-hour group session (Krakow, Kellner, Pathak, & Lambert, 1995) or four weekly 2-hour group sessions (Krakow & Zadra, 2006b). Nonetheless, we still observe many of these nightmare patients in need of further dream interpretation, related psychodynamic work, or other types of psychotherapy following their course of behavioral nightmare treatment, which aligns with our rationale for advocating IRT as an adjunctive therapy. That is, even when PTSD patients' chief complaints are chronic nightmares, we do not offer IRT as the treatment for their PTSD; we treat their nightmares, anticipate posttraumatic stress symptoms will decrease to a degree, and then refer them back to their mental health providers for additional treatments.

In recent workshop trainings conducted at U.S. military bases, I learned that some mental health providers are implementing IRT as the first mental health treatment for trauma survivors with nightmares, after which standard exposure therapy is offered to treat PTSD. The anecdotal reports provided to me specifically mentioned that treating nightmares first achieved at least two benefits for their patients prior to initiating exposure therapy. First, by treating nightmares, these patients began sleeping better. Second, IRT was accepted as an easier pathway to begin some degree of PTSD treatment in general, and in several cases these patients progressed more rapidly through the specific use of exposure protocols.

Overall, because successfully treated nightmare patients are able to gain a better night's sleep, we speculate they are more alert and capable of making clearer decisions about additional therapies. In addition, having overcome the burden of nightmares, patients may improve their capacity to focus on the need to treat residual distress symptoms. These points are key and may serve as the bridge that helps various professionals—encumbered by paradoxically competing perspectives—to realize the relevance and importance of direct nightmare treatment. For example, consider the following paragraph extracted from the AASM practice parameters regarding nightmare morbidity: "The presence of nightmare disorder can impair quality of life, resulting in sleep avoidance and sleep deprivation, with a consequent increase in the intensity of the nightmares. Nightmare disorder can also predispose to insomnia, daytime sleepiness, and fatigue. It may also cause or exacerbate underlying psychiatric distress and illness. Nightmare disorder can be associated with waking psychological dysfunction, with the frequency of nightmares being inversely correlated with measures of well-being and measures of nightmare distress being associated with psychopathology such as depression and anxiety" (Aurora et al., 2010, p. 391).

I suspect most mental health professionals do not perceive or appreciate the impact of "nightmares as a distinct disorder" on quality of life. Yet even the cited paragraph is too general, and it underestimates the critical importance of nightmare effects on mental and physical health. For example, most mental health professionals are likely unfamiliar with numerous research papers demonstrating the consistent association between nightmare problems and suicidality, all of which point to the potential for nightmare treatment to modify a salient risk factor for this dangerous condition (Agargun et al., 2007; Bernert & Joiner, 2007; Sjostrom, Hetta, & Waern, 2009). Few practitioners may know that nearly one-third of patients with alcohol-use disorders reported self-medicating behavior at bedtime to alleviate nightmares (Hershon, 1977); and finally, from our extensive years of research on treatment-seeking nightmare patients, few would suspect that a large proportion of these patients suffer from comorbid obstructive sleep apnea (Krakow et al., 2002a).

An encouraging development among military mental health professionals, however, suggests some practitioners are already engaging nightmare patients in light of these salient perspectives. As mentioned earlier regarding my training experiences at various U.S. military bases, I observed these specific cohorts of mental health professionals were increasingly aware of the comorbidity described earlier: that is, nightmare patients often manifested comorbid insomnia and sleep apnea. Part of the training, which uses our Sleep Dynamic Therapy^{TM} model, (Krakow et al., 2002c; Krakow, 2007) expands on their capacity to assess and treat sleep disorders in service members with PTSD or other mental health problems. The objective is to teach these professionals how to approach sleep disorders from the perspective of a sleep medicine specialist. The general framework of the 3-day training program focuses on the four major disorders of insomnia, nightmares, sleep apnea, and leg movement disorders. One full day of the program delves into the specific application of the IRT method for chronic nightmares.

During the IRT training day, we briefly discuss the advent of Prazosin as an expedient treatment pathway not only because it may decrease disturbing dreams, but some research indicates it will reduce posttraumatic stress symptoms as well. In the military, this drug is in common use. Still, the medication may not work for some patients, and other patients prefer non-pharmacologic treatments. When introducing IRT, I learned that nearly 80 to 90% of attendees had already heard about IRT for nightmares, and anywhere from 10% to 50% were already applying IRT steps in their clinical practices. At the locations where IRT was in more frequent use, individual practitioners described the approach of offering a patient a starting point with either IRT for nightmares or exposure therapy for PTSD. Some providers had found PTSD patients most receptive to starting with IRT, after which they reported how nightmare treatment appeared to pave the way forward as described above. The same phenomenon was also described in offering cognitive-behavior therapy for insomnia (CBT-I) prior to initiating exposure therapy for PTSD, and again some patients preferred insomnia treatment first. In both instances, whether it was nightmare or insomnia treatment, mental health providers reported that patients who were sleeping better before starting exposure therapy appeared more receptive, willing, or able to enter this more intensive form of therapy. Some providers reported this approach was becoming a mainstay in their practice, because so many patients were more eager to initiate sleep treatments prior to PTSD treatments.

This progression toward a sleep-oriented perspective in managing mental health patients with nightmares or nightmares and insomnia appears to be setting the stage for an even greater infusion of evidence-based sleep treatments into mental health practices. In addition, as I discussed with these mental health providers at the training, the fields of psychology and psychiatry are not only natural allies to the specialty of sleep medicine, but the practitioners in these fields represent the most sophisticated healthcare providers in terms of dealing with behavioral problems in general. Thus, these individuals have the clear potential to rapidly learn how to assess and treat sleep disorders in their mental health patients. It has been most satisfying that our landmark paper in *JAMA* has been described by so many researchers and clinicians as one that helped to open the doorway into this new perspective; to wit, treating a sleep disorder just might facilitate treatment of a mental health disorder, directly or indirectly.

Nightmares and Sleep Breathing

Most recently, we have defined an additional purpose for evaluating nightmares based on our clinical work and research in which we describe the Nightmare Triad Syndrome wherein we detect the unusual and unexpected co-morbidity among nightmares, insomnia and sleep apnea (McIver et al., 2013a; McIver et al.,

2013b). Although we first learned about this triad in the mid-1990s in the sample of sexual assault survivors who we eventually reported on in the *JAMA* article, we were not clear on the pathophysiological relationship among these disorders until more recently. Basically, in the 1990s and early 2000s, we examined successive series of trauma survivors including those exposed to sexual assault, other criminal assault, or a disaster (urgent fire evacuees) (Krakow et al., 2000a; Krakow et al., 2001b; Krakow et al., 2002b; Krakow et al., 2004; Krakow et al., 2006), all of whom reported high frequencies of nightmares and insomnia and also reported many symptoms consistent with undiagnosed sleep apnea.

In these studies, we commonly saw patients presenting with a complaint of nightmares, but who were also nearly always suffering from the other two conditions, insomnia and sleep apnea. In a paper published on crime victims seeking treatment for nightmares and insomnia, the sleep apnea rate exceeded 90% (40 of 44 patients objectively tested) (Krakow et al., 2001b). In all other samples, this extremely high objective rate was observed regardless of whether the patients presented with the standard sleep apnea symptoms (sleepiness, snoring, loud snoring, choking or gasping in sleep, witness apneas) or the less well-known, end-organ symptoms (dry mouth, morning headache, nocturia) (Krakow et al., 2006).

Immediately, we could not help but wonder whether these findings were coincidental or whether cause and effect relationships would emerge. The truth remains to be discovered, but there is a very small but growing interest in the impact of sleep fragmentation influences on the stability of the human upper airway, and this research first described by Series, Roy, and Marc suggests any form of sleep fragmentation may worsen upper airway collapsibility (Series, Roy, & Marc, 1994; Series, 2009). This finding is quite provocative in that sleep disorders such as nightmares or insomnia clearly fragment sleep in myriad ways. More speculatively, once we began to notice this high rate of sleep apnea in nightmare patients, we became increasingly curious to learn more details from our patients about their experiences during a middle of the night awakening. Although we can only report anecdotally, it was quite interesting to recall so many patients describing the classic sensation of shortness of breath upon awakening from a nightmare and now wondering whether this experience might be a breathing event as well as an anxiety response. Still, this point remains highly speculative and will no doubt prove difficult to study in light of Hartmann's seminal work on the general lack of nightmare experiences reported in the sleep lab environment (Hartmann, 1984).

Naturally, we wanted to look at whether or not the treatment of sleep apnea would decrease nightmares, and in 2000 we published the first retrospective case series describing patients with nightmares and sleep apnea undergoing various forms of treatment such as positive airway pressure therapy (PAP), dental devices and one case of obesity treatment. Although the sample was small, the results clearly showed a significant association between the treatment of sleep apnea and improvements in nightmare frequency, posttraumatic stress symptoms, and sleep quality (Krakow et al., 2000b). Since then, two studies were recently published. One study in 2012 comprised 99 nightmare patients who showed an association for nightmare reduction in obstructive sleep apnea (OSA) patients using their PAP devices compared to no changes in dreams among OSA patients not undergoing treatment for the sleep breathing condition. Nightmares disappeared in 91% of the patients who used PAP (50 of 55 patients) compared with only a 36% decrease (16 of 45) among those who refused to use PAP ($p < 0.001$) (BaHammam, Al-Shimemeri, Salama, & Sharif, 2013). Tamanna and colleagues have published the most recent study, examining changes in nightmare frequency in PTSD patients with OSA. Working with 69 patients, divided into two groups based on either REM-predominant or NREM-predominant OSA, nightmare frequency dropped nearly 50% in both groups and was clearly associated with greater compliance with PAP devices. A 10% improvement in compliance was associated with a mean decrease of one nightmare per week (Tamanna, Parker, Lyons, & Ullah, 2014).

It cannot go without saying, however, that PAP therapy is viewed by many patients as a "nightmare" treatment in and of itself. All the physiological hassles with the device involving adaptation to pressurized air blown into the nose or mouth and the need to fastidiously fit the best mask to the face (nasal pillows, over the nose, over the nose and mouth) may require considerable time, money, and effort before a patient experiences obvious benefits. In our own experience working at a sleep center that specializes in mental health patients with sleep disorders, we found standard issue CPAP (continuous pressure), a device that delivers one stream of pressurized air at a set level during inhalation and exhalation, rarely works in patients with any degree of anxiety. Thus, for nightmare patients we have found more expedient results by prescribing dual-pressure systems that adjust the airflow settings to more comfortably address the physiological sensations and distinct pressure needs that accompany the different phases of breathing (Krakow, Ulibarri, Romero, Thomas, & McIver, 2013).

Conclusions

In sum, nightmare effects are extensive and intensive, and more systematic efforts are needed to triage patients to the appropriate lines of therapy. In the general population alone, chronic nightmares are a common problem thought to affect at minimum 4% of adults (Zadra & Donderi, 2000), albeit there is no research that clarifies how many of these patients would benefit from treatment. More relevant are the increasing numbers of PTSD patients, including many with likely nightmare conditions, among military personnel returning from combat operations (Hoge et al., 2004). Actual rates of PTSD may exceed 20% (Thomas et al., 2010), although the rate of nightmare problems is unknown. These patients threaten to overwhelm current mental health facilities, and as noted in the introduction, this dilemma is compounded because most psychiatrists and therapists still view the nightmare problem through the framework of PTSD, which does not consistently lead patients to successful treatments for their nightmare problems. Not only does the research literature align with this conventional viewpoint (i.e. treat PTSD and the patient's nightmares should go away), but also and ironically most studies on evidence-based treatment of PTSD do not even mention whether or not the therapy was effective in decreasing chronic nightmares (Spoormaker & Montgomery, 2008).

If we are to help these patients overcome the problem of the nightmare disorder, it remains unclear how many therapists and psychiatrists are available to provide dream interpretation approaches and psychoanalytic (e.g. Jungian) approaches or how many behavioral sleep specialists are available to provide IRT or related imagery or desensitization techniques. Instead, what we might anticipate in the near future is that a majority of these PTSD patients with nightmares will receive an inferior nightmare therapy in the form of medication for PTSD while some will receive a Grade A medication treatment in the form of Prazosin, but which might require lifelong usage. (See these references for prescribing guidelines: Calohan, Peterson, Peskind, & Raskind, 2010; Taylor, Freeman, & Cates, 2008; Thompson, Taylor, McFall, Barnes, & Raskind, 2008.) Regardless of how things unfold in the short term, it is imperative to find ways to disseminate self-empowering treatments to patients with nightmares, because it appears likely either IRT or dream interpretation therapy create clear-cut opportunities for cures. These approaches are likely to yield extremely high efficacy when administered by an expert sleep or mental health professional, but it remains to be seen how to strategically implement these types of programs to create greater accessibility. The wild card is whether or not many of these patients need sleep testing sooner to evaluate for comorbid sleep apnea and how many will see their nightmares decrease with sleep apnea treatment, notably PAP therapy.

Many valuable and efficacious therapies are emerging for the treatment of nightmares, yet it remains fair to say that we are still in an evolving process in which these treatments remain largely unavailable to the patients and unused by their healthcare providers. It thus remains one of those odd circumstances in health care of a "cure in search of a patient."

Additional Reading and Resources

Krakow, B. (2003). Imagery rehearsal therapy for chronic posttraumatic nightmares: a mind's eye view. In R. Rosnar (Ed.), *Dreams & Cognitive Therapy*. New York: Springer Publishing.

Krakow, B. (2010). Imagery rehearsal therapy for adolescents. In M. Perlis, M. Aloia, & B. R. Kuhn (Eds.), *Behavioral Treatments for Sleep Disorders: A Comprehensive Primer of Behavioral Sleep Medicine Interventions*. Waltham, MA: Elsevier/Academic Press.

Krakow, B., & Zadra, A. (2010). Imagery rehearsal therapy: principles and practice In J. F. Pagel (Ed.), *Dreaming and Nightmares, An Issue of Sleep Medicine Clinics*. Philadelphia, PA: Elsevier/Saunders.

Krackow, Barry. (2002). *Turning Nightmares into Dreams*. Workbook and audio series. Albuquerque, NM: Maimonides Sleep Arts and Sciences. Website: www.nightmaretreatment.com.

References

Agargun, M. Y., Besiroglu, L., Cilli, A. S., Gulec, M., Aydin, A., Inci, R., et al. (2007). Nightmares, suicide attempts, and melancholic features in patients with unipolar major depression. *Journal of Affective Disorders, 98,* 267–270.

Aurora, R. N., Zak, R. S., Auerbach, S. H., Casey, K. R., Chowdhuri, S., Karippot, A., et al. (2010). Best practice guide for the treatment of nightmare disorder in adults. *Journal of Clinical Sleep Medicine, 6,* 389–401.

BaHammam, A. S., Al-Shimemeri, S. A., Salama, R. I., & Sharif, M. M. (2013). Clinical and polysomnographic characteristics and response to continuous positive airway pressure therapy in obstructive sleep apnea patients with nightmares. *Sleep Medicine, 14,* 149–154.

Bernert, R. A. & Joiner, T. E. (2007). Sleep disturbances and suicide risk: A review of the literature. *Neuropsychiatric Disease and Treatment, 3,* 735–743.

Brewin, C. R., Lanius, R. A., Novac, A., Schnyder, U., & Galea, S. (2009). Reformulating PTSD for DSM-V: life after Criterion A. *Journal of Traumatic Stress, 22,* 366–373.

Calohan, J., Peterson, K., Peskind, E. R., & Raskind, M. A. (2010). Prazosin treatment of trauma nightmares and sleep disturbance in soldiers deployed in Iraq. *Journal of Traumatic Stress, 23,* 645–648.

Diagnostic and Statistical Manual of Mental Disorders. (2000). 4th ed. Washington, DC: American Psychiatric Association.

Dierks, M. R., Jordan, J. K., & Sheehan, A. H. (2007). Prazosin treatment of nightmares related to posttraumatic stress disorder. *Annals of Pharmacotherapy, 41,* 1013–1017.

Hartmann, E. (1984). *The Nightmare: The Psychology and Biology of Terrifying Dreams.* New York: Basic Books.

Hershon, H. I. (1977). Alcohol withdrawal symptoms and drinking behavior. *Journal of Studies on Alcohol, 38,* 953–971.

Hoge, C. W., Castro, C. A., Messer, S. C., McGurk, D., Cotting, D. I., & Koffman, R. L. (2004). Combat duty in Iraq and Afghanistan, mental health problems, and barriers to care. *New England Journal of Medicine, 351,* 13–22.

Kellner, R., Neidhardt, J., Krakow, B., & Pathak, D. (1992). Changes in chronic nightmares after one session of desensitization or rehearsal instructions. *American Journal of Psychiatry, 149,* 659–663.

Krakow, B. (2007). *Sound Sleep, Sound Mind: 7 Keys to Sleeping through the Night.* Hoboken, NJ: John Wiley & Sons, Inc.

Krakow, B., Germain, A., Tandberg, D., Koss, M., Schrader, R., Hollifield, M., et al. (2000a). Sleep breathing and sleep movement disorders masquerading as insomnia in sexual-assault survivors. *Comprehensive Psychiatry, 41,* 49–56.

Krakow, B., Haynes, P. L., Warner, T. D., Santana, E., Melendrez, D., Johnston, L., et al. (2004). Nightmares, insomnia, and sleep-disordered breathing in fire evacuees seeking treatment for posttraumatic sleep disturbance. *Journal of Traumatic Stress, 17,* 257–268.

Krakow, B., Hollifield, M., Johnston, L., Koss, M., Schrader, R., Warner, T. D., et al. (2001a). Imagery rehearsal therapy for chronic nightmares in sexual assault survivors with posttraumatic stress disorder: a randomized controlled trial. *Journal of the American Medical Association, 286,* 537–545.

Krakow, B., Kellner, R., Neidhardt, J., Pathak, D., & Lambert, L. (1993). Imagery rehearsal treatment of chronic nightmares: with a thirty month follow-up. *Journal of Behavioral Therapy & Experimental Psychiatry, 24,* 325–330.

Krakow, B., Kellner, R., Pathak, D., & Lambert, L. (1995). Imagery rehearsal treatment for chronic nightmares. *Behaviour, Research and Therapy, 33,* 837–843.
Krakow, B., Kellner, R., Pathak, D., & Lambert, L. (1996). Long term reductions in nightmares treated with imagery rehearsal. *Behavioural and Cognitive Psychotherapy, 24,* 135–148.
Krakow, B., Lowry, C., Germain, A., Gaddy, L., Hollifield, M., Koss, M., et al. (2000b). A retrospective study on improvements in nightmares and post-traumatic stress disorder following treatment for co-morbid sleep-disordered breathing. *Journal of Psychosomatic Research, 49,* 291–298.
Krakow, B., Melendrez, D., Johnston, L., Warner, T. D., Clark, J. O., Pacheco, M., et al. (2002a). Sleep-disordered breathing, psychiatric distress, and quality of life impairment in sexual assault survivors. *Journal of Nervous and Mental Disease, 190,* 442–452.
Krakow, B., Melendrez, D., Johnston, L., Warner, T. D., Clark, J. O., Pacheco, M., et al. (2002b). Sleep-disordered breathing, psychiatric distress, and quality of life impairment in sexual assault survivors. *Journal of Nervous and Mental Disease, 190,* 442–452.
Krakow, B., Melendrez, D., Pedersen, B., Johnston, L., Hollifield, M., Germain, A., et al. (2001b). Complex insomnia: insomnia and sleep-disordered breathing in a consecutive series of crime victims with nightmares and PTSD. *Biological Psychiatry, 49,* 948–953.
Krakow, B., Melendrez, D., Warner, T. D., Clark, J. O., Sisley, B. N., Dorin, R., et al. (2006). Signs and symptoms of sleep-disordered breathing in trauma survivors: a matched comparison with classic sleep apnea patients. *Journal of Nervous and Mental Disease, 194,* 433–439.
Krakow, B., & Neidhardt, E. J. (1992). *Conquering Bad Dreams & Nightmares.* New York: Berkley Books.
Krakow, B., Ulibarri, V. A., Romero, E. A., Thomas, R. J., & McIver, N. D. (2013). Adaptive servo-ventilation therapy in a case series of patients with co-morbid insomnia and sleep apnea. *Journal of Sleep Disorders: Treatment & Care, 2 epub.*
Krakow, B. & Zadra, A. (2006a). Clinical management of chronic nightmares: imagery rehearsal therapy. *Behavioral Sleep Medicine, 4,* 45–70.
Krakow, B. & Zadra, A. (2006b). Clinical management of chronic nightmares: imagery rehearsal therapy. *Behavioral Sleep Medicine, 4,* 45–70.
Krakow, B. J., Melendrez, D.C., Johnston, L. G., Clark, J. O., Santana, E. M., Warner, T. D., et al. (2002c). Sleep Dynamic Therapy for Cerro Grande Fire evacuees with posttraumatic stress symptoms: a preliminary report. *Journal of Clinical Psychiatry, 63,* 673–684.
McIver, N. D., Krakow, B., Krakow, J., Baade, R., Cox, M., Rafferty, M., et al. (6–1–2013a). Nightmare Triad Syndrome in at-risk adolescents in a public charter high school. *Sleep, 36.* A367 Abstract.
McIver, N. D., Krakow, B., Krakow, J., Baade, R., Cox, M., Rafferty, M., et al. (2013b). Nightmare Triad Syndrome in At-Risk Adolescents in a Public Charter High School. Poster Presentation, June 5, 2013. SLEEP, the 27th Annual Meeting of the Associated Professional Sleep Societies LLC. Baltimore, MD.
Miller, W. R. & DiPilato, M. (1983). Treatment of nightmares via relaxation and desensitization: a controlled evaluation. *Journal of Consulting and Clinical Psychology, 51,* 870–877.
Parker-Pope, T. (2010, July 27). Should nightmares have happy endings? *New York Times.*
Series, F. (2009). Can improving sleep influence sleep-disordered breathing? *Drugs, 69 Suppl 2,* 77–91.

Series, F., Roy, N., & Marc, I. (1994). Effects of sleep deprivation and sleep fragmentation on upper airway collapsibility in normal subjects. *American Journal of Respiratory and Critical Care Medicine, 150,* 481–485.

Sjostrom, N., Hetta, J., & Waern, M. (2009). Persistent nightmares are associated with repeat suicide attempt: a prospective study. *Psychiatry Research, 170,* 208–211.

Spoormaker, V. I. & Montgomery, P. (2008). Disturbed sleep in post-traumatic stress disorder: secondary symptom or core feature? *Sleep Medicine Reviews, 12,* 169–184.

Tamanna, S., Parker, J. D., Lyons, J., & Ullah, M. I. (2014). The effect of continuous positive air pressure (CPAP) on nightmares in patients with posttraumatic stress disorder (PTSD) and obstructive sleep apnea (OSA). *Journal of Clinical Sleep Medicine, 10,* 631–636.

Taylor, H. R., Freeman, M. K., & Cates, M. E. (2008). Prazosin for treatment of nightmares related to posttraumatic stress disorder. *American Journal of Health-System Pharmacy, 65,* 716–722.

Thomas, J. L., Wilk, J. E., Riviere, L. A., McGurk, D., Castro, C. A., & Hoge, C. W. (2010). Prevalence of mental health problems and functional impairment among active component and National Guard soldiers 3 and 12 months following combat in Iraq. *Archives of General Psychiatry, 67,* 614–623.

Thompson, C. E., Taylor, F. B., McFall, M. E., Barnes, R. F., & Raskind, M. A. (2008). Non-nightmare distressed awakenings in veterans with posttraumatic stress disorder: response to prazosin. *Journal of Traumatic Stress, 21,* 417–420.

Zadra, A. & Donderi, D.C. (2000). Nightmares and bad dreams: their prevalence and relationship to well-being. *Journal of Abnormal Psychology, 109,* 273–281.

13

POSITIVE ASPECTS OF THE CLASSIC NIGHTMARE

J. F. Pagel

ASSOCIATE CLINICAL PROFESSOR UNIVERSITY OF COLORADO SCHOOL OF MEDICINE—SOUTHERN COLORADO FAMILY MEDICINE RESIDENCY PROGRAM—PUEBLO, COLORADO AND—SLEEP DISORDERS CENTER OF SOUTHERN COLORADO, PARKVIEW MEDICAL CENTER, PUEBLO, COLORADO

Among the clay tables inscribed with the first decipherable script is a nightmare reported by the King Gilgamesh more than 4,000 years ago in Mesopotamia. This nightmare is one of the oldest of recorded stories:

> I took hold of a wild bull of the wilderness. He bellowed and kicked up earth; dust made the sky dark. I ran from him. With terrible strength he seized my flank. He tore out. . . . Besides my first dream I saw a second dream. In my dream, a mountain toppled. It laid me low and took hold of my feet. The glare was overpowering. . . . A man appeared, the handsomest in the land. . . . From under the mountain he pulled me out, gave me water to drink. . . . I saw a third dream and the dream I saw was in every way frightening. The heavens cried out; earth roared. Daylight vanished and darkness issued forth. Lightening flashed, fire broke out, clouds swelled; it rained death. The glow disappeared, the fire went out, and all that had fallen turned to ashes. (Gardner & Maier, 1984, p. 134)

This classic nightmare has consistent characteristics as described by Macnish (1834) in one of the first of modern texts to address sleep:

> Imagination cannot conceive the horror it frequently gives rise to, or language describe them in adequate terms. They are a thousand times more frightful than the visions conjured up by necromancy or diablerie . . . The whole mind, during the paroxysm is wrought up to a pitch of unutterable despair . . . the modifications which nightmare assumes are infinite, but one passion is almost never absent—that of utter and incomprehensible dread. (p. 138)

The Anglo Saxon/Indo-Germanic term *nightmare* is derived from Sanskrit roots and the concept of night-fiend or incubus/succubus—a creature able to suck out your soul during your sleep (Jones, 1923). Few other waking or sleeping experiences have such a negative reputation. It seems quite illogical that there could anything good about a state as horrible as a nightmare. Based on reputation, etymology, and experience, nightmares are sometimes viewed as adverse psychological events needing to be changed or eliminated (Krakow & Neidhart, 1992). It seems quite illogical that there could anything good about such a horrible state as a nightmare.

Negative Dreams and Nightmares

Bizarre negative dreams occurring during sleep are not always classic nightmares. Dreams from all sleep stages include negative content. Sleep-onset hallucinations and the deep-sleep parasomnias, especially night terrors, can be remarkably bizarre, including dream content that parodies that of the classic rapid eye movement (REM) sleep–associated nightmare (Pagel, 2014). Classic nightmares have the same typical narratives, but are usually of greater length and detail. They are also more likely to be perceived as terrifyingly real. But even such apparently classic nightmares can occur outside REM sleep, particularly in individuals with the diagnosis of posttraumatic stress disorder, or PTSD (Pagel & Neilsen, 2005). There is no clear correlate between REM sleep and dreaming. Dreams occur at high frequency outside REM sleep and twenty percent of REM sleep is dreamless (Foulkes, 1985). Nightmares, however, are more closely tied to REM sleep than are other dreams. For most of us, the vivid and classic nightmare of dread and imminent danger from which there is no escape except by waking is a REM sleep–associated dream.

Nightmare Incidence

Most of us occasionally experience nightmares. Nightmares are so common as to be considered "normal" experiences. On average, most of us will report the recall of dreams somewhere between once and three times a week, while most of us will experience at least one nightmare a month. In our sleep lab studies, 70.4% of patients report having at least one nightmare each month: N = 1,150, Mean Age = 49.6, Gender = 1.56 (F = 1 M = 2). (Pagel & Kwaitkowski, 2003; Pagel & Shocknasse, 2007; Pagel, 2010). But not everyone had nightmares. Individuals were significantly more likely to report never having experienced a nightmare (29.6%) than to report never having dreamed (9.6%). The dreamers reporting only positive dreams were slightly older but otherwise comparable to those with nightmares. Nightmares continue to be experienced on a regular basis even into extreme old age (Figure 13.1). Those individuals reporting very frequent nightmares (every night) are more likely to be female, and more likely to be young (Pagel & Vann, 1992).

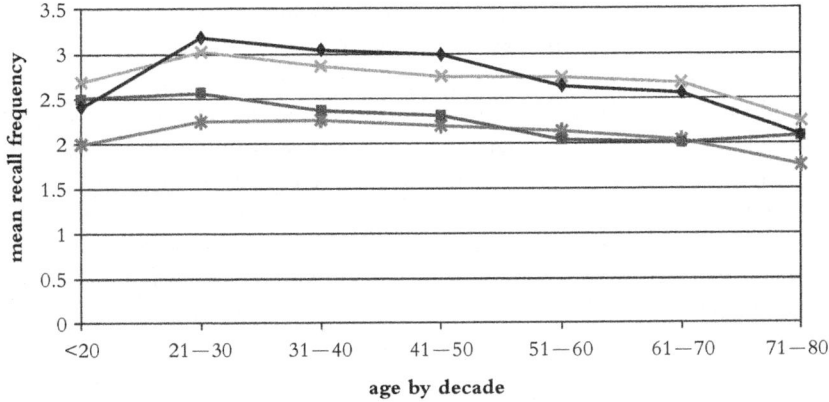

FIGURE 13.1 Reported dream recall by decade (diamond = female; cross = male) and nightmare recall (square = female; complex cross = male). Recall frequency is reported on a Likert scale in which never = 1, monthly = 2, weekly = 3, biweekly = 4, and nightly = 5.

The Nightmare as a Marker for Objectively Normal Sleep Insomnia

Insomnia is the complaint of difficulty initiating or maintaining sleep or the complaint of nonrestorative sleep that is associated with negative effects on waking function (Edinger et al., 2004). Nightmares often induce arousals and difficulty returning to sleep and, particularly in individuals with PTSD, can occur shortly after sleep onset and interfere with the initiation of sleep (Belicki et al., 1997). Most studies indicate that individuals with the complaint of insomnia are also more likely to report a higher frequency of nightmares (Ohayon & Morselli, 1994). Very few of these studies have evaluated by polysomnography, which would provide objective support for the subjective complaint of insomnia. In our sleep laboratory Shocknasse and I used polysomnography to access the objective sleep parameters of sleep latency, total sleep time (TST), sleep efficiency, wake after sleep onset (WASO), as well as sleep stage percentages (Pagel & Shocknasse, 2007). As in the other studies, the group complaining of insomnia reported a significantly higher frequency of nightmares. However, when we looked at the sleep laboratory data, this finding was not reflected in the objective data. Nightmare frequency was significantly higher for those with the best sleep who had longer sleep time, increased REM sleep time, increased light sleep (Stages 1 and 2), better sleep efficiency, and lower amounts of wake after sleep onset. Among individuals complaining of insomnia, the report of nightmares actually turned out to be a marker for better objective sleep. Nightmare recall was lowest in those with the lowest total sleep time, those who slept for less than 65% of the night, and for those who had the most time awake after sleep onset. Nightmare recall was also significantly lower among patients with the lowest amounts of REM sleep time. This study indicates that as sleep quality deteriorates, significantly fewer nightmares are reported, suggesting that in order for nightmares to occur, there must be a framework of sufficient sleep. That framework is likely to require at least some REM sleep if nightmares are to occur. Clinically, insomnia is most often a symptom, a complaint of poor, nonrestorative sleep rather than an objective lack of sleep that can be demonstrated in the sleep laboratory; as such, our findings remain consistent with other studies indicating that individuals with the complaint of insomnia report a higher incidence of nightmares. It is the complaint of poor-quality sleep rather than an objective decline in the measured amount and quality of sleep that is associated with increased nightmare frequency.

Sleep Apnea

Patients with sleep apnea will occasionally report nightmares of suffocation. Such reports were included among the earliest "scientific" descriptions of nightmares:

> The Nightmare generally seizes people sleeping on their backs, and often begins with frightful dreams, which are soon succeeded by a difficult respiration, a violent oppression of the breast, and a total privation of voluntary motion. In this agony they sigh, groan, utter indistinct sounds, and remain in the jaws of death, till, by the utmost efforts of nature, or some external assistance, they escape out of that dreadful torpid state. As soon as they shake off that vast oppression, and are able to move the body, they are affected with a strong Palpitation, great Anxiety, Languor, and Uneasiness; which symptoms gradually abate, and are succeeded by the pleasing reflection of having escaped such imminent danger. (Bond, 1753, p. 2)

However, such nightmares are not common. Among the many thousands of patients that we have evaluated in our sleep laboratory for sleep apnea, and asked for the content of their dreams and nightmares, a few have reported nightmares that could be ascribed to the experience of stopping breathing, based on content such as being buried alive or drowning. Perhaps the most specific was a nightmare of being stuffed into a stoppered bottle in which the patient turned blue. Yet few patients with sleep apnea have such nightmares. Most patients with severe apnea stop breathing for many seconds, some for minutes, before startling arousals that end with the loud snoring of resumed sleep. Sleep is resumed without conscious awakening and without reported nightmares.

Greater than 90% of our sleep laboratory patients are being evaluated for sleep apnea. When we asked these individuals how often they experienced nightmares, those with the worse sleep apnea (the most respiratory events and apneas during sleep) had the lowest incidence of nightmares (Pagel, 2010). Sleep laboratory

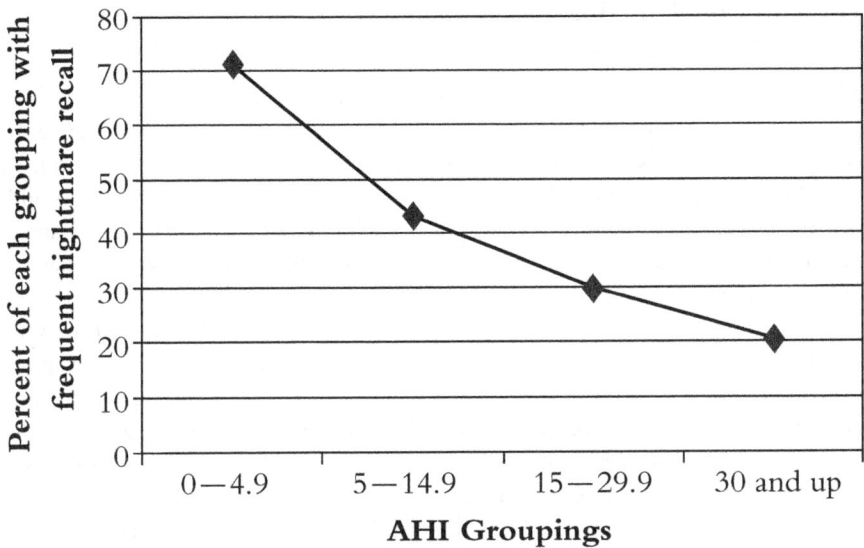

FIGURE 13.2 Nightmare recall by AHI groupings

patients reporting few dreams and nightmares (<1/month) had a significantly higher apnea hypopnea index (AHI) (mean 40.3) and apnea index (AI) (mean 21.0) compared to those reporting frequent nightmares (>1/week) (AHI 24.6 and AI 9.4) (p-value 0.000). For individuals reporting rare nightmares, the severity of sleep-disordered breathing as determined by AHI and AI was significantly worse. Apnea severity had no significant affect on their reported frequency of dream recall. The individuals meeting criteria for severe sleep apnea (an AHI greater than 30 per hour) had very few nightmares. The percentage of individuals reporting frequent nightmares (>1/week) declined significantly (p-value 0.000) with increasing AHI (Figure 13.2). I suspect that this finding is in part secondary to the reduced amount of REM sleep, since in patients with severe apnea sleep is so disrupted by the breathing disturbance that very little REM sleep can occur. With less REM sleep, it is apparently more difficult to have REM sleep–associated nightmares.

The insomnia and sleep apnea studies indicate that a basic framework, amount, and quality of sleep is necessary if nightmares are to occur. Individuals with objectively poor sleep as well as those with severe sleep apnea rarely report nightmares. From this perspective, nightmares can be a marker for good or better sleep. Patients with severe sleep apnea and objective insomnia have fewer nightmares. That does not mean that in any way that the nightmares of good sleep are less distressing than the nightmares of poor sleep. However, if you don't sleep, or if your sleep is of exceedingly poor quality, it is difficult to have nightmares.

The Potential Function for Nightmares in Emotional Processing

The high incidence and almost ubiquitous nature of the nightmare experience argues for the nightmare being a "normal" rather than pathologic experience. It also supports the possibility that nightmares could have a cognitive function. It would be extremely unusual for any species to preserve an apparently useless and negative psychological and physiological behavior through the many years since the beginnings of recorded history, if that behavior did not on some level have a survival function.

It has been suggested that nightmares might have an evolutionary function, simulating during sleep potential threats that are likely to occur during waking (Revonsuo, 2003). It is possible that such nightmares helped early humans to survive by rehearsing threat perception and avoidance without any biological cost. Living on the plains of Africa, among larger and more dangerous predatory species, early human life experience is likely to have been defined by the recurrent experience of trauma affecting both sleep and waking behavior. Today, however, it is less apparent how nightmares might have value in assisting us to avoid threats (Malcolm-Smith & Solms, 2004).

Nightmares are uncomfortable and distressing experiences. For some, particularly those with PTSD, nightmares can disrupt sleep and negatively affect the mood and behavior of the waking day. For individuals with the diagnosis of PTSD, that affect is often one of waking distress (Zadra & Donderi, 2000). For traumatized individuals, nightmares seem overwhelmingly negative—the essence of fear and the memory of a disturbing experience. Nightmares, among the most impactful and significant of all dreams, will often affect our next-day mood and waking behavior. Sigmund Freud (1916/1951) suggested that symptoms characteristic of PTSD most often occur after the experience of a trauma of indigestible intensity:

> We describe as "traumatic" any excitations from outside which are powerful enough to break through the protective shield. It seems to me that the concept of trauma necessarily implies a connection of this kind with a breach in an otherwise efficacious barrier against stimuli. Such an event as an external trauma is bound to provoke a disturbance on a large scale in the functioning of an organism's energy and to set in motion every defensive measure ... there is no longer any possibility of preventing the mental apparatus from being flooded with large amounts of stimulus (p. 14).

The association of nightmares with PTSD suggests that the emotional processing functioning during normal dreaming is overwhelmed by such trauma, resulting in recurrent, distressing nightmares (Kramer, 1993).

It has been suggested that REM sleep dreams such as nightmares may have a functional role in the processing of the emotions associated with negative life experiences (Levin & Nielsen, 2007). After sleep that includes dreaming, waking emotional mood is known to change. Pre-sleep mood is different from post-sleep mood, with the variability and intensity of emotion decreasing across the night (Cartwright, Luten, Young, Mercer, & Bears, 1998; Kramer, 2007). For many dreamers, this change in affect is in the positive direction. In individuals with PTSD, however, the change is in the opposite direction, with negative dreams potentially producing nighttime insomnia and waking distress (Levin & Nielsen, 2007). PTSD is a condition that clearly alters REM sleep, inducing increased REM sleep pressure (i.e., a higher tendency to go into REM sleep when able to sleep). Imaging studies indicate that the areas processing fear and negative emotions have increased activity during REM sleep (Nofzinger, 2004). This REM sleep/PTSD association supports the postulate that REM sleep functions in emotional regulation. Levin and Nielsen (2007) have proposed that PTSD nightmares are secondary to the failure of a system of fear-memory extinction that functions during REM sleep dreaming. Trauma-related nightmares that persist over time and continue to generate distress could reflect a failure of this process.

There are, however, known aspects of the nightmare experience that fit poorly into this theoretic construct: (1) Almost all dreams from all stages of sleep include emotional content. Since emotional dreams occur in all stages of sleep, it is doubtful that emotional neural-processing is limited to REM sleep. While it is possible that the processing of negative emotions during sleep is restricted to REM sleep, there is little other evidence supporting the theoretic postulate (Pagel, 2014). (2) PTSD nightmares often occur outside REM sleep, also supporting this contention that emotional processing during sleep is not restricted to REM sleep. It is likely that PTSD nightmares are secondary to an individual's inability to process severe and overwhelming experiences of trauma. That emotional processing does not appear to be limited to a particular stage of sleep (Pilar, Malhotra, & Lavie, 2000). (3) Nightmares are reported to occur regularly (>1/month) by up to 70% of the population (Pagel & Kwaitkowski, 2003; Pagel & Shocknasse, 2007; Pagel, 2010). Occasional nightmares are a "normal" experience. Nightmares are, however, also reported by patients with a variety of psychiatric illnesses. While the evidence is far form clear, there are suggestions that nightmares are reported more often by patients with diagnoses including insomnia, depression, neuroticism, schizotypy, psychosis, and PTSD (Li et al., 2014). The number of published studies on particular associations between nightmares and psychiatric illnesses has tended to follow the generally accepted theoretic perspectives of nightmares. During the time periods when nightmares were viewed as hallucinatory/psychotic experiences, published studies suggested that nightmares were more common in patients with psychosis and schizotypy (Claridge, Clark, & Davis, 1997). More recently studies have focused on the association of nightmares with trauma; this work emphasizes the concomitant presence of nightmares in suicidal individuals as well as in those with PTSD (Nadorff, Nazem, & Fiske, 2014).

The distress associated with the experience of the nightmare can sometimes be profound, leading to suggestions that treating nightmares might be helpful in the treatment of both PTSD and depression (Pigeon, Campbell, Possemato, & Ouimette, 2014). But even for individuals with severe trauma-associated PTSD, the nightmare is a symptom rather than a cause of the disorder. What we most clearly understand of dream content, including nightmares, is its continuity with waking experience. Individuals with psychiatric diagnoses by definition have a waking experience that is both difficult and distressing. It is unsurprising that their dreams should be difficult and distressing as well.

In the popular medical press the theoretic perspective that REM sleep has a primary function in emotional processing has been extended to the suggestion that any medication that suppresses REM sleep is likely contraindicated in patients with PTSD (Walker, 2009b). Quoting Matthew Walker, "one of the functions of REM sleep is to tell the brain to sift through the days events, process the negative emotions attached to them, then strip it away from memories" (Walker 2009a). This somewhat simplistic view of a complex postulate suggests that REM sleep somehow acts as a filter during sleep to strain out the negative emotions of waking life experience. The medications most likely to suppress REM sleep include benzodiazepines and antidepressants. These are currently among the few drugs that have shown positive results in the treatment of PTSD. Currently we are faced with a "suicide epidemic" among soldiers suffering form PTSD who are returning home from conflict. It seems disingenuous to suggest that drugs used to treat their anxiety and depression should be discontinued based on such an unproven theoretic construct.

The history of the association of PTSD with nightmares is a cautionary tale. Therapists became convinced, based on their training and the prevalent theoretic perspectives, that frequent nightmares indicated the presence of underlying suppressed trauma even in individuals with no obvious history of trauma. That trauma was most often presumed to be unremembered and suppressed childhood sexual abuse. Intensive exploratory psychotherapy was initiated in order to identify the hidden traumatic origin of the reported nightmares. This approach led to therapeutic support for memories, sometimes false, that could have produced the experienced nightmares. Treatment frequently included family confrontation and resultant disarray. This approach is clearly inappropriate when applied to individuals with nightmare disorder, who have frequent nightmares and no history of trauma. For most individuals who have nightmares, they are neither a marker nor an indication that significant trauma, physical, psychiatric, or spiritual disorders are present. By far, the majority of us will at least occasionally experience a nightmare. For most of us, nightmares are a "normal" experience.

Nightmare Use in the Creative Process

Nightmares from throughout our recorded history of being human have been incorporated into some of our greatest narrative and pictorial art. The cave art found in southern Europe suggests that this is a process that likely extends

35,000 years ago into the Paleolithic era. There are nightmares in our most ancient literature, nightmares incorporated into our holy books, our ancient myths, and the Icelandic sagas. Grimm's fairy tales form an index of Germanic nightmares. Beowulf, for the Danes, is a description of a monster likely to have come from a nightmare. Coleridge worked from his nightmares, as did Poe, Robert Louis Stevenson, and perhaps most famously Mary Shelley (Buckley, 2009). Nightmare art forms an artistic genre, extending from the skewered bodies and human/animal combinations of cave art and rock petroglyphs of prehistory, to Hieronymus Bosch, Goya, Fussili, Picasso, and Salvador Dali, and into the art of our present day (Van de Castle, 1994).

Nightmares appear likely to have at least one important function, in what is perhaps humanity's most important species survival characteristic—our creativity. Nightmares, those horrifying dreams of fear and despair, when used in creative process can sometimes contribute to a remarkably beneficial effect on the achieved results of that work. Individuals with artistic and flexible personal approaches to their exterior world are those most likely to experience nightmares. Indeed, there are suggestions, beyond Freud, that nightmares can be used in creativity, potentially contributing to the diversity and extent of individual experience. Nightmares provide the dreamer access to the dark side of this world. The nightmare experience can be the concrete metaphor of horror, or a version of reflective fantasy. As James Hillman (1972) points out, even experiences of apparent psychopathology such as nightmares can be essential for "normal" functioning in our psychological lives:

> Concretism obscures the light and blocks the movement of fantasy. . . . From this perspective, a pure spark of reflective life must be kept intact at all costs. A spontaneous insight gives the freedom to move away from nature's oppression and igniting the capacity to imagine life and not only to be driven by it. (p. 55)

The Sundance Filmmaker Studies

At the Sundance film labs, my colleagues and I worked with successful filmmakers, actors, and screenwriters. When we began these studies, we were aware of Ernest Hartmann's work indicating that artistic personality types were more likely to have frequent nightmares (Hartmann, 1984, 1991, 1998) and anecdotal reports suggesting that dreaming might have a role in the creative aspects of filmmaking. At Sundance, questionnaires and interviews indicated that these successful filmmakers recalled and used their dreams and nightmares at an even higher frequency than we had expected (Pagel, Kwiakowski, & Broyles, 1999). Since filmmaking is a group endeavor requiring diverse roles, we were able to compare the responses of individuals in working roles (support crew, drivers, and assistants) to the responses from technically trained professionals (cinematographers, producers, editors, executive producers, and script supervisors) and from the individuals in what we considered to be the most highly creative roles (actors, screen writers, and directors). Individuals in creative roles turned out to have significantly higher nightmare recall compared to the working group. The responses from the professionals were somewhere in between. Overall dream/nightmare use was significantly higher for the creative group compared to the working group. When we compared these results to those from our earlier general population studies, we found that dream/nightmare use for all filmmaking groups was significantly higher (Pagel & Vann, 1992; Pagel et al., 1999). While overall, creative process was one of the highest responses, the affects of dreaming on behavior were not limited to the creative aspects of these individuals' work. The incorporation of dreams into waking life was global, with responses significantly higher for 12 of the 17 waking behaviors queried. This waking use of dreams and nightmares varied in part based on creative role, and the increased use was associated with an increase in both dream and nightmare recall (Pagel et al., 1999). The Sundance studies indicated that individuals successful in their creative roles report a higher frequency of nightmares and are more likely to use them in their creative process. Almost all of these successfully creative individuals had nightmares and used them in their work.

We expanded on this study by asking individuals in our sleep laboratory population to describe their creative process as well as to rate their levels of creative interest on a 0–5 scale ranging from 0 = "no creative process" to 5 = "income-producing life focus" (Pagel & Kwiakowski, 2003). The results of this study indicated that individuals reporting any creative interest were significantly more likely to use their dreams and nightmares than those reporting no creative interest. The group with creative interest (N = 424) also had a significantly higher incidence of nightmares when compared to the grouping reporting no creative interest (N = 58). Their use of nightmares extended into many aspects of waking behavior beyond their use in creativity. We compared the 26% of our laboratory patients who (at least on questionnaire) reported never having had a nightmare to the 10% who reported at least two nightmares each week. Individuals with frequent nightmares were more likely to use their dreams in their waking behaviors—particularly in their relationships, setting goals, adapting to stress, and in planning for the future.

Positive Aspects of the Classic Nightmare: Conclusion

It is an ancient and persistent view that nightmares are indicative of underlying spiritual and/or psychiatric illness. Nightmares are often reported by individuals who score abnormally on psychological tests as well as on screening tests for the diagnoses of insomnia, depression, neuroticism, schizotypy, psychosis, and PTSD (Krakow et al., 2001; Li et al., 2014; Claridge et al., 1997). The theoretical perspective that nightmares reflect a functional failure in emotional processing also supports the pathological role for nightmares (Levin & Nielsen, 2007). These studies have led to suggestions that nightmares be treated in otherwise psychiatrically and spiritually healthy individuals in order to help in preventing the onset of potential psychiatric illness (Krakow et al., 2006; Erman 1995). There is evidence suggesting that nightmares can be a symptom of some psychiatric illnesses. But these nightmares are associated with the illnesses; they are not the cause of these illnesses. There is no evidence suggesting that treating nightmares can prevent psychiatric illness.

Nightmares require a basic framework, amount, and quality of sleep if they are to occur. Individuals with objectively poor sleep as well as those with severe sleep apnea rarely report nightmares. From this perspective, having nightmares is a marker for objectively better sleep. If you don't sleep, or if your sleep is of exceedingly poor quality, it is difficult to have nightmares (Pagel & Shocknasse, 2007; Pagel, 2010).

Nightmares have a role in creativity. Individuals with nightmares are more likely than others to have a creative or artistic focus in their daily lives (Hartmann, 1984, 1991, 1998). There is little question that writers, painters, and filmmakers use their nightmares as inspiration for their work (Pagel et al., 1999). Sometimes they successfully utilize these nightmares in creative careers (Pagel & Kwiakowski, 2003). Individuals with a higher frequency of nightmares also have higher levels of dream recall, and they are more likely to use both their dreams and nightmares in a wide spectrum of waking behaviors (Pagel & Vann, 1992; Pagel et al., 1999; Pagel & Kwiakowski, 2003). Nightmares are uncomfortable and distressing experiences, even for the artists who use nightmares as their muse, yet nightmares can be utilized in a positive fashion when used in a creative process.

Most of our dreams include negative content (Kramer, 2007). Some of the most negative dreams are those that we call nightmares. For many of us, one of the psychodynamics of sleep can be an opportunity to escape from the unresolved problems of the day. In the nightmare, however, we wake to escape from the unresolved horrors and problems of the night (Hillman, 1972). If we are very lucky, we will never experience the same level of negative cognitive or behavioral stress during waking that we commonly experience during the amazing and remarkable dreams that we call our nightmares.

References

Belicki K, Chambers E, Ogilvie R. Sleep quality and nightmares. Sleep Research 1997:26;63.
Bond J. An Essay on the Incubus or Nightmare. 1753.
Buckley K. Dreaming and the World's Religions, New York, New York University Press, 2009.
Cartwright R, Luten A, Young M, Mercer P, Bears M. Role of REM sleep affect in overnight mood regulation: a study of normal volunteers. Psychiatry Research 1998:81; 1–8.

Claridge G, Clark K, Davis C. Nightmares, dreams and schizotypy. British Journal of Clinical Psychology 1997:36;377–386.

Edinger J (Chair); Work group members: Bonnet M, Bootzin R, Doghramp K, Dorsey C, Espie C, Jamieson A, McCall W, Morin C, Stepanski E. Derivation of research diagnostic criteria for insomnia: Report of an American Academy of Sleep Medicine work group. Sleep 2004;27;1567–1592.

Ermann M. Die Traumerinnerinnerung bei Patienten mit psychogenen Schlafstorungen: Empirische Befunde und einige Folgerungen fur das Verstandis des Traumens. In W Leuschner, S Hau (Eds.), Traum und Gedachtnis: Neue Ergebisse aus psychologischer, psychoanalytischer, und neurophysiologischer Forschung. Munster, LIT Verlag, 1995, pp. 165–86.

Foulkes D. Dreaming: A Cognitive-Psychological Analysis. Hillsdale, NJ, Lawrence Erlbaum Associates, 1985.

Freud S. Beyond the Pleasure Principle, Vol 18, The Standard Edition. J. Strachey, (Trans. & Ed.), London, Hogarth, 1916/1951, p. 14.

Gardner J, Maier, J (Trans.). Gilgamesh. New York, Knopf, 1984.

Hartmann E. The Nightmare. New York, Basic Books, 1984.

Hartmann E. Boundaries in the Mind: A New Psychology of Personality. New York, Basic Books, 1991.

Hartmann E. Dreams and Nightmares: The New Theory on the Origin and Meaning of Dreams. New York, Plenum Trade, 1998.

Hillman J. Pan and the Nightmare, Putnam, Connecticut, Spring. 1972.

Jones E. On the Nightmare. London, Hogarth Press, 1923, p.320–339.

Krakow B. Nightmare complaints in treatment-seeking patients in clinical sleep medicine settings: diagnostic and treatment implications. Sleep 2006:29;1313–1319.

Krakow B, Melendrez D, Pedersen B, et. al. Complex insomnia: insomnia and sleep-disordered breathing in a consecutive series of crime victims with nightmares and PTSD. Biological Psychiatry 2001:49;948–53.

Krakow B, Neidhart E. Conquering Bad Dreams and Nightmares: A Guide to Understanding Interpretation and Cure. New York, Berkley Books, 1992.

Kramer M. The selective mood regulatory function of dreaming: an update and revision, In A Moffitt, M Kramer, R Hoffmann (Eds.), The Functions of Dreaming. Albany, State University of New York Press, 1993, p. 139–196.

Kramer M. The Dream Experience: A Systematic Exploration. New York, Routledge, 2007, p. 102.

Levin R, Nielsen T. Disturbed dreaming, posttraumatic stress disorder, and affect distress: A review and neurocognitive model. Psychological Bulletin, 2007:133;482–528.

Li S. Yu M. Lam S. Zhang J. Li A. Lai K. Wing Y. Frequent nightmares in children: Familial aggregation and associations with parent reported behavioral and mood problems. Sleep 2014:34;487–493.

Macnish R. The Philosophy of Sleep. Glasgow, WR McPhun,1834.

Malcolm-Smith S, Solms M. Incidence of threat in dreams: A response to Revonsuo's threat simulation theory. Dreaming 2004:14;220–229.

Nadorff M, Nazem S, Fiske A. Insomnia symptoms, nightmares, and suicidal ideation in a college student sample. Sleep 2014:34;93–98.

Nofzinger E. What can neuroimaging findings tell us about sleep disorders? Sleep Medicine 5 (suppl 1) 2004:S16–S22.

Ohayon M, Morselli N. Nightmares: Their relation with insomnia, mental illness and diurnal functioning. Sleep Research 1994:23;171.

Pagel JF. The nightmares of sleep apnea: Nightmare frequency declines with increasing Apnea Hypopnea Index (AHI). Journal of Clinical Sleep Medicine 2010:6;69–74.

Pagel JF. Dream Science: Exploring the Forms of Consciousness. Oxford, UK, Academic Press, 2014.

Pagel JF, Kwiatkowski CF. Creativity and dreaming: Correlation of reported dream incorporation into awake behavior with level and type of creative interest. Creativity Research Journal 2003:15;199–205.

Pagel JF, Kwiatkowski C, Broyles K. Dream use in film making. Dreaming 1999:9;247–296.

Pagel JF, Nielsen T. Parasomnias: Recurrent nightmares. In The International Classification of Sleep Disorders: Diagnostic and Coding Manual (ICD-11). Darien, IL, American Academy of Sleep Medicine, 2005.

Pagel JF, Shocknasse S. Dreaming and insomnia: Polysomnographic correlates of reported dream recall frequency. Dreaming 2007:17;140–151.

Pagel JF, Vann B. The effects of dreaming on awake behavior. Dreaming 1992:2;229–237.

Pigeon W, Campbell C, Possemato K, Ouimette P. Longitudinal relationships of insomnia, nightmares and PTSD severity in recent combat veterans. Journal of Psychosomatic Research 2014:75;546–550.

Pilar G, Malhotra A, Lavie P. Post-traumatic stress disorder and sleep—what a nightmare! Sleep Medicine Review 2000:4;183–200.

Revonsuo A. The reinterpretation of dreams: An evolutionary hypothesis of the function of dreaming. In E Pace-Schott, M Solms, M Blagrove, S Harnad (Eds.) Sleep and Dreaming: Scientific Advances and Reconsiderations. Cambridge, UK, Cambridge University Press, 2003, pp. 85–111.

Van de Castle R. Our Dreaming Mind: A Sweeping Exploration of the Role that Dreams have Played in Politics, Art, Religion and Psychology, from Ancient Civilizations to the Present Day. New York, Ballantine Books, 1994.

Walker MP. The role of sleep in cognition and emotion. Annals of the New York Academy of Sciences 2009a:1156;168–97.

Walker M: Interview, Staples T. Wish fulfillment? No. But dreams do have meaning. Time. June 15, 2009b. www.time.com/time/health/article/0,8599,190451,00.html last accessed 8/11/2009.

Zadra A, Donderi D. Nightmares and bad dreams: Their prevalence and relationship to well-being. Journal of Abnormal Psychology 2000:109;273–281.

14

THE CONTRASTING EFFECTS OF NIGHTMARES, EXISTENTIAL DREAMS, AND TRANSCENDENT DREAMS

Don Kuiken

UNIVERSITY OF ALBERTA

The Contrasting Effects of Nightmares, Existential Dreams, and Transcendent Dreams

Bert States (1997) proposed that *some* dreams have "magnitude" (p. 238). His term superficially resembles Jung's reference to "big" dreams (e.g., Jung, 1966, p. 117), which involve mythological motifs (e.g., encounters with spiritual beings), abstract geometric patterns (e.g., mandalas), and transcendent otherness (e.g., a numinous presence). But for States, magnitude more nearly resembles the "size" that Aristotle (1998) attributed to tragic predicaments, which involve the core of a person's prospects for well-being (e.g., irreconcilable moral conflicts), an acute sense of human vulnerability (e.g., exposed limitations), and cathartic pity and terror (e.g., restorative grief). States (1997, pp. 246–250) compares the magnitude of the following dream with the concluding scene from *King Lear*:

> I was running along a path toward a house where some friends were having an afternoon gathering. . . . I was joining the group with very positive expectations. Then suddenly, on a path parallel to my own, slightly below it, I saw a finch speeding along on the ground in the opposite direction, much like the Roadrunner in the cartoon. The finch was a brilliant green-yellow color, as delicate as a Christmas ornament, and it seemed mechanically propelled. Inexplicably, I found a large pebble in my hand and I tossed it back over my head, almost aimlessly, in the bird's direction. No sooner was the pebble in flight than I conceived the consequence, and I shouted, "No!" But the bird was already squeaking aloud in pain; the pebble had clearly severed one of its wings and it was vainly flapping the other wing in a pathetic effort to right itself. I now saw that the bird was made of flesh and there was no undoing the damage I had done. I began to howl. (States, 1997; pp. 238–239)

After extended reflection, including comparison with the moment of his sister's death and with Lear's plaintive words for the dead Cordelia, States concludes that his dream was "grief incarnate" (p. 245). While differentiable from the numinous rapture of Jung's big dreams, the nature of this dream's magnitude remains ambiguous. The desperate "No," the painful "squeaking," and the agonizing "howl" suggest *nightmarish* dread. And yet, the agonizing *sadness* that concludes States's dream is unlike the stark *fear* that normally enfolds nightmare imagery (Robert & Zadra, 2014). So, is the "magnitude" of States' dream merely an alternative term for nightmare "intensity"? Or is it qualitatively different? In the context of contemporary dream studies, this is not an idle question.

During the last two decades, nightmare-centred threat, fear, and defence have virtually defined theories of dream formation and function. Hartmann (1998) argued that nightmares after trauma are "prototypic" of "the same process [that] occurs in all dreams" (p. 33). Revonsuo (2000) stressed the centrality of a threat-triggered mnemonic system that regulates "fear or defensive responses" (p. 887). Domhoff (2003) placed repetitive posttraumatic nightmares at one end of a continuum that "fits with the persistence of negative memories stored in the vigilance/fear system" (p. 28). Nielsen and Levin (2007) emphasized that dreaming reflects the construction of extinction memories through which fear memories, including their emotional concomitants, become inhibited. Even without denying the importance of posttraumatic dreams and nightmares, the preceding models overemphasize traumatic distress and potentially overlook the influence of other emotion-coordinating systems on dreaming and dream function. At the very least they do not address the effects of the separate system that mediates separation distress (Panksepp, 2005)—and that may mediate dreams expressive of "grief incarnate."

Overgeneralized models of traumatic stress exacerbate the problem. Much contemporary research has characterized traumatic stress as a common response to threat and violence (e.g., physical abuse) *and* separation and loss (e.g., death of a parent; Figley, Bride, & Mazza, 1997; Green, 2000). However, it is increasingly clear that the traumatic stress model assimilates loss to trauma at the expense of research and clinical understandings of bereavement (Raphael & Martinek, 1997; Stroebe & Schut, 2005–2006). Although both involve intrusive thoughts in *some* form (e.g., repetitive thoughts about the trauma or loss) and avoidance in *some* form (e.g., staying away from reminders of the trauma or loss), the role of hyperarousal within traumatic distress is distinctively associated with amygdala-mediated vigilance. The role of hyperarousal in dreams involving traumatic distress is differentiable from the role of separation distress (e.g., the sense of a foreshortened future) in the generation of very differently expressive dream patterns (Kuiken, Chudleigh, & Racher, 2010).

Similar conceptual tension is evident in the definition of nightmares in the *Diagnostic and Statistical Manual of Mental Disorders, Fifth Edition (DSM-5)* (APA, 2013), especially in the symptom descriptions for Posttraumatic Stress Disorder

(PTSD) and Separation Anxiety Disorder. First, nightmares are generically defined as "story-like sequences of dream imagery that . . . incite anxiety, fear, or *other dysphoric emotions*" (italics mine, p. 404). Then, symptoms of PTSD are said to include nightmares "*thematically related to the major threats* involved in the traumatic event" (italics mine, p. 282), while symptoms of Separation Anxiety Disorder purportedly include nightmares involving "the *theme of separation*" and "*separation anxiety*" (italics mine, pp. 191–192). Reference to "other dysphoric emotions" in the generic definition of nightmares seems a (clumsy) conceptual extension enabling nightmares thematically related to separation distress to be included in the same category as nightmares thematically related to traumatic distress.

Monothetic and Polythetic Oneiric Categories

Throughout the literature just mentioned, attempts to define nightmares have involved search for a minimal set of attributes (e.g., dream imagery, dysphoric emotion, immediate awakening with recall) each of which is necessary and the combination of which is sufficient for identifying nightmares (cf. Robert & Zadra, 2014). Such *monothetic* approaches to definitional specificity run several risks: (1) the minimal set of attributes of the class often excludes other relevant attributes (e.g., the frequency of physical aggression in nightmares); (2) selection of that minimal set of attributes often reflects investigator presuppositions, rather than empirical observation (e.g., the "invisibility" of sadness in nightmares); and (3) stipulation of an "essential" set of attributes often leads to false negatives. The latter problem is evident in attempts to distinguish "nightmares" from "bad dreams" on the basis of whether intensely disturbing emotions induce immediate awakening and recall. Hasler and Germain (2009) point out that differences between nightmare intensity and bad dream intensity are small and that the reported absence of immediate awakening with recall after bad dreams is subject to distortion. More telling, though, is that bad dreams involve *different* emotions (e.g., anger) and themes (e.g., interpersonal conflict) than do nightmares (Robert & Zadra, 2014), suggesting that current monothetic definitions of nightmares and bad dreams potentially obscure qualitatively different phenomena. Thus, although the search for monothetic definitional specificity is commonplace in nightmare studies (and throughout neo-positivist psychological science), it may be as ill-suited to its definitional (and classificatory) objectives as it historically has been in taxonomic studies in the biological sciences. The search for a monothetic definition of nightmares (or, for that matter, bad dreams) is much like asking for the "operational definition" of a dolphin.

In general, a contrasting *polythetic* approach to definitional specificity has guided the emergence of biological taxonomies and perhaps should be considered in attempts to attain definitional precision in dream studies. For example, the approach to identifying nightmares might well be guided by classificatory objectives according to which (cf. Beckner, 1959):

1. Each instance of the category "nightmare" is expected to have a large number of distinctive (or at least differentiating) attributes;
2. Each attribute in that array is expected to be an attribute of many instances of the category "nightmare"; and
3. No attribute in that array is expected to be an attribute of every instance of the category "nightmare."

By virtue of the third criterion, no attribute is strictly invariant (necessary); by virtue of the second criterion, each attribute is only more-or-less invariant; and by virtue of the first criterion, the systematic *comparison* of entities across a large number of their attributes becomes the empirical mode of access to these categories. Such comparative category articulation requires the assessment of degrees of similarity, primarily because the degree of similarity between two or more category instances depends upon how *many* parts of each are "the same." This orientation toward category articulation is also found in phenomenological philosophy (Husserl, 1948/1973, §45, p. 193), affirming the relevance of this orientation for the study of *experiential* narratives in the psychological sciences (Kuiken & Miall, 2001).

To some extent, the *polythetic* approach to category articulation has also guided the evolution of diagnostic categories in the *DSM-5* (APA, 2013, p. 733). The diagnostic criteria for PTSD illustrate the structure of a polythetic class: the enduring and disturbing conjunction of (1) at least one of four kinds of exposure to actual or threatened death, injury, or violence; (2) at least one of five types of intrusion symptoms; (3) at least one of two forms of avoidance symptoms; (4) at least two of seven altered mood or cognition symptoms; and (5) at least two of six hyperarousal symptoms. It is not difficult to imagine comparably structured *polythetic* definitional specificity for nightmares, although the taxonomic procedures that facilitate articulation of polythetic categories are not routinely included in nightmare investigators' methodological repertoire. Nonetheless, rather than stipulating monothetic category boundaries, it is important to delineate empirically the polythetic boundaries of the category "nightmare"—as well as other categories of dreams that are "big," "intense," or have "magnitude."

Classificatory Studies of Impactful Dreams

The *polythetic* approach to definitional specificity has shaped the design of a series of classificatory studies of impactful dreams conducted at the University of Alberta. In the first such study, Kuiken and Sikora (1993) asked participants to describe dreams that continued to influence their thoughts and feelings even after awakening. Then, similarly expressed meanings were identified through systematic close reading and comparison of the dream narratives (e.g., descriptions of sudden scene shifts, descriptions of recurrent attempts to avoid harm), rather than according to a priori conceptions (cf. Kuiken & Miall, 2001; Kuiken, Schopflocher, & Wild, 1989).

The presence or absence of these similarly expressed meanings was combined with participant ratings (e.g., of emotion) to create matrices that, when cluster analyzed, yielded polythetic categories. Thus, instances of each category shared a substantial number of experiential attributes; each attribute described many instances of the category; and no attribute was invariant across instances of each category.

These classificatory procedures revealed three types of impactful dreams, each distinguishable by coherent profiles of attributes involving emotions, sensory phenomena, movement characteristics, motives and goals, and dream endings. A category called "nightmares" included dreams with vivid tactile-kinesthetic imagery, vivid or unusual sounds, physical metamorphoses, energetic activity, harm avoidance, and intense fear during the transition to wakefulness; a category called "existential dreams" included dreams with vivid tactile-kinesthetic imagery, light/dark contrasts, ineffectual movement (fatigue), separation and loss, spontaneous affective shifts, and intense sadness during the transition to wakefulness; and a category called "transcendent dreams" included dreams with vivid tactile-kinesthetic imagery, spreading warmth, unusual sources of light, felt vitality, flying and floating, magical accomplishment, perspective shifts, and awe and ecstasy during the transition to wakefulness. Nightmares, existential dreams, and transcendent dreams all differ from mundane dreams; involve intense affect at the moment of awakening; and include imagery that seems "real" even after awakening.

Busink and Kuiken (1996) replicated the Kuiken and Sikora study, using the recurrently expressed meanings identified in the first study as content analytic categories, and found the same three polythetic dream categories (nightmares, existential dreams, and transcendent dreams). Later, Kuiken, Lee, Eng, and Singh (2006) identified these three dream types by cluster analyzing questionnaire items based on the recurrent expressed meanings and rating scales that differentiated the basic dream types in the first two studies. Most recently, Lee and Kuiken (in press) estimated the average attribute profile for each dream category, enabling use of a profile-matching strategy to identify dream types in a new sample. In sum, across this series of studies, the same three polythetic dream categories (nightmares, existential dreams, and transcendent dreams) have consistently been observed.

Emotion Contrasts Across Polythetic Dream Categories

Because of the pivotal role of emotion intensity in generic definitions of nightmares, it is useful to examine more closely the emotions that differentiate nightmares, existential dreams, and transcendent dreams from each other (and from mundane dreams). In doing so, it is also useful to move beyond (1) the usual nightmare-centered characterization of emotion categories (e.g., "anxiety, fear, [and] other dysphoric emotions"; *DSM-5*), (2) the restricted array of emotions that dreamers *spontaneously* describe in open-ended dream reports (e.g., Robert & Zadra, 2014), and (3) the presupposition that a single primary emotion characterizes each dream category. In a recent study of 174 impactful dreams reported online immediately

TABLE 14.1 Distinctive Feelings and Emotions for Each Polythetic Dream Category

	Mundane dreams (n = 54)	Transcendent dreams (n = 22)	Nightmares (n = 41)	Existential dreams (n = 57)
Scared/terrified	0.30^d	1.91^c	*3.34^a*	2.72^b
Sad/downhearted	0.82^c	1.32^{bc}	1.32^b	*3.44^a*
Ecstatic/in awe	0.83^b	*2.64^a*	0.46^b	0.51^b
Vulnerable/helpless	0.96^c	1.73^b	*3.17^a*	*3.11^a*
Nervous/anxious	1.24^c	1.91^b	*3.02^a*	*2.91^a*
Guilty/ashamed	0.35^b	0.18^b	0.63^b	*2.02^a*
Despair/discouraged	0.70^c	0.96^{bc}	1.49^b	*2.81^a*
Angry/frustrated	0.85^c	1.14^{bc}	1.73^b	*2.51^a*
Lost/disoriented	1.02^c	1.59^b	*2.32^a*	*2.44^a*
Inadequate/failed	0.67^{bc}	0.18^c	0.88^b	*1.53^a*
Disgusted/repulsed	0.46^b	0.59^b	0.71^b	*1.32^a*
Powerful/competent	0.85^b	*1.68^a*	0.20^c	0.26^c
Happy/joyful	1.69^a	1.68^a	0.34^b	0.19^b
Hopeful/optimistic	1.57^a	1.55^a	0.22^b	0.28^b
Peaceful/calm	1.50^a	1.32^a	0.22^b	0.25^b
Longing/yearning	1.04^a	1.00^a	*0.22^b*	1.37^a
Relieved/made safe	1.02^a	1.23^a	0.49^b	0.39^b
Affectionate/loving	1.26^a	1.32^a	0.20^b	0.47^b

Note. Means with different superscripts within rows differ significantly from each other ($p < .05$; LSD).

after awakening, participants rated the intensity of each of the 18 emotions (e.g., scared/terrified, sad/downhearted; from 0 = "not at all" to 4 = "extremely") used in Hartmann's (2013) scheme for assessing central image intensity. As indicated in Table 14.1, this approach reveals a level of emotional complexity that would not otherwise be evident.

Nightmare Emotions

As expected (because it is one of the attributes that defines this polythetic category), scared/terrified was a *distinctive* nightmare attribute. No other emotion category differentiated nightmares from existential dreams, transcendent dreams, *and* mundane dreams. This pattern is broadly compatible with the results of prior studies of nightmare emotions (cf. Table 1 in Robert & Zadra, 2014). However, two emotions sometimes attributed to nightmares were *not* distinctively nightmarish. Specifically, nervous/anxious was equally characteristic of nightmares *and* existential dreams (which at least complicates the generic definition of nightmares in *DSM-5*), and vulnerable/helpless was equally characteristic of nightmares and existential dreams (which complicates Hartmann's [1998] attribution of this emotion to nightmares).[1]

Finally, yearning/longing is an emotion whose *absence* is distinctively characteristic of nightmares. Although the absence of an attribute is not usually considered a useful definitional criterion, this possibility becomes salient in the comparative procedures used to identify polythetic dream categories. In this case, an absence is informative; the distinctive absence of yearning/longing in nightmares may help to explain their *lack* of quasi-therapeutic benefit. Clinical wisdom and psychotherapy research (e.g., Diamond, Rochman, & Amir, 2010) suggest that anxious anger *without* shifts to unexpressed sadness is incompatible with progress in psychotherapy. The absence of yearning/longing, then, is consistent with other evidence (see the discussion of Contrasting Carryover Effects on pp. 182–184) that nightmares are *not* endogenous "quasi-therapeutic" events.

Existential Dream Emotions

As expected (because it is one of the attributes that defines this polythetic category), sad/downhearted was a *distinctive* attribute of existential dreams. Two other emotion categories also differentiated existential dreams from nightmares, transcendent dreams, *and* mundane dreams. First, guilty/ashamed was associated with existential dreams, a finding consistent with prior classificatory studies (Busink & Kuiken, 1996; Kuiken & Sikora, 1993; Kuiken et al., 2006). Second, inadequate/failed was associated with existential dreams, which is congruent with prior evidence that, in existential dreams, the dreamer is tired, weak, or unable to move and unable to attain his/her goals. Whether inadequate/failed should be considered a kinaesthetic aspect of movement ineffectuality, a negative outcome of dream actions, and/or an emotion requires closer consideration.

Finally, the distinctively high ratings for guilty/ashamed, despair/discouraged, and disgusted/repulsed in existential dreams suggest that *moral* inadequacy and failure become salient within that dream type. Guilt is explicitly mentioned in the following example:

> In my dream, from my recollection, I was nowhere. I wasn't inside or outside. I was crying but I didn't know why. Then my close friends appeared and tried to take me with them. I was hesitant to follow them; I remember feeling guilty. My family members showed up, all but my Mom. Then it hit me: We were all upset because my Mom had passed away. I don't know how, when, or how; I just know I was feeling a lot of pain. Next thing I knew people kept appearing and consoling me. I was then woken up because I was crying and I had a horrible feeling in my stomach.

Transcendent Dream Emotions

As expected (because it is one of the attributes that defines this polythetic category), ecstatic/in awe was a *distinctive* attribute of transcendent dreams. Only one other emotion category differentiated transcendent dreams from nightmares, existential dreams, *and* mundane dreams (powerful/competent), a finding consistent with prior evidence that, in transcendent dreams, the dreamer feels energetic and alive and possesses an exceptional (perhaps magical) ability to attain his/her goals (Busink & Kuiken, 1996; Kuiken & Sikora, 1993; Kuiken et al., 2006). Whether powerful/competent should be understood as a kinaesthetic aspect of movement efficacy (including flying or floating), a positive outcome of dream actions, and/or an emotion requires further study.

Finally, for two reasons, transcendent dreams cannot simply be described as dreams with positive emotions (cf. Hartmann, 2013; Robert & Zadra, 2014). First, ratings of happy/joyful, hopeful/optimistic, peaceful/calm, and relieved/made safe in transcendent dreams do *not* differ from ratings of those emotions in *mundane* dreams. In addition, ratings of nervous/anxious are *higher* in transcendent dreams than in mundane dreams. Thus, a subtle blend of anxiety and elevation (Keltner & Haidt, 2003) distinguishes this dream type, as affirmed by the following example:

> I saw a few beautiful birds; they were flying around my house [and] then went down in my background. They were so beautiful that I want[ed] to touch them. Suddenly, one of them [was dead] because of me. I [was] very sad, so I tried to find out [whether] that was caused by me or not. Then, I came to a monk and ask[ed] him that. He told me just one sentence: "Don't worry, maybe you are dreaming." I woke up after he told me that.

General Comments

The attributes that identify each of the three basic impactful dream types involve not only complex variations in emotion, as just described, but also sensory phenomena, movement characteristics, motives and goals, and dream endings. Further articulation of these polythetic dream categories requires consideration of each level in this multileveled array. Although all three impactful dream types involve emotion that is especially intense just before awakening, considerable complexity would be sacrificed by simply characterizing nightmares as frightening dreams that initiate immediate awaking, existential dreams as sad dreams that initiate immediate awakening, and transcendent dreams as involving positive emotions that initiate immediate awakening.

Although 41% of the dreamers just described had recently experienced significant loss (including traumatic loss) and 27% had recently experienced significant trauma, the occurrence of such emotional complexity in the dreams of individuals diagnosed with PTSD or Separation Anxiety Disorder has not been studied. The prevalence of these particular emotion profiles among individuals diagnosed with Nightmare Disorder also warrants closer study.

The Contrasting Carryover Effects of Impactful Dreams

Distinguishing between nightmares, existential dreams, and transcendent dreams invites reconsideration of both dream formation and dream function. A comprehensive theory of dreaming would move beyond traumatic stress and (nightmare-centred) threat and fear (e.g., Hartmann, 1998; Revonsuo, 2000; Domhoff, 2003; Nielsen & Levin, 2007) to address the distinctive effects of loss and sadness (existential dreams), as well as the distinctive effects of ascent and ecstasy (transcendent dreams). The only attempt to begin this theoretical task is Hunt's (1989) dream typology (nightmares, titanic dreams, archetypal dreams), which roughly corresponds to the preceding empirical classification (nightmares, existential dreams, transcendent dreams). However, Hunt was especially concerned with the formation and effects of transcendent (archetypal) dreams, while my colleagues and I (Kuiken, 1999; Kuiken & Sikora, 1993; Kuiken et al., 2006) have been especially concerned with the formation and effects of existential dreams. Even so, our complementary efforts converge in one important respect. Hunt suggested that the visual-spatial imagery (e.g., flying and floating) of transcendent (archetypal) dreams *metaphorically* reasserts the motifs characteristic of Jung's (1966) big dreams, including their *aesthetic* aspects. We have suggested that the tactile-kinesthetic imagery (e.g., movement ineffectuality) of existential dreams *metaphorically* reasserts the affective themes characteristic of dreams with magnitude (States, 1997), including their *aesthetic* aspects. Theorists often argue that dreaming is metaphoric, suggesting the figurative origins of such aesthetic outcomes.

Theories of Dream Metaphor

According to one family of theories, metaphors are formed and comprehended by a process of *comparison*. For example, according to the structure-mapping theory proposed by Gentner, Bowdle, Wolff, and Boronat (2001), metaphoric commonalities are found by mapping or transferring features of a metaphoric vehicle onto a metaphoric topic. Thus, the 5-year-old child in Foulkes's (1999) studies who said, "I dreamed I was in the bathtub asleep," metaphorically sensed that "My bed *is like* a bathtub." According to another family of theories, metaphors are formed and comprehended by a process of categorization. According to the class-inclusion theory proposed by Glucksberg (2001), metaphor comprehension occurs when the topic is understood as a member of an *ad hoc* category for which the vehicle is an exemplar—while the topic constrains the attributes that are relevant. Thus, Foulkes's 5-year-old dreamer metaphorically sensed that "My bed *is* a bathtub," which enables "seeing" a bathtub as a place for sleeping (even though, like a bed, it is a place that is dry, not wet).

Both comparison and class inclusion theories of metaphor describe a mode of thinking that requires higher level executive functions (metacognition) than are typically available during dreaming (i.e., systematic comparison, qualified class inclusion). However, the *ad hoc* class inclusion part of the class inclusion model may be all that is needed to describe dream thought as at least *quasi*-metaphoric. Subsuming the vehicle and topic within a single *ad hoc* category (the *is* part; "My bed *is* a bathtub") may be precisely what remains of metaphoric thinking when the higher-level executive function that can constrain it (the *is not* part; "My bath-tub bed *is* dry, *not* wet) has been diminished by the deactivation of the dorsolateral prefrontal cortex that occurs during REM sleep. An array of comparably passive semantic conflations has recently become the focus of research in psycholinguistics: modifier-modified compounds that are not conventionally figurative but that similarly generate category transformation. By this account, Foulkes's 5-year-old may have dreamed a noun-noun compound (bathtub-bed) that is analogous to many conventional (e.g., beach-ball) and creative (e.g., knifing-winds) modifier-modified compound phrases (Mather, Jones, & Estes, 2014). Moreover, an analysis of literary stylistics provided by Mukarovský (1940/1976) suggests that such quasi-metaphoric "crossings" are at the core of *literary* poetics. If this formulation can be generalized to an *oneiric* poetics, dreaming—at least certain types of dreaming—may have aesthetic effects comparable to reading poetry.

The Aesthetic Effects of Impactful Dreams

The viability of this proposal was initially bolstered by studies comparing the effects of nightmares, existential dreams, and transcendent dreams on self-perceptual depth. First, while nightmares consistently evoke postawakening distress such as lingering vigilance, inability to resume sleep, feared return of disturbing images (Belicki, 1992; Miró & Martínez, 2005), existential dreams consistently evoke postawakening distress *and* self-perceptual depth (sensitivity to aspects of life usually ignored, reaffirmation of personal convictions; Busink & Kuiken, 1996; Kuiken & Sikora, 1993; Kuiken et al., 2006). Second, transcendent dreams, unlike either nightmares or existential dreams, evoke a form of self-perceptual depth that has spiritual import (attunement to preternatural phenomena; Kuiken et al., 2006). The self-perceptual depth evoked by existential dreams and by transcendent dreams may be two versions of the same basic aesthetic phenomenon.

Specifically, existential dreams may evoke a form of sublime feeling that combines self-perceptual depth with affective disquietude (sadness, inadequacy) and an inexpressible sense of finitude; transcendent dreams may evoke a form of sublime feeling that combines self-perceptual depth with affective enthrallment (ecstasy, power) and an inexpressible sense of reverence. This proposal is risky but not reckless. The term "sublime" names an experience that resists articulation—sufficiently so to motivate even sympathetic scholars to argue that a theory of the sublime is not possible (Forsey, 2007; Sircello, 1993). Yet literary theories of the sublime, however well-suited to their objectives, have persisted beyond their 18th and 19th century romantic versions (e.g., Kant, Coleridge) to include 20th and 21st century modern (Mallarmé, Woolf) and postmodern renderings (Lyotard, Celan).

One risk in this proposed alliance between literary and psychological theory is that the latter may motivate attention to subjective feelings toward or judgments about "objectively" sublime things such as the Grand Canyon (Konečni, 2011), rather than to a conception of sublimity that integrates subjectivity and objectivity. Kant's (1790/1987) *Critique of Judgment*, which has contributed to discussions of the romantic, modern, and postmodern sublime, remains relevant because it provides just such an integrated conception. According to the present construal of Kant's aesthetics, sublime feeling involves: (1) abrupt recognition of limited conceptual access to an elusive, incongruous, or overwhelming "object"; (2) simultaneous recognition of a partial (preconceptual) grasp of that "object"; and (3) awareness of the expressive mode of engagement through which that "object" has become further (but still partially) disclosed.

So, in the empirical manner of a psychologist—and much to the chagrin of colleagues in literary studies and philosophy—Kuiken, Campbell, and Sopčák (2012) devised empirical indices of (1) sublime enthrallment (the interactive combination of questionnaire subscales that assess wonder, reverence, inexpressible realizations, and self-perceptual depth) and (2) sublime disquietude (the interactive combination of questionnaire subscales that assess disquietude, finitude, inexpressible realizations, and self-perceptual depth). In two recent studies of literary reading (Kuiken et al., 2012), the preceding index of sublime enthrallment was predictably greater following, for example, in-depth engagement with Coleridge's "Frost at Midnight," Shelley's "Mont Blanc," and Rilke's "First Duino Elegy." The preceding index of sublime disquietude was predictably greater following, for example, in-depth engagement with Celan's "Death Fugue," Owen's "Exposure," and Levi's "The Black Stars."

The aesthetic parallel between reading poetry and dreaming plausibly includes correspondence between the forms of sublime feeling that occur in both domains. Consistent with this possibility, in two studies of impactful dreams recorded at home using online procedures, Kuiken (2014) recently found that existential dreams were followed by reports of sublime disquietude; transcendent dreams were followed by sublime enthrallment; and nightmares were followed *by neither form of sublime feeling*. Like engagement with literature that portrays and perhaps induces sublime disquietude (e.g., Celan's "Death Fugue"), existential dreams primarily evoke disquietude (finitude) at the limits of expressibility. In addition, like engagement with literature that portrays and perhaps induces sublime enthrallment (e.g., Shelley's "Mont Blanc"), transcendent dreams primarily evoke wonder (reverence) at the limits of expressibility. The carryover effects of these two impactful dream types—but not nightmares—involve a "touch" of sublimity.

Implications

Just as lingering with a poem can bring a reader to the limits of expressibility, so, too, can some impactful dreams. The magnitude of existential dreams is a form of sublimity that combines self-perceptual depth with disquietude (sadness, insufficiency) and (existential) finitude; the magnitude of transcendent dreams is a form of sublimity that combines self-perceptual depth with enthrallment (ecstasy, elevation) and (spiritual) reverence. Interestingly, *DSM-5* acknowledges that the former occurs during bereavement: "dysphoric dreams may occur during bereavement but typically involve loss and sadness and are followed by self-reflection and insight, rather than distress, on awakening" (APA, 2013, p. 406). Although some evidence (Kuiken, 1993) affirms that separation anxiety during bereavement predicts existential dreams, Cartwright's (2010) studies of dreams that allude to disrupted family relations after divorce suggest that bereavement is not the only form of separation that generates existential dreams, their self-perceptual shifts, and their aesthetic effects.

Despite their agonizing sadness, the self-perceptual shifts and aesthetic effects of existential dreams may contribute to their perceived value. Despite their *angst*, sublime disquietude is not despair; by virtue of the animated engagement that supports *partial* disclosure they are potentially restorative. For this reason, it is crucial to differentiate existential dreams from nightmares within interventions designed to reduce "nightmare" distress (cf. Krakow & Zadra, 2010). Dreamers may be reluctant to let go of diagnosed "nightmares" that in fact involve the sublime magnitude of existential dreams. Their reluctance may reflect a combination of "inappropriate" reluctance to let go of actual *nightmares* and an "appropriate" reluctance to let go of the *existential dreams* (and even transcendent dreams) whose magnitude not only awakens them but also transports them to the limits of aesthetic expressibility.

Note

1. Hartmann actually scored this set of dreams using his criteria for central image intensity. In his assessment, 42% of dreams scored for scared/terrified were also scored for vulnerable/helpless emotion. Only 22% of dreams scored for sad/downhearted and only 5% of dreams scored for nervous/anxious were also scored for vulnerable/helpless emotion.

References

American Psychiatric Association (APA). (2013). *Diagnostic and statistical manual of mental disorders, fifth edition*. Washington, DC: American Psychiatric Association.
Aristotle. (1998). *Aristotle's poetics* (S. H. Butcher, Trans.). New York: Hill and Wang.
Beckner, M. (1959). *The biological way of thought*. New York: Columbia University Press.
Belicki, K. (1992). Nightmare frequency versus nightmare distress: Relations to psychopathology and cognitive style. *Journal of Abnormal Psychology, 101*, 592–597.
Businck, R., & Kuiken, D. (1996). Identifying types of impactful dreams: A replication. *Dreaming, 6*(2), 97–119.
Cartwright, R. D. (2010). *The twenty-four hour mind: The role of sleep and dreaming in our emotional lives*. Oxford, New York: Oxford University Press.

Diamond, G. M., Rochman, D., & Amir, O. (2010). Arousing primary vulnerable emotions in the context of unresolved anger: "Speaking about" versus "speaking to." *Journal of Counseling Psychology, 57*(4), 402–410.

Domhoff, G. W. (2003). *The scientific study of dreams: Neural networks, cognitive development, and content analysis.* Washington, DC: American Psychological Association.

Figley, C. R., Bride, B. E., & Mazza, N. (1997). *Death and trauma: The traumatology of grieving.* Washington, DC: Taylor & Francis.

Forsey, J. (2007). Is a theory of the sublime possible? *Journal of Aesthetics and Art Criticism, 65*(4), 381–389.

Foulkes, D. (1999). *Children's dreaming and the development of consciousness.* Cambridge, MA.: Harvard University Press.

Gentner, D., Bowdle, B., Wolff, P., & Boronat, C. (2001). Metaphor is like analogy. In D. Gentner, K. Holyoak, & B. Kokinov (Eds.), *Analogical mind: Perspectives from cognitive science* (pp. 199–253). Cambridge, MA: MIT Press.

Glucksberg, S. (2001). *Understanding figurative language: From metaphors to idioms.* New York: Oxford University Press.

Green, B. L. (2000). Traumatic loss: Conceptual and empirical links between trauma and bereavement. *Journal of Personal and Interpersonal Loss, 5,* 1–17.

Hartmann, E. (1998). *Dreams and nightmares: The origin and meaning of dreams.* Cambridge, MA: Perseus Publishing.

Hartmann, E. (2013). Thymophor in dreams, poetry, art, and memory: Emotion translated into imagery as a basic element of human creativity. *Imagination, Cognition and Personality, 33*(1), 165–191.

Hasler, B. P., & Germain, A. (2009). Correlates and treatments of nightmares in adults. *Sleep Medicine Clinics, 4*(4), 507–517.

Hunt, H. T. (1989). *The multiplicity of dreams: Memory, imagination, and consciousness.* New Haven: Yale University Press.

Husserl, E. (1948/1973). *Experience and judgment* (James S. Churchill & Karl Ameriks, Trans.). Evanston, IL: Northwestern University Press.

Jung, C. G. (1966). *The collected works of C. G. Jung.* (H. E. Read, Ed.) (Vol. 17). Princeton, NJ: Princeton University Press.

Kant, I. (1790/1987). *Critique of judgment* (W. Pluhar, Trans.). Indianapolis: Hackett Publishing Company.

Keltner, D., & Haidt, J. (2003). Approaching awe, a moral, spiritual, and aesthetic emotion. *Cognition & Emotion, 17*(2), 297–314.

Konečni, V. J. (2011). Aesthetic trinity theory and the sublime. *Philosophy Today, 55*(1), 64–73.

Krakow, B., & Zadra, A. (2010). Imagery rehearsal therapy: Principles and practice. *Sleep Medicine Clinics, 5*(2), 289–298.

Kuiken, D. (1993, June). Dreams and stress: Loss and dream impact. Paper presented at the Conference of the Association for the Study of Dreams, Santa Fe, New Mexico.

Kuiken, D. (1999). An enriched conception of dream metaphor. *Sleep and Hypnosis, 1,* 112–121.

Kuiken, D. (2014, June). Impactful dreams, sublime feeling, and reflective awareness. Paper presented at the Conference of the International Association for the Study of Dreams, Berkeley, California.

Kuiken, D., Campbell, P., & Sopčák, P. (2012). The Experiencing Questionnaire: Locating exceptional reading moments. *Scientific Study of Literature, 2*(2), 243–272.

Kuiken, D., Chudleigh, M., & Racher, D. (2010). Bilateral eye movements, attentional flexibility and metaphor comprehension: The substrate of REM dreaming? *Dreaming, 20*(4), 227–247.

Kuiken, D., Lee, M.-N., Eng, T., & Singh, T. (2006). The influence of impactful dreams on self-perceptual depth and spiritual transformation. *Dreaming, 16*(4), 258–279.

Kuiken, D., & Miall, D. S. (2001). Numerically aided phenomenology: Procedures for investigating categories of experience. *Forum Qualitative Sozialforschung/Forum: Qualitative social research, 2*(1). Online journal available at: http://qualitative-research.net/fqs/fqs-eng.htm.

Kuiken, D., Schopflocher, D., &Wild, T. C. (1989). Numerically aided phenomenological methods: A demonstration. *Journal of Mind and Behavior, 10*, 373–392.

Kuiken, D., & Sikora, S. (1993). The impact of dreams on waking thoughts and feelings. In A. Moffitt, M. Kramer, & R. Hoffmann (Eds.), *The functions of dreaming* (pp. 419–476). Albany: State University of New York Press.

Lee, M-N., & Kuiken, D. (in press). Continuity of reflective awareness across waking and dreaming states. *Dreaming*.

Mather, E., Jones, L. L., & Estes, Z. (2014). Priming by relational integration in perceptual identification and Stroop colour naming. *Journal of Memory and Language, 71*(1), 57–70.

Miró, E., & Martínez, M. P. (2005). Affective and personality characteristics in function of nightmare prevalence, nightmare distress, and interference due to nightmares. *Dreaming, 15*, 89–105.

Mukarovský, J. (1940/1976). *On poetic language.* J. Burbank & P. Steiner (Trans.). Lisse, The Netherlands: Peter de Ridder Press.

Nielsen, T., & Levin, R. (2007). Nightmares: A new neurocognitive model. *Sleep Medicine Reviews, 11*(4), 295–310.

Panksepp, J. (2005). Affective consciousness: Core emotional feelings in animals and humans. *Consciousness and Cognition, 14*, 30–80.

Raphael, B. & Martinek, N. (1997). Assessing traumatic bereavement and posttraumatic stress disorder. In J. P. Wilson & T. M. Keane (Eds.), *Assessing psychological trauma and PTSD* (pp. 373–395). New York: Guilford.

Revonsuo, A. (2000). The reinterpretation of dreams: An evolutionary hypothesis of the function of dreaming. *Behavioral and Brain Sciences, 23*(6), 877–901.

Robert, G., & Zadra, A. (2014). Thematic and content analysis of idiopathic nightmares and bad dreams. *Sleep, 37*(2), 409–417.

Sircello, G. (1993). How is a theory of the sublime possible? *Journal of Aesthetics and Art Criticism, 51*(4), 541–550.

States, B. O. (1997). *Seeing in the dark: Reflections on dreams and dreaming.* New Haven, CT: Yale University Press.

Stroebe, M. & Schut, H. (2005–2006). Complicated grief: A conceptual analysis of the field. *Omega: Journal of Death and Dying, 52*, 53–70.

15
CROSS-CULTURAL ASPECTS OF EXTRAORDINARY DREAMS

Jacquie Lewis and Stanley Krippner

SAYBROOK UNIVERSITY

In the book *Life on the Mississippi* (1883/2013), Mark Twain relates a dream where he observes a metal coffin with his brother Henry in it. Atop Henry's chest was a bouquet of flowers, all white, save one red one in the middle. A few days later Henry died in a riverboat accident. When Twain went to his brother, he lay in a metal coffin, rather than the standard wooden coffin that others from the accident had been placed in, and a woman was bringing a bouquet of flowers to place on Henry's chest, the same as those in Twain's dream.

Extraordinary dreams appear to occur around the world, yet are rarely reported or studied (Krippner, Bogzaran, & de Carvalho, 2002; Krippner & de Carvalho, 1998). Some people who experience extraordinary dreams may be frightened or worry that they are symptoms of mental illness. Still others find them filled with meaning and direction but do not tell anyone about them for fear of social censure. In either event, it is important that clinicians are aware of this type of dream and take care not to pathologize them.

These unusual or extraordinary dreams include, among others, *creative dreams, lucid dreams, healing dreams, dreams within dreams, out-of-body dreams, telepathic dreams, mutual (and shared) dreams, clairvoyant dreams, precognitive dreams, past-life dreams, initiation dreams,* and *visitation dreams*.

There are waking life analogues to most of these dreams, but the fact that they occur during sleep provides researchers with clues as to how they can be studied. The available data indicate that they are especially common in fantasy-prone individuals and people with flexible psychological boundaries. Therefore, they are examples of the continuity hypothesis: dream life reflects waking life. An artist who manifests creativity while awake may continue creative work while asleep. An individual who has spontaneous or deliberate out-of-body experiences while awake might also engage in "astral travel" while asleep. At the same time, there are those who report these extraordinary experiences only while asleep and thus are taken by surprise—they may doubt their sanity.

The Old Testament is rife with examples of extraordinary dreams, most of them prophetic in nature (Noegel, 2001). And as far back as 350 BCE Aristotle (1952) stated that these dreams were likely to be coincidental rather than the result of divine intervention. In the modern era Freud (Fodor, 1951) believed that telepathic dreams existed and, along with Jung (1974), acknowledged that they were worthy of investigation. Freud felt that their dynamics resembled those of more ordinary dreams while Jung posited that they supported his concept of a collective unconscious.

Although the body of research on extraordinary dreams is small, experimental studies of putative telepathic, clairvoyant, and precognitive dreams have been outlined by Roe and Sherwood (2009) and by Krippner (2007a). Anecdotal cases have also been discussed by Krippner et al., (2002) and an overview of both anecdotal and laboratory studies has been surveyed by Krippner (2007b). Whereas previous laboratory studies of dream telepathy, dating back to the 1960s, have used art prints or photographs as target pictures, a more recent study used video clips. It was found that participants were more likely to achieve direct hits when the video clips were emotionally negative rather than when they were positive or neutral (Sherwood, Dalton, Steinkamp, & Watt, C., 2000). Krippner (2006) has also speculated that telepathic and precognitive dreams may be affected by the earth's geomagnetic field. LaBerge (2007, 2013) has also outlined the history, since the 1970s, of lucid dreaming research in the laboratory.

There are several books, most of them popular rather than professional, which discuss extraordinary dreams (e.g., Guiley 1998; Van de Castle, 1994), including creative dreams (Delaney, 1991), lucid dreams (Gackenbach & Bosveld, 1989), healing dreams (Barasch, 2000; Garfield, 1991), mutual dreams (Magallon, 1997), and precognitive dreams (Ryback & Sweitzer, 1988). Kelly Bulkeley's book, *Spiritual Dreaming* (1995), contains separate chapters on creative dreams, lucid dreams, healing dreams, precognitive dreams, initiation dreams, and visitation dreams. This list is not exhaustive; there are other dream categories that could be described as "archetypal" (Jung, 1974), "sexual" (Paley, 1990), "impactful" (Kuiken & Smith, 1993), or "numinous"—those in which there is an encounter with "that which is beyond the sphere of the usual, the intelligible, and the familiar" (Bulkeley, 1995, p. 2).

The purpose of this chapter is to outline the most notable study of extraordinary dreams, spanning seven countries, conducted by Krippner and Faith (2001). It is hoped that this will expand the cross-cultural literature of dreams to include those dream reports that can be described as extraordinary, thus helping to dispel any fears or misconceptions individuals may have about them. On occasions, extraordinary dreams may be part of a pathological syndrome, but more commonly they reflect normal, albeit unusual, processes of mental functioning.

Method

The research participants were members of dream seminars that Krippner conducted between 1990 and 1998. These events were held in various parts of Argentina, Brazil, England, Russia, Japan, Ukraine, and the United States. The age span ranged from people in their 20s to their 70s (as determined from registration information and informal conversations), with a few individuals even younger or older. Middle and upper middle income groups were overrepresented because there were entrance fees for most of the seminars; however, a few scholarships were available for lower income individuals. Because most of the events were held at colleges, universities, and cultural centers, the educational level of the participants was higher than would have been found in the general population. The dream seminars did not focus on extraordinary dreams but on ways in which dream work could be practically applied to problems in daily life. Hence "demand characteristics" were kept at a minimum. It was ascertained, whenever possible, that research participants had lived for at least three years in the country to which they were assigned for comparative purposes. Attendees were asked to write down a recent dream and leave it on a nearby table; most of them did so, and many hoped that their dream report would be selected for teaching purposes later in the seminar. Only one dream from each of the research participants was utilized.

For a dream report to be scored as a *creative dream,* an actual problem from waking life had to be solved. To be scored as a *lucid dream,* the dream report had to specifically state that the dreamer was aware that he or she was dreaming before awakening. To be scored as a *healing dream,* the dream report content had to assist in ameliorating or preventing physical, emotional, or spiritual distress following the dream experience. To be scored as *a dream within a dream,* the dream report mentioned entering a different state of consciousness within the dream or the dreamer appeared to wake from the dream only to discover, upon their "false awakening," that the dream was still going on. To be scored as an *out-of-body dream,* the dreamer needed to report the sensation of leaving his or her body while the dream was going on. For scoring as a *telepathic dream,* the dreamer needed to claim that a dream matched the mental content of a distant person in external reality that was confirmed sometime after the dreamer awoke. For a dream report to be scored as a *mutual* or *shared dream,* the dreamer and someone else had to claim that they had experienced similar dreams on the same night. For a dream report to be scored as a *clairvoyant dream,* it needed to match a distant event, and a purported confirmation of this match was made during wakefulness. A *precognitive dream* needed to provide specific information about a future event that supposedly matched information about that event. To be scored as a *past-life dream,* the dreamer had to report taking on a different identity than his or her ordinary identity, one subjectively associated with a purported former lifetime or "incarnation." To be scored as an *initiation dream,* the dream report had to describe the introduction of the dreamer to a nonordinary reality, to membership in an esoteric social group, or to a previously unexplored vocational path; in each case, this initiation needed to be agreeable and meaningful. It is not unusual for people to dream about dead friends and relatives, but to be scored as a *visitation dream,* the deceased person or an entity from another reality had to provide counsel or direction that the dreamer found of comfort or value. Purported visits from outer-space aliens were placed in this category if the purpose of their visit was to bring instructive information to the dreamer.

It was kept in mind that these were dream reports, not the experienced dreams themselves. Any number of distortions and omissions can occur between the time a dream is experienced and the time the dream is reported. As a result no external attempt was made to determine whether a purported clairvoyant dream actually matched the event in waking life about which the dreamer claimed to dream. No attempt was made to verify precognitive or telepathic dreams. These attempts have been made under controlled conditions (Ullman, Krippner, with Vaughan, 1989), but were considered beyond the scope of this study.

When a dream contained elements of two categories, it was scored for both categories; for tabulation purposes, half a point was given for each category. Two raters, Yuko Suzuki and Laura Faith, categorized each dream; interrater reliability was .95. In cases of disagreement, Krippner made the final decision.

Results

The total number of dream reports collected for analysis was 1,871 (1,014 from women and 857 from men). Table 15.1 presents the data for each country.

Female dreamers reported 77 extraordinary dreams (7.0% of all female dream reports), while male dreamers reported 58 extraordinary dreams (6.8% of all male reports). Chi square statistics were applied to gender differences, which were not found to be statistically significant.

Table 15.2 presents the breakdown of these dream reports into the categories utilized in the study, while Table 15.3 presents the percentage of anomalous dream reports per country.

TABLE 15.1 Gender Breakdown for Dream Reports from Seven Countries

Country	Female	Male	Total
Argentina	111	101	212
Brazil	136	103	239
England	104	101	205
Japan	66	70	136
Russia	140	105	245
United States	353	277	630
Ukraine	104	100	204
Totals	1,014	857	1,871

TABLE 15.2 Breakdown of Anomalous Dreams for Total Sample

Category	Number	Percent
Clairvoyant	5	0.3
Creative dreams	4.5	0.24
Dreams within dreams	11.5	0.6
Healing	3	0.16
Initiation	15	0.8
Lucid dreams	31.5	1.67
Mutual or shared	2	0.1
Out-of-body	24	1.28
Past-life	6.5	0.3
Precognitive	17	1.0
Telepathic	2	0.1
Visitation	21	1.1
Total	143	7.65%

TABLE 15.3 Breakdown of Anomalous Dreams per Country

Country	Anomalous Dreams (in percent)
Argentina	8.6
Brazil	10.9
England	3.9
Japan	8.1
Russia	12.7
United States	5.7
Ukraine	5.9

The country with the highest percentage of extraordinary dreams was Russia (12.7%), followed by Brazil (10.9%), Argentina (8.6%), Japan (8.1%), Ukraine (5.9%), the United States (5.7%), and England (3.9%). There were a few statistically significant differences: Russian dreamers reported significantly more extraordinary dreams than dreamers from Ukraine, the United States, and England.

Dream Report Examples

An Argentine man reported a **creative dream**: *I was with a former teacher of mine who had come to my office to give me some help with a project I am doing for our business* *in waking life. I welcome his interest and assistance. He knew exactly what advice I needed; between the two of us, we finished the project successfully. When I awakened, I put his advice to good use in a project on which I was working.*

An Argentine woman submitted an **out-of-body** dream report: *I felt as if I were dying but it was not as traumatic as I had imagined. I felt peaceful and relaxed, almost incorporeal. It was a profound sensation. There was an appearance of vivid white light.*

A Russian woman reported a **lucid dream**: *I am on the balcony of my home, and I am aware that I am dreaming. Everything around me is brightly colored.*

Another Russian woman rendered a report scored as a **healing dream**: *A small black snake appears and bites me on the right side of my neck. I squeeze it with three fingers and it opens its mouth. I squeeze the poison out of it. When I wake up I use that squeeze when I have headaches. They have almost disappeared.*

A Brazilian woman had the following **telepathic dream:** *I was with a woman who I had met a few days earlier in waking life. She works with vibrations and wanted to enlist me for a session. During the session, she said "Your friend Yussara has cancer, and you must ask her about this." The other day I telephoned Yussara and told her my dream. She told me that she had just been to a physician who told her she has cancer.*

An English man reported a **dream within a dream:** *I am on a train and fall asleep. I wake up just as they are serving breakfast. I recall having a dream about Jesus. I am trying to remember the details because I have very good feelings about the dream. Then I really wake up. I realize that I was still asleep when I was served breakfast.*

Two Japanese women reported **mutual dreams** from the same night. The first woman dreamed: *I am in the lobby of a big hotel. There is a large pillar made of marble. My friend is there and I stab her with a knife. I don't know why I stab her. Nobody seems to notice what I have done.* The second woman reported: *I am in a hotel lobby. There is a big pillar there and I am standing by it. My younger sister comes in. She walks right up to me and stabs me with a knife. I died from the stabbing.*

Another Japanese woman dreamed: *I was a young beggar somewhere in Europe. Two other beggars and I came back from begging on the street. We had no food or money. My clothes were dirty and I had long, curly, brown hair. I had not bathed in a long time. I opened a heavy wooden door at a gate of a thick stone fortress. In the fortress there was an area for miserable beggars to sleep. An ugly old woman found me and other beggars trying to keep warm by a fire. She hit one of us and dashed a container of liquid on the head of the other one. I think it was the tenth or the eleventh century. I was not Japanese. It might have been a former lifetime.* This report was scored as a **past-life dream.**

A Russian man reported a **clairvoyant dream**: *I am in an empty room. I try to pass through the wall. It is solid and I cannot go through it. There is a slogan on the wall, "If you are brave go through it." A business associate of mine appears. Then I wake up. Later, I ask him if I can visit his house. When I enter, I see the same wall but there is no slogan on it.*

A dream report of a Russian man was scored as **precognitive**: *I was walking down the street. I saw a beautiful woman approaching me. As she came closer I could see her face. She smiled at me and I fell in love with her. I wanted to marry her and have a child* with her. *A short time later, I saw the same woman in my graduate class in St. Petersburg; we are married now.*

Another Russian man's report was scored as an **initiation dream**: *Deities told me that I needed to transform myself to become a healer. It seemed as if I had died, and then I was reborn again. The deities told me that I needed to advance one more level, to learn about external kindness but also to be kind to myself. Once I learned this lesson, I would be able to start healing people. I went through three cycles of death and rebirth, and when I awakened, I felt that my initiation was complete. Later, I began to study healing with a local practitioner.*

Sometimes dreams represented two categories. A Japanese woman reported the following dream: *My father, who died in World War II, appears to me. He gives me advice about my artwork, what to paint and how to do it. He tells me the topics, what brushes to use, and what colors to use. When I wake up, I follow his advice, and I sell the pictures!* This report qualified as a **creative dream**. However, it was also scored as **a visitation dream** because her father, dead at the time of the dream, gave valuable counsel to the dreamer.

Discussion

This study revealed that Russian participants reported significantly more extraordinary dreams as dreamers from the United States or England, while the difference between percentages of extraordinary dreams reported by Ukrainian, Brazilian and Argentinian participants was in between these extremes, with Japan, England, and the United States reporting the least. The percentage of extraordinary dreams in the Ukraine was much closer to that in the United States rather than in Russia, despite the geographic proximity of Ukraine and Russia.

The question arises as to what characteristics of a particular culture may be associated with the incidence and significance of extraordinary dreams. A number of studies indicate that gender, age, education, religion, ethnic background, and socioeconomic status influence the likelihood of reporting unusual experiences. It is of interest that Joseph Glicksohn (1990) found a correlation between participants' belief systems and the incidence of occurrence of various types of unusual subjective experiences, such as lucid dreaming and out-of body experience. In this connection, cultural belief systems appear to be the most likely parameters to be explored in future studies about the consequences of extraordinary dreams. It will be recalled that the ratio of extraordinary Ukrainian dreams resembled the U.S. ratio more closely than the Russian ratio, despite their geographical proximity and the large number of Russian-speaking people in Ukraine.

Clinical Implications

Some extraordinary dreams can be life changing for individuals. For this reason, they should not be ignored but could be investigated to determine under what conditions they occur, what constitutes a legitimate extraordinary dream versus wishful thinking on the part of the dreamer, what personality types are more prone to extraordinary dreams, and whether such dreams can occur at will.

The Krippner and Faith database indicates that visitation and past-life dreams can be of therapeutic value for the dreamer. The following visitation dream, by an American woman, appears to have contributed to the dreamer's self confidence in her waking life: *I am visited by a friend of mine from waking life. He has been murdered in waking life and we discuss the conditions under which he was killed. He can fly and I want to fly too. My friend takes me to a street where I can rent wings for 25 cents. I am able to fly with these wings, but then I realize it is my confidence that is keeping me in the air. My friend has taught me a great lesson.*

The following example illustrates the therapeutic value of a past-life dream. A Brazilian woman dreamed: *I'm in a bedroom and I look at a man who is kneeling by a bed that is between the two of us. He asks me if I am going to see a doctor. Before I can answer him, he says that it is no use to see a doctor because there is no treatment for what is wrong with me. He asks me if I want to know why I am so ashamed. I say "yes" and he says, "Dive in me to see your life before this one." So I kneel by the bed in front of him, go out of my body, and dive into his chest. At this moment, I am upside down and in a dark area. I feel a stroke on my back at the heart level and realize that I am in another life. In this past life, I wanted to hurt a man. To provoke him, I got into an accident and paralyzed myself. So I was in a wheelchair. I couldn't move and had no control of the lower part of my body. And that is why I am still ashamed of that part of my body.* The dreamer's self-esteem and body concept reportedly improved following this dream, even though there was no assurance that the past-life report was veridical.

Limitations

This study was delimited to self-selected participants from seven countries. No attempt was made to generalize these findings to the population of these countries as a whole, or to other parts of the world.

These samples of dream reports had particular characteristics that were both advantageous and disadvantageous for a study of gender and national differences. The participants were self-selected; this fact limits the generalizability of these findings. Even though participants were merely asked for a "recent dream," it is possible that they selected an especially dramatic or puzzling dream, hoping it would be selected for group discussion. But it is also possible that they selected an ordinary dream that would not be personally revealing, omitting a more recent dream that would have evoked embarrassment.

The samples were also not directly comparable. The Ukrainian sample was largely composed of university students while the samples from the United States and Argentina were almost entirely from professionals. The samples from the United States, Russia, England, and Brazil were distributed from around the country, while those from Argentina and Japan represented large urban centers.

Nonetheless, this study helps lay groundwork for further investigations into extraordinary dreams. Hopefully, it will also help dispel any claims that extraordinary dreams are necessarily abnormal or pathological. On occasion, psychologically healthy individuals can experience extraordinary dreams and put them to constructive use.

Acknowledgements

The research reported in this chapter was supported by the Saybrook University Chair for the Study of Consciousness.

References

Aristotle (1952). *On prophesying by dreams*. In R. M. Hutchins (Ed.), *Aristotle* (Vol. 2; pp. 707–709). Chicago, IL: Encyclopedia Britannica.

Barasch, M. I. (2000). *Healing dreams: Exploring the dreams that can transform your life*. New York, NY: Riverhead/Penguin.

Bulkeley, K. (1995). *Spiritual dreaming: A cross-cultural and historical journey*. Mahwah, NJ: Paulist Press.

Delaney, G. (1991). *Breakthrough dreaming*. New York, NY: Bantam Books.

Fodor, N. (1951). *New approaches to dream interpretation*. New Hyde Park, NY: University Books.

Gackenbach, J., & Bosveld, J. (1989). *Control your dreams*. New York, NY: Harper & Row.

Garfield, P. (1991). *The healing power of dreams*. New York, NY: Simon & Schuster.

Glicksohn, J. (1990). Belief in the paranormal and subjective paranormal experience. *Personality and Individual Differences, 11*, 675–683.

Guiley, R. E. (1998). *Dreamwork for the soul: A spiritual guide to dream interpretation*. New York, NY: Berkley Books.

Jung, C. G. (1974). *Dreams*. Princeton, NJ: Princeton University Press.

Krippner, S. (2006). Geomagnetic field effects in anomalous dreams and the Akashic field. *World Futures, 62*, 103–113. doi: 10.1080/02604020500412741

Krippner, S. (2007a, June). *Investigating anomalous experiences in dreams*. Paper presented at preconference workshop for the annual convention of the International Association for the Study of Dreams, Sonoma State University, Rohnert Park, CA.

Krippner S. (2007b). Anomalous experiences and dreams. In D. Barrett & P. McNamara (Eds.), *The new science of dreaming: Content, recall, and personality correlates* (Vol. 2; pp. 285–306). Westport, CT: Praeger.

Krippner, S., Bogzaran, F., & de Carvalho, A. P. (2002). *Extraordinary dreams and how to work with them*. Albany, NY: State University of New York Press.

Krippner, S., & de Carvalho, A. P. (1998). *Sonhos exoticos* [Exotic dreams]. Sao Paulo, Brazil: Summus.

Krippner, S. & Faith L. (2001). Exotic dreams: A cross-cultural study. *Dreaming, 11*(2), 73–82.

Kuiken, D., & Smith, L. (1993). Impactful dreams and metaphor generation. *Dreaming, 1*, 135–145.

LaBerge, S. (2007). Lucid dreaming. In D. Barrett & P. McNamara (Eds.), *The new science of dreaming: Content, recall, and personality correlates* (Vol. 2; pp. 307–328). Westport, CT: Praeger.

LaBerge, S. (2013). Lucid dreaming: Paradoxes of dreaming consciousness. In E. Cardena, S. J. Lynn, & S. Krippner (Eds.), *Varieties of anomalous experiences: Examining the scientific evidence* (pp. 145–173). Washington, DC: American Psychological Association.

Magallon, L. L. (1997). *Mutual dreaming: When two or more people share the same dream.* New York, NY: Pocket Books.

Noegel, S. (2001). Dreams and dream interpreters on Mesopotamia and in the Hebrew Bible [Old Testament]. In K. Bulkeley (Ed.), *Dreams: A reader on the religious, cultural, and psychological dimensions of dreaming* (pp. 45–71). New York, NY: Palgrave.

Paley, K. S. (1990). Dreamers do it in their sleep. In S. Krippner (Ed.), *Dreamtime and dreamwork: Decoding the language of the night,* (pp. 161–168). New York, NY: Tarcher/Perigee.

Roe, C. A., & Sherwood S. J. (2009). Evidence for extrasensory perception in dream content: A review of experimental studies. In S. Krippner & D. J. Ellis (Eds.), *Perchance to dream: The frontiers of dream psychology* (pp. 211–238). New York, NY: Nova Science.

Ryback, D., with Sweitzer, L. (1988). *Dreams that come true.* New York, NY: Dolphin/Doubleday.

Sherwood, S. J., Dalton, K., Steinkamp, F., & Watt, C. (2000). Dream clairvoyance study II using dynamic video-clips: Investigation of consensus voting judging procedures and target emotionality. *Dreaming, 10*(4), 221–236.

Twain, M. (1883/2013). *Life on the Mississippi.* Hazelton, PA: The Electronic Classics Series. Retrieved from www2.hn.psu.edu/faculty/jmanis/twain/lifeonmr.pdf

Ullman, M., & Krippner, S., with Vaughan, A. (1989). *Dream telepathy: Experiments in nocturnal ESP* (2nd ed.). Jefferson, NC: McFarland.

Van de Castle, R. L. (1994). *Our dreaming mind.* New York, NY: Ballantine.

16

LUCID DREAMING

Metaconsciousness During Paradoxical Sleep

Stephen LaBerge

In the course of everyday life, we rarely reflect on our global reality orientation and state of consciousness. Even less do we question whether we are awake or not. By way of illustration, if I were to ask *you*, the reader, if you knew you were awake when you started to read this paragraph, you'd probably respond "of course!" But if pressed for details ("Were you actually consciously aware of your state?"), you'd have to admit that you weren't thinking about it until just now. So we may implicitly *presume* that we are awake, not because we are normally explicitly metaconsciously aware of being in any particular state of consciousness, but because we tacitly accept the default assumption of *real until proven otherwise.*

As William James (1890) perspicuously observed, everything we experience seems real, and for us, *is real,* until we have another *contradictory* experience that forces us to test and choose among conflicting experiences, which are more, and which are less coherent with what else we know (or think we do) about the world, and thus which to keep, and which to discard as *unreal.*

Likewise, while dreaming, we do not usually notice that we are dreaming. However, there is a significant exception to this: During what are usually called *lucid dreams* (LDs) (van Eeden, 1913), we take explicit note or *cognizance* of the fact that we *are* dreaming. This means that we not only know that we are dreaming, we also know that we know it. This reflection on our state of consciousness typically comes about, analogously as it does in waking life, when experiential anomalies occur that give rise to the question of how to resolve contradictory evidence. For example, suppose I am talking to Sigmund Freud himself (according to the testimony of my senses), yet I know Dr. Freud is as dead as psychoanalysis. I may decide that Freud is only a ghost, or lives on in his books, or in a moment of oneiric confabulation, a sort of "Freudian slip," and so on, and continue to dream non-lucidly. Or I may realize that the correct explanation of the "hallucinated Freud" is that *I am now dreaming*. This thought may be in passing and forgotten in a moment, or by a process of recursive conscious reflection may lead to a sustained LD lasting many minutes in which metaconsciousness of dreaming is retained while the LD lasts (Kahan & LaBerge, 1994).

During such cognizant dreams, experience and experiments show that to a much greater extent than previously assumed, expert lucid dreamers can reason rationally, remember the conditions of waking life, and act voluntarily within the dream upon reflection or in accordance with plans decided upon before sleep,— all while remaining soundly asleep, vividly experiencing a dream world that can appear astonishingly real (Green, 1968; LaBerge & DeGracia, 2000; van Eeden, 1913). This all obviously contradicts the widespread misconception of (non-lucid) dreams as necessarily lacking reflection, attentional control, or true volition (Hobson, 2009; Rechtschaffen, 1978; Voss, Holzmann, Tuin, & Hobson, 2009).

It is difficult to determine the precise prevalence of LDs for several reasons. First, LDs vary from the minimal thought "this is just a dream" in passing, to extended peak experiences. Second, lucid dreaming is a learnable skill (LaBerge, 1980b), and intentional practice can increase the frequency and quality of LDs. Under ordinary conditions, most dreams are probably not lucid, and most spontaneous LDs are not completely lucid (Barrett, 1992; LaBerge & DeGracia, 2000). Keeping in mind that many of the LDs reported here and elsewhere are of unknown duration and lucidity. A sample of 2,665 visitors to www.lucidity.com (LaBerge, 2014) reported average dream recall (two or three dreams per week) and a median LD rate of twice a year; 25% reported monthly and 10% claimed twice-weekly LDs (i.e., about 1.5% of all dreams). A subset of 902 with nightly or better dream recall reported 50% monthly, and 25% reported weekly LDs. This represents about 2.5% of all dreams.

Before eye-movement signaling provided objective proof of its existence, few dream researchers were willing to credit subjective reports of lucid dreaming at face value, as reports of dreaming *during* sleep. Havelock Ellis (1922) shows this attitude was at least 60 years old:

> I have never detected in my own dreams any recognition that they are dreams. I may say, indeed that I do not consider that such a thing is really possible, though it has been born witness to by many philosophers and others from Aristotle . . . and Gassendi onwards. *The phenomenon occurs; the person who says to himself that he is dreaming believes that he is still dreaming, but one may be permitted to doubt that he is.* It seems far more probable that he has for a moment, without realising it, emerged at the waking surface of consciousness. . . . It may even occur that a person partly wakes up, perceives what is going on around him, converses about it, falls asleep again, and imagines in the morning that the whole episode was a dream. (p. 65)

Probably this attitude derived from the vague notion that *being asleep means being unconscious.* Unconscious of what? Presumably, the environment. But in this muddled light, claiming to be conscious of anything at all during sleep, especially that one *is* asleep, or dreaming, might seem contradictory (LaBerge 1985, 1990), though not to the extremely lucid Pierre Gassendi, the 17th-century philosopher dismissed by Ellis, who thought that for the understanding to realize that one is dreaming required nothing more than being able to think that one is thinking, an endogenous mental capacity that does not involve the external senses and thus does not depend on being awake (LaBerge, 1985).

Unfortunately, 300 years after Gassendi, a behaviorist philosopher notoriously contended that when anyone says, "I had a dream," the "dream" they refer to is *the story they tell after waking,* not some hypothetical and unobservable experience during sleep. Thus it was nonsense even to *say* "I am dreaming," making lucid dreaming not only impossible, but impossible to even *think about.*

The answer to this sort of theoretical philosophy must be actual experimental evidence, and studies began to appear in the late 1970s suggesting that LDs occur during REM sleep. Based on standard sleep recordings of two subjects who reported a total of three LDs upon awakening from REM periods (REMPs), Ogilvie, Hunt, Sawicki, and McGowan (1978) cautiously concluded that "it may be that lucid dreams begin in REM" (p. 165). Their caution was probably appropriate because they couldn't prove that the reported LDs had in fact occurred *during* the REM sleep immediately preceding the awakenings and reports, rather than in any of the several alternatives hypothesized by skeptics—such as *during* the awakening in a hypnopompic state, or *after* awakening in a REM-like state of sleep inertia, or *not at all!* This last alternative is bizarrely dreamlike: Suppose, mused Dennett (1976), we aren't having experiences during REM sleep that we later report on awakening; perhaps, instead false memory "cassettes" are being spliced together à la the sci-fi film *Total Recall*, and these confabulated "cassettes" are loaded into memory upon awakening, ready for recall as "dreams." Thus, "[i]f asked what it is like to dream one ought to say (because it would be the truth): 'it is not like anything.' I go to sleep and when I wake up I find I have a tale to tell, a 'recollection' as it were" (Dennett, 1976, p. 139). Dennett's point was that there was no way to distinguish the "cassette theory" from the standard "experience during sleep theory" of dreaming, because there was no way to know what the dreamer was or wasn't experiencing while still asleep.

Dennett was using a *reductio ad absurdum* to challenge the standard "experience during sleep theory" of dreaming by showing that there was no way to distinguish it from the absurd "cassette theory," because presumably there was no way to know what the dreamer was or wasn't experiencing while still asleep. But this presumption is wrong; there *is* a way to know, and this happened to be just what was needed to prove that LDs occur during sleep: a voluntary response by the subject marking the exact time the LD was taking place.

Lucid Dreaming Verified by Volitional Communication During REM Sleep

My colleagues and I (LaBerge, Nagel, Dement & Zarcone, 1981a,b) provided the necessary verification by tasking lucid dreamers to induce and time stamp the onset and offset of LDs by means of specific voluntary dream actions expected to produce corresponding physiological responses observable on a polygraph (e.g., patterns of eye movements or fist clenches). Using this approach, we recorded seven subjects (from 2–23 nights), who during the 52 nights, reported 50 LDs, in 44 of which they reported signaling. Of these, we were able to blindly match 40 signal-verified lucid dreams (SVLDs), all of which occurred during epochs of unambiguous REM sleep scored according to the conventional criteria (Rechtschaffen & Kales, 1968). Note that these SVLDs were not brief interludes of lucidity or "semi-wakefulness": they usually lasted several minutes (mean: 115 sec, range: 5–490 sec). Figure 16.1 shows one of several examples that should have definitively settled the question "Can lucid dreams occur during REM sleep?" in 1981. Given that if only *one* of these 40 LDs was correctly scored as REM sleep, logic requires rejecting the hypothesis that reflective consciousness cannot occur during sleep. It is odd indeed to read revisionist claims that "many" or "most" dream researchers were not convinced by this evidence that LDs really can occur in real time during REM sleep (Hobson, 2009; cf. LaBerge, 2010).

Moreover, multiple studies in our own and more than a dozen other independent laboratories have replicated the association of lucid dreaming with REM sleep using eye-movement signals, obtaining essentially the same results (Armstrong-Hickey, 1988; Brylowski, Levitan, & LaBerge, 1989; Dane, 1984; Dresler, et al., 2011; Erlacher & Schredl, 2008; Hearne, 1978, 1983; Holzinger, Levitan, & LaBerge, 2006; Price & Cohen, 1988; Ogilvie, Hunt, Kushniruk, & Newman, 1983; Schatzman, Worsley, & Fenwick, 1988; Voss et al., 2009; and Watanabe, 2003). It is noteworthy that no other dream content dimension has been shown to occur so exclusively in REM compared to non-REM sleep, as persistent lucid dreaming and the voluntary action required by SVLDs.

However, demonstrations that signaling of LDs occurs during REM sleep raises another kind of question: What exactly do we mean by the assertion that lucid dreamers are "asleep"? Perhaps these "dreamers" are not really dreamers, as some argued in the last century; or perhaps this "sleep" is not really sleep, as some have argued in this century. How do we know that lucid dreamers are "really asleep" when they signal? If we consider perception of the external world as a criterion of being awake (to the external world), we can conclude that they are actually asleep (to the external world) because although they know they are in the laboratory, this knowledge is a matter of memory, not perception. While in the LD, they typically experience themselves being totally embodied within the dream world and not in sensory contact with the external world. Their metaconsciousness

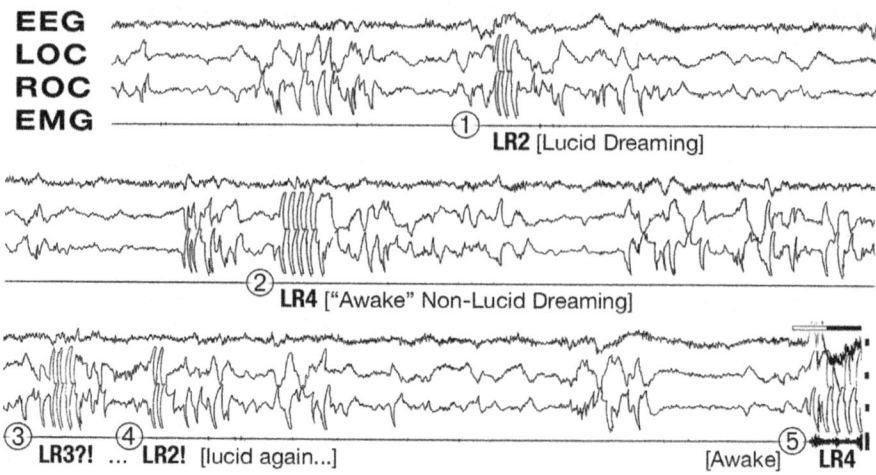

FIGURE 16.1 Voluntary eye-movement signals (VEMS) validate report of lucid dreaming during uninterrupted REM sleep. A standard polysomnogram [EEG, left and right EMs (LOC and ROC), and chin muscle tone (EMG)] shows the last 6 minutes of a 30-minute REM period. Before sleep, the subject (RK) agreed to mark two events with distinct VEMS: *On Lucid Dream Onset* (LDO) with two pairs of left-right EMs (LR2); and *On Awakening* with four pairs (LR4). VEMS followed the script: "Look at your left ear, right ear, etc." This assured full-scale VEMS, without head movement. On awakening, RK reported the VEMS labeled 1–5. LDO is localized by the ANS "surprise response" (biphasic HR and scalp SPR), just before the LR2 signal (1). In the next 90 seconds, RK "flew about, exploring" until he concluded (falsely) he'd awakened, and signaled LR4 (2). [N.B., this signal, made while RK was *non-lucid*, shows the precise correspondence between EOG and gaze is not limited to LDs.] RK began recording his dream, until "a lab tech" started rudely ripping off his electrodes! He began signaling: LRLRLR . . . (3) but stopped short; he'd been signing LR4, the wrong signal! He paused, then corrected his error with LR2 (4), and went on exploring his LD for another 90 seconds. Finally, he awoke, signaled LR4 (5), and recorded his dream. Calib.: 10 sec., 50μV. [Figure revised from LaBerge et al. 1981b]

(Kahan & LaBerge, 1994) informs them that the dream world in which they seem to be contained is actually contained *in their minds*. But they don't see themselves in two places at once—only one, in the dream. This point is worth emphasizing because some researchers mistakenly believe that lucid dreamers are in "a dissociated state" in which they characteristically see themselves "from the outside" or "as if on a screen" (Voss et al., 2014). This sounds more like hypnagogic imagery than a full-blown REM LD; in any case, *none* of the more than 100 REM SVLDs we have content-analyzed have this feature (Levitan, LaBerge, DeGracia, & Zimbardo, 1999).

It might be objected that lucid dreamers might be awake but simply not be attending to the environment; rather than being asleep, perhaps they are merely absorbed in their private fantasy worlds as, for example, when deeply immersed in a novel or daydream. However, according to their reports (LaBerge, 1980a, 1985), if lucid dreamers deliberately attempt to feel the bedcovers under which they know they are sleeping, or listen for the ticking of the clock they know is beside their bed, they typically fail to feel or hear anything except what they find in their dream worlds. So lucid dreamers can metaconsciously note *the absence of sensory input* from the external world; therefore, on empirical grounds, they conclude that they are asleep.

If, in a contrary case, subjects were to claim to have been awake while showing physiological signs of sleep, or vice versa, we might have cause to doubt their subjective reports. However, when our subjects reported being certain that they were asleep they showed physiological indications of unequivocal REM sleep (LaBerge, Nagel, Dement, & Zarcone, 1981a). Some critics have suggested that "demand characteristics" might account for our results. It is true that our subjects were under demand to have, signal, and report LDs, but how could demand alone account for them doing all three things without having been lucid in the first place?

Physiological Characteristics of Lucid Dreaming

My colleagues and I analyzed psychophysiological data from 76 SVLDs of 13 subjects (LaBerge, Levitan, & Dement, 1986). We divided each SVLD into 30-second epochs aligned with the signals marking lucidity onset (LDO). For each epoch, we scored sleep stage (Rechtschaffen & Kales, 1968), counted REMs (REMd adjusted to REMs per minute) and scalp skin-potential responses (SPR per minute), and, for SVLDs recorded with corresponding measures, we also calculated heart rate (HR, beats per minute) and respiration rate (RR, breaths per minute).

For the first lucid epoch, beginning with the initiation of the signal, the sleep stage was unequivocal REM in all cases (Rechtschaffen & Kales, 1968). Physiological comparison of REMd, HR, RR, and SPR showed that the lucid epochs of the SVLD REMPs had significantly higher levels of physiological activation than the preceding epochs of non-lucid REM from the same REMP. Similarly, H-reflex amplitude is lower during lucid REM (including *during* signaling) compared to non-lucid REM sleep (Brylowski, Levitan, & LaBerge, 1989).

Physiological data were also collected for 61 control non-lucid REMPs, derived from the same 13 subjects, in order to allow comparison with SVLDs. Mean values for REMd and SPR were significantly higher for REMPs with LDs than non-lucid control REMPs (RR and HR did not differ).

Given the finding that LDs reliably occur during activated (phasic) REM, measures of central nervous system activation, such as REMd, should positively correlate with LD distribution. Since it had been previously observed that REMd starts at a low level at the beginning of REMPs and increases until it reaches a peak after approximately five to seven minutes (Aserinsky, 1971), we (LaBerge et al., 1986) hypothesized that LD probability should follow a parallel development. We accordingly found that mean REMd correlated positively and significantly with LD probability ($r = .66$, $p < .01$). Similarly, Kramer (2011) found dream content to intensify with time into REMPs.

Lucid dreams have been frequently reported to occur most commonly late in the sleep cycle (Green, 1968; Moers-Messmer, 1938; van Eeden, 1913). My colleagues and I (LaBerge et al., 1986) tested this hypothesis by first determining, for each of their 12 subjects, the time of night that divided their total REM time into two equal parts. All but one of the subjects had more LDs in the second half of their REM time than in the first half (binomial test; $p < .01$). For the combined sample, LD probability was calculated for REMPs one through six of the night by dividing the total number of LDs observed in a given REMP by the corresponding total time in stage REM for the same REMP. A regression analysis showed that LD probability linearly increased with ordinal REMP number ($r = .98$, $p < .0001$). This is in accordance with studies showing intensification of dream content with time of night (for review, see Kramer, 2011).

There are two distinct ways in which LDs are initiated. In the usual case, subjects report having been in the midst of a dream when a bizarre occurrence causes sufficient reflection to yield the realization that they are dreaming. In the other, less frequent case, subjects report having briefly awakened from a dream and then falling back asleep directly entering the dream with no (or very little) break in consciousness (Green, 1968; LaBerge 1985). Here is an example of a wake-initiated LD:

> I was lying awake in bed late in the morning listening to the sound of running water in the adjoining bathroom. Presently an image of the ocean appeared, dim at first like my usual waking imagery. But its vividness rapidly increased while, at the same time, the sound of running bathwater diminished; the intensity of the internal image and external sound seemed to alter inversely (as if one changed a stereo balance control from one channel to the other). In a few seconds, I found myself at the seashore standing between my mother and a girl who seemed somehow familiar. I could no longer hear the sound of the bath water, but only the roar of the dream sea. (LaBerge, 1980a, p. 85)

Note that the subject is continuously conscious during the transition from wakefulness to sleep. This fact suggests that Foulkes (1985) is overstating the case by claiming that it is "a necessary part of the experience we call 'sleep' that we lose a directive and reflective self. You can't fall asleep, or be asleep, if your waking self is still regulating and reflecting upon your conscious mental state" (p. 42).

Since LDs initiated in these two ways ought to differ physiologically in at least one respect (viz., an awakening preceding one but not the other), the SVLDs were dichotomously classified as either "wake-initiated" (WILD) or "dream-initiated" (DILD), depending on whether or not the reports mentioned a transient awakening in which the subject consciously perceived the external environment before reentering the dream state. Fifty-five (72%) of the SVLDs were classified as DILDs and the remaining 21 (28%) as WILDs. For all 13 subjects, DILDs were more common than WILDs (binomial test, $p < .0001$). Compared to DILDs, WILDs were more frequently preceded by physiological indications of awakening (Chi-squared = 38.3, 1df, $p < .0001$) supporting the validity of classifying LDs in this manner.

To summarize, an elevated level of central nervous system activation seems to be a necessary condition for the occurrence of LDs. Evidently the high level of metacognitive function involved in lucid dreaming requires a correspondingly high level of cortical activation and working memory (WM). Becoming lucid (i.e., metaconscious) (Kahan & LaBerge, 1994) requires adequate WM to reflect long enough when anomalies occur to allow their interpretation as *dreamsigns*, in accordance with the pre-sleep intention to recognize that one is dreaming. This level of cortical and cognitive activation is not always available during sleep, but normally only during periods of phasic REM. While LD onset may depend on random fluctuations of brain-stem arousal, the fact that cortical activation remains high during sustained LDs lasting from hundreds to thousands of seconds implies a forebrain mechanism of top-down regulation of arousal.

Psychophysiological Studies of Dreaming I: Classic Paradigm

The psychophysiological approach was responsible for the Golden Age of dream research in the decades following the discovery of REM sleep (Aserinsky & Kleitman, 1953) and the subsequent association of REM with dreaming (Dement & Kleitman, 1957). Although the psychophysiological paradigm of dream research was fruitful for many years (see Arkin, Antrobus, & Ellman, 1978), it possesses a fatal flaw: as long as the subjects are non-lucid, there is no way to be certain that they will dream about what the researcher might like to study. Ironically, just at the time we were applying the psychophysiological method to prove LDs occurred in REM sleep, some researchers were declaring it "not to be a wise place for dream psychology to continue to commit much of its limited resources" (Foulkes, 1981, p. 249). Moffitt and Hoffman's (1987) view was in striking contrast:

> ... with LaBerge's proof traditional dream psychophysiology has proved useful in demonstrating that the traditional scientific and psychoanalytic view of dreams of dreaming were, if not incorrect, then limited in ways that have fundamental implications for ... dream [and] cognitive psychology,

and, finally, cognitive and ecological epistemology. That is worth the cost of 30 years of psychophysiological research. (p. 154)

The fact that trained lucid dreamers can remember to perform predetermined actions and signal to the laboratory overcame the basic difficulty of the old methodology and suggested a new paradigm for dream research (LaBerge, 1980a): lucid dreamers, I proposed, "could carry out diverse dream experiments marking the exact time of particular dream events, allowing the derivation of precise psychophysiological correlations and the methodical testing of hypotheses" (LaBerge et al., 1981a, p. 727).

A prerequisite for this or any other application is access to the state. I have demonstrated that lucid dreaming is a learnable skill (LaBerge, 1980b) and there are a variety of techniques available for inducing LDs (LaBerge & Rheingold, 1990; Price & Cohen, 1988). My colleagues and I have experimented with methods for helping dreamers to realize that they are dreaming by means of various external cues (voice, vibrations, and light) applied during REM sleep, which if incorporated into dreams, can remind dreamers that they are dreaming (LaBerge, 1980a; LaBerge, 1985; LaBerge & Rheingold, 1990). The most effective cues were flashes of light (LaBerge & Levitan, 1995). Additional factors increasing LD probability include sleep cycle interruption (LaBerge, Phillips, & Levitan, 1994) and REM intensification via pre-sleep acetylcholinesterase inhibitor supplementation (LaBerge & LaMarca, 2014).

Psychophysiological Studies of Dreaming II: Lucid Paradigm

The eye movement signaling methodology forms the basis for a more powerful approach to dream research than previously available methods: trained subjects can induce LDs and then remember to carry out pre-planned dream experiments, marking the exact time of particular dream events with eye movement signals, allowing much more efficient study of correlations between the dreamer's subjective reports and recorded physiology.

My colleagues and I employed this strategy in a series of studies at Stanford University that demonstrated a striking degree of psychophysiological parallelism during lucid REM dreaming. In a study of dream time, subjects estimated 10-second intervals during their LDs. Signals marking the beginning and end of the subjective intervals allowed comparison with objective time. In all cases, time estimates during the LDs were within standard errors of time estimates while awake and likewise close to the actual time between signals. In short, it takes as long to do something in a dream as it does in waking life (LaBerge, 1980a, 1985).

In another study, we asked four trained lucid dreamers to either breathe rapidly or to hold their breath (in their LDs), marking the interval of altered respiration

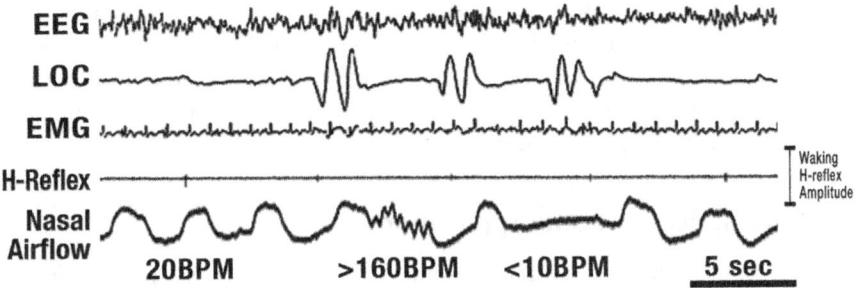

FIGURE 16.2 Voluntary control of respiration during REM lucid dreaming. The lucid dreamer participant observer (LDPO) performs a protocol agreed upon before sleep. After becoming lucid, the LDPO signals LRLR (see Figure 16.1), then breathes as rapidly as possible for 5 seconds, again signals LRLR, holds his breath for 5 sec, and ends with a final LRLR. During the tachypnea phase, his respiration rate increased 800% compared to immediately before the task. Just as obviously, he did not breath during the apnea segment. This recording also elicited H-reflex (a measure of spinal reflex excitability) every five seconds. As can be seen in the figure, compared to Waking (calibration at far right), H-reflex is very strongly suppressed during the LD, supporting the idea that lucid dreams occur during a deepened and intensified variety of paradoxical sleep rather than a lighter state of near-waking (Brylowski, Levitan, & LaBerge, 1989).

with eye movement signals (LaBerge & Dement, 1982). Respiration exactly corresponded to the reported patterns (Figure 16.2).

Other studies demonstrated that dreamed movements result in corresponding patterns of muscle twitching, and that dreamed sexual activity is associated with physiological responses very similar to those associated with actual sexual activity (LaBerge, Greenleaf, & Kedzierski, 1983).

We also found that we could distinguish dreaming and imagination physiologically by means of a visual tracking task (LaBerge & Zimbardo, 2000). We asked subjects to give the usual signal when they realized they were dreaming, then to slowly and smoothly move their finger, held at arms length, in a circle about 20 degrees wide, centered in the visual field, while tracking the tip of the finger. They also did the tracking task while awake with eyes open ("perception") and eyes closed ("imagination"). Imagination was much more likely to show rapid, saccadic eye movements, while dreaming and perception showed predominately slow, smooth tracking eye movement. The statistically significant differences in tracking presumably reflect corresponding differences in visual vividness, with dreaming and waking perception both being more subjectively vivid than visual imagination.

The results of these and other similar studies can be summarized as follows: dreamed experiences produce effects on the dreamer's brain (and to a lesser extent, body) remarkably similar to the physiological effects that are produced by actual experiences of the corresponding events while awake. If it were not for the fact that most of our muscles are paralyzed during REM sleep, we would actually do what we are doing in the dream. Perhaps this explains in part why we are so inclined to mistake our dreams for reality: to the brain processes that construct our experiential model of the world, dreaming of perceiving or doing something is equivalent to actually perceiving or doing it.

Clinical Implications and Applications

Insofar as LDs are experienced as interesting, exciting, and relatively pleasant, mood elevations would be expected to ensue upon awakening (LaBerge, 1985). As predicted, in a study of dream content and overnight changes of mood, my colleagues and I found significantly more positive mood following LDs than NLDs (Levitan and LaBerge, 1993). In contrast to NLDs, which are typically accompanied by mild anxiety, emotions in LDs are usually positive, ranging from mild exhilaration to deeply meaningful, ecstatic peak experiences.

Lucid dreaming may have other positive effects. For example, Gruber, Steffen, and Vonderhaar (1995) concluded "that frequent lucid dreamers, characterized by the unusual degree of control they often exhibit within the dream state, are also better able to manage or control various aspects of cognitive, emotional, and social functioning while awake" (p. 7). A possible example may be provided by an Israeli study reporting evidence that frequent LDs may increase resilience in the face of exposure to terrorism (Soffer-Dudek, Wertheim, & Shahar, 2011).

Lucid dreaming has often been said to possess unique psychotherapeutic potential (e.g., Garfield, 1979; LaBerge, 1985). More than 150 years ago, the Marquis Hervey de Saint-Denys used lucidity to cure himself of a terrifying recurrent nightmare (Saint-Denys, 1867/1982):

> One night, . . . when the dream returned for the fourth time, at the moment my persecutors were about to renew their pursuit, a feeling of the truth of the situation was suddenly awakened in my mind; and the desire to combat these illusions gave me the strength to overcome my instinctive terror. Instead of fleeing, . . . I resolved to contemplate with the closest attention the phantoms that I had so far only glimpsed rather than seen. . . . I fixed my eyes on my principal attacker, who somewhat resembled the grinning, bristling demons which are sculpted in cathedral porticos, and as the desire to observe gained the upper hand over my emotions, . . . I watched as the monster lost its fantastic frightening detail and collapsed into an empty costume, a bundle of rags . . . and then awoke. The nightmare did not recur thereafter. (pp. 58–59)

Tholey (1988) also observed that when the dreamer courageously and openly looks at hostile dream figures, their appearance often becomes less threatening.

Indeed, most people say that becoming lucid in a nightmare makes them feel better afterwards more often than not. In a survey study of 698 college students, my colleagues and I found that of the 505 who reported having had both LDs and nightmares, most (59%) claimed that becoming lucid in a nightmare usually improved the outcome; about a third thought it usually made no difference; and 8% said it made things worse (Levitan & LaBerge, 1990). Lucidity was about seven times more likely to make nightmares better than worse, supporting the notion that lucid dreaming is generally a good thing—but, remembering the 8%, not necessarily all the time or for everyone. Holzinger (2014) makes a similar point. Finally, anyone who worries because lucid dreams can sometimes be upsetting should consider the alternative—non-lucid dreams, which not are not-uncommonly disturbing enough to be called "nightmares." For most people in most circumstances, lucidity will do more good than harm.

Several case studies (Brylowski, 1990; Zadra & Pihl, 1997) and a randomized controlled study (Spoormaker & van den Bout, 2006) have provided support for the claim that lucid dreaming can be an effective treatment of nightmares. The fact that children can learn and apply lucid dreaming to overcoming nightmares (Armstrong-Hickey, 1988) is clearly worthy of further study (e.g., see LaBerge & Rheingold, 1990).

Tholey (1988) has researched the effect of various attitudes towards hostile dream characters, concluding that a conciliatory approach—through engaging in dialogs with hostile dream characters—is most likely to result in a positive outcome. He found that when dreamers tried to reconcile with hostile figures, the figures often transformed from "lower" order into "higher" order creatures, meaning from beasts or mythological beings into humans, and that these transformations frequently allowed the dreamers to immediately understand the meaning of their dreams. Furthermore, conciliatory behavior towards threatening figures would generally cause them to look and act in a more friendly manner. For example, Tholey (1988) himself dreamt:

> I became lucid, while being chased by a tiger, and wanted to flee. I then pulled myself back together, stood my ground, and asked, "Who are you?" The tiger was taken aback but transformed into my father and answered, "I am your father and will now tell you what you are to do!" In contrast to my earlier dreams, I did not attempt to beat him but tried to get involved in a dialogue with him. I told him that he could not order me around. I rejected his threats and insults. On the other hand, I had to admit that some of my father's criticism was justified, and I decided to change my behavior accordingly. At that moment my father became friendly, and we shook hands. I asked him if he could help me, and he encouraged me to go my own way alone. My father then seemed to slip into my own body, and I remained alone in the dream. (p. 265)

I reported that the proportions of LDs triggered by anxiety significantly decreased in each of the first four years included in my dissertation study, from 15/62 (36%), to 17/111 (19%), 10/215 (5%), and finally 2/150 (1%) (LaBerge, 1980a). The striking decrease in proportion (and absolute frequency in the last two years) of anxiety-initiated LDs with time was probably related to the psychotherapeutic techniques that I was practicing, primarily seeking to face, work through, and accept dream figures or situations that I had been avoiding (LaBerge, 1985; see also Tholey, 1988), as the following quote illustrates:

> I was in the middle of a riot in a classroom; a furious mob was raging about, throwing chairs and fighting with each other. A huge repulsive barbarian with a pock-marked face, . . . had me hopelessly locked in an iron grip from which I was desperately trying to free myself. At this point, I became lucid, and remembering what I had learned from past LDs, I stopped struggling . . . and tried to project loving acceptance as I faced this "ogre."
>
> At first, I failed utterly, feeling overwhelming repulsion and disgust. He was simply too ugly to love: thus spoke my visceral reactions. So I tried again, but first I remembered to seek love within my own heart. Finding it, I looked my ogre in the eyes, and trusting my intuition, beautiful words of compassionate acceptance flowed out of me, and as they did, he melted into me. As for the riot, it had vanished without a trace; the dream was over and I awoke, feeling wonderfully calm. (LaBerge & DeGracia, 2000, p. 279)

Note the image of incorporation that occurs in both of these dreams of integration, in which hostile rejected images (tiger, father, and ogre, Jungian "shadow" figures all) are integrated into the model of the self (the dream-ego). This illustrates the unique and important power of lucid dreaming to further self-integration.

I believe a major mechanism whereby nightmares become recurrent is the following process: First, you wake from a nightmare in a state of intense anxiety and fear; the nightmare was so unpleasant that it exceeds your ability to cope. You don't want to even think about it; presumably you also hope it never happens again! But, by an *ironic mental process* (Wegner, 1994), the wish to avoid at all costs the events of the nightmare *ensures that they will be remembered*. (Think of how maladaptive it would be to walk down a certain path, fall in a snake pit, eventually climb out, and decide to just forget about it.) Later, you experience something that again causes you to dream about a situation similar to the original nightmare. In the dream you recognize (perhaps unconsciously) the similarity, and thus expect the same thing to happen again. Thus, expectation causes the dream to follow the first plot, and the more the dream recurs, the more likely it is to recur in an increasingly stereotyped form. Looking at recurrent nightmares in this way suggests a simple treatment: you need to conceive of a new response to the dream situation to weaken the expectation that it has only one possible outcome. Imaginatively reexperiencing the dream *as a dream* allows you to develop more adaptive responses to the particular dream situation should it reoccur. This provides a plan to cope with the situation and releases you from the vicious cycle of ironic motivation. For details and several case studies, see LaBerge and Rheingold (1990).

Another promising clinical application is the use of lucid dreaming as a means to resolve "unfinished business" such as in the case of the death of a loved one (for examples, see LaBerge & Rheingold, 1990; and Tholey, 1988). Lucid dreaming therapy may be especially helpful in cases of pathological grief, allowing an otherwise impossible, as-if-real, and potentially healing encounter with the deceased that can facilitate letting go.

Finally, an intriguing speculation is that lucid dreaming might help the terminally ill to approach their impending death with equanimity, acceptance, and sometimes something more (LaBerge, 1985; LaBerge & Rheingold, 1990). This is a major reason Tibetan Buddhists give for developing proficiency in (lucid) dream yoga (LaBerge, 2003). The Tibetans believe that practice of LD yoga provides essential preparation for being lucid in the dreamlike after-death state, allowing a higher level of choice about what happens next: a "favorable rebirth," "enlightenment," or simply a return to the Nothing from which we came, perhaps what Westerners would call "a good death."

We have seen that lucid dreaming is an experiential and physiological reality. But whether we should consider it a paradoxical form of sleep, or a paradoxical form of waking, or something else entirely, still seems too early to tell. Terms like *sleep, waking,* and *dreaming* may be too coarse a net to capture the finer structures of consciousness. Our vocabulary for describing states of consciousness is still too undeveloped. But for now, lucid dreaming should remind us not to prematurely close our accounts on the possibilities of human consciousness and the paradoxical sleeping brain.

References

Arkin, A., Antrobus, J., & Ellman, S. (1978). (Eds.) *The mind in sleep.* Hillsdale, NJ: Lawrence Erlbaum Associates.

Armstrong-Hickey, D.A. (1988). The validation of lucid dreams in school-age children. *Sleep Research, 17,* 114.

Aserinsky, E. (1971). Rapid eye movement density and pattern in the sleep of young adults. *Psychophysiology, 8,* 361–375.

Aserinsky, E., & Kleitman, N. (1953). Regularly occurring periods of eye motility and concomitant phenomena during sleep. *Science, 118,* 273–274.

Barrett, D. (1992). Just how lucid are lucid dreams: An empirical study of their cognitive characteristics. *Dreaming, 2,* 221–228.

Brylowski, A. (1990). Nightmares in crisis: Clinical applications of lucid dreaming techniques. *Psychiatric Journal of the University of Ottawa, 15,* 79–84.

Brylowski, A., Levitan, L., & LaBerge, S. (1989). H-reflex suppression and autonomic activation during lucid REM sleep: A case study. *Sleep, 12,* 374–378.

Dane, J. (1984). An empirical evaluation of two techniques for lucid dream induction. Unpublished doctoral dissertation, Georgia State University.

Dement, W., & Kleitman, N. (1957). Cyclic variations in EEG during sleep and their relation to eye movements, body motility, and dreaming. *EEG and Clinical Neurophysiology, 9*, 673–690.

Dennett, D. C. (1976) Are dreams experiences? *Philosophical Review, 73*, 151–171.

Dresler, M., Koch, S., Wehrle, R., Spoormaker, V., Holsboer, F., Steiger, A., Sämann, P., Obrig, H. & Czisch, M. (2011). Dreamed movement elicits activation in the sensorimotor cortex. *Current Biology, 21*, 1833–1837.

Ellis, H. (1922). *The world of dreams*. Boston and New York: Houghton Mifflin.

Erlacher, D., & Schredl, M. (2008). Cardiovascular responses to dreamed physical exercise during REM lucid dreaming. *Dreaming, 18*, 112–121.

Foulkes, D. (1981). Dreams and dream research. In W. Koella (Ed.), *Sleep 1980* (pp. 246–257). Basel: Karger.

Foulkes, D. (1985). *Dreaming: A cognitive-psychological analysis*. Hillsdale, NJ: Lawrence Erlbaum Associates.

Garfield, P. (1979). *Pathway to ecstasy*. New York: Holt, Rhinehart, & Winston.

Green, C. (1968). *Lucid dreams*. London: Hamish Hamilton.

Gruber, R. E., Steffen, J. J., & Vonderharr, S. P. (1995). Lucid dreaming, waking personality, and cognitive development. *Dreaming, 5*, 1–12.

Hearne, K. M. T. (1978). Lucid dreams: An electrophysiological and psychological study. Unpublished doctoral dissertation, University of Liverpool.

Hearne, K. M. T. (1983). Electrophysiological aspects of lucid dreams: More detailed findings. *Journal of Lucid Dream Research, 1*, 21–47.

Hobson, J. A. (2009). The neurobiology of consciousness: Lucid dreaming wakes up. *International Journal of Dream Research, 2*, 41–44.

Holzinger, B. (2014). Lucid dreaming in psychotherapy. In R. Hurd & K. Bulkeley (Eds.), *Lucid dreaming: New perspectives on consciousness during sleep, Vol. 1* (pp. 37–61). Santa Barbara, CA: Praeger.

Holzinger, B., LaBerge, S., & Levitan, L. (2006). Psychophysiological correlates of lucid dreaming. *Dreaming, 16*, 88–95.

James, W. (1890). *The principles of psychology, Vol. 2*. New York: Dover Publications.

Kahan, T. L., & LaBerge, S. (1994). Lucid dreaming as metacognition: Implications for cognitive science. *Consciousness and Cognition, 3*, 246–264.

Kramer, M. (2011). REM sleep and dreaming: The nature of the relationship. In B. N. Mallick, S. R. Pandi-Perumal, R. W. McCarley, & A. R. Morris (Eds.), *REM sleep: Regulation and function* (pp. 40–48). Cambridge: Cambridge University Press.

LaBerge, S. (1980a). Lucid dreaming: An exploratory study of consciousness during sleep. Doctoral dissertation, Stanford University. University Microfilms International No. 80-24,691.

LaBerge, S. (1980b). Lucid dreaming as a learnable skill: A case study. *Perceptual and Motor Skills, 51*, 1039–1042.

LaBerge, S. (1985). *Lucid dreaming*. Los Angeles: Tarcher.

LaBerge, S. (1990). Lucid dreaming: Psychophysiological studies of consciousness during REM sleep. In R. R. Bootsen, J. F. Kihlstrom, & D. L. Schacter (Eds.), *Sleep and cognition* (pp. 109–126). Washington, DC: American Psychological Association.

LaBerge, S. (2003). Tibetan dream yoga and lucid dreaming: A psychophysiological perspective. In B. A. Wallace (Ed.) *Buddhism and science* (pp. 233–258). New York: Columbia University Press.

LaBerge, S. (2010). Signal-verified lucid dreaming proves that REM sleep can support reflective consciousness. *International Journal of Dream Research, 3(1)*, 26–27.

LaBerge, S. (2014). Lucid dreaming: Paradoxes of dreaming consciousness. In E. Cardeña, S. J. Lynn, & S. Krippner (Eds.), *Varieties of anomalous experience: Examining the scientific evidence* (2nd Ed.) (pp. 145–172). Washington, DC: American Psychological Association.
LaBerge, S. & DeGracia, D. J. (2000). Varieties of lucid dreaming experience. In R. G. Kunzendorf & B. Wallace (Eds.), *Individual differences in conscious experience* (pp. 269–307). Philadelphia: John Benjamins.
LaBerge, S. & Dement, W. C. (1982). Voluntary control of respiration during REM sleep. *Sleep Research, 11*, 107.
LaBerge, S., Greenleaf, W. & Kedzierski, B. (1983). Physiological responses to dreamed sexual activity during lucid REM sleep. *Psychophysiology, 20*, 454–455.
LaBerge, S. & LaMarca, K. (2014, April). Pre-sleep treatment with acetylcholinesterase inhibitors enhances memory, cognition, and metaconsciousness (lucidity) in dreaming. Presentation at the 10th biennial meeting of the Toward a Science of Consciousness Conference, Tucson, AZ.
LaBerge, S., & Levitan, L. (1995). Validity established of DreamLight cues for eliciting lucid dreaming. *Dreaming, 5*, 159–168.
LaBerge, S., Levitan, L. & Dement, W. C. (1986). Lucid dreaming: Physiological correlates of consciousness during REM sleep. *Journal of Mind and Behavior, 7*, 251–258.
LaBerge, S., Nagel, L., Dement, W.C., & Zarcone, V., Jr. (1981a). Lucid dreaming verified by volitional communication during REM sleep. *Perceptual & Motor Skills, 52*, 727–732.
LaBerge, S., Nagel, L., Dement, W.C., & Zarcone, V., Jr. (1981b). Evidence for lucid dreaming during REM sleep. *Sleep Research, 10*, 148.
LaBerge, S., Phillips, L., & Levitan, L. (1994). An hour of wakefulness before morning naps makes lucidity more likely. *NightLight, 6(3)*, 1–5.
LaBerge, S., & Rheingold, H. (1990). *Exploring the world of lucid dreaming*. New York: Ballantine.
LaBerge, S. & Zimbardo P. G. (2000). Smooth tracking eye-movements discriminate both dreaming and perception from imagination. Toward a Science of Consciousness Conference IV, Tucson, April 10, 2000. <http://lucidity.com/Tucson2000abs.html>.
Levitan, L. & LaBerge, S. (1990). Beyond nightmares: Lucid resourcefulness vs. helpless depression. *NightLight, 2(4)*, 1–6.
Levitan, L. & LaBerge, S. (1993). Day life, night life: How waking and dreaming experiences relate. *NightLight, 5(1)*, 4–6.
Levitan, L., LaBerge, S., DeGracia, D. J. & Zimbardo, P. G. (1999). "Out-of-body experiences," dreams, and REM sleep. *Sleep and Hypnosis, 1*, 186–196.
Moers-Messmer, H. von, (1938). Träume mit der gleichzeitigen Erkenntnis des Traumzustandes [Dreams with simultaneous cognizance of the dream state], *Archiv für Psychologie, 102*, 291–318.
Moffitt, A. & Hoffman, R. (1987). On the single-mindedness and isolation of dream psychophysiology. In J. Gackenbach (Ed), *Sleep and dreams: A sourcebook* (pp. 145–186). New York: Garland Publishing.
Ogilvie, R., Hunt, H., Kushniruk, A. & Newman, J. (1983). Lucid dreams and the arousal continuum. *Sleep Research, 12*, 182.
Ogilvie, R., Hunt, H., Sawicki, C., & McGowan, K. (1978). Searching for lucid dreams. *Sleep Research, 7*, 165.
Price, R. F. & Cohen, D. B. (1988). Lucid dream induction: An empirical evaluation. In J. Gackenbach & S. LaBerge (Eds.) *Conscious mind, sleeping brain* (pp. 105–154). New York: Plenum Press.

Rechtschaffen, A. (1978). The single-mindedness and isolation of dreams. *Sleep, 1,* 97–109.

Rechtschaffen, A. & Kales, A. (Eds.) (1968). *A manual of standardized terminology, techniques and scoring system for sleep stages of human subjects.* Los Angeles: UC Brain Information Service.

Saint-Denys, H. D. (1867/1982). *Dreams and how to guide them* (M. Schatzman, Trans.). London, England: Duckworth.

Schatzman, M., Worsley, A., & Fenwick, P. (1988). Correspondence during lucid dreams between dreamed and actual events. In J. Gackenbach & S. LaBerge (Eds.), *Conscious mind, sleeping brain* (pp. 155–179). New York: Plenum.

Soffer-Dudek, N., Wertheim, R., & Shahar, G. (2011). Lucid dreaming and resilience in the face of exposure to terrorism. *Journal of Traumatic Stress, 24,* 125–128.

Spoormaker, V. I., van den Bout, J. (2006). Lucid dreaming treatment for nightmares: A pilot study. *Psychotherapy-and-Psychosomatics, 75,* 389–394.

Tholey, P. (1988). A model for lucidity training as a means of self-healing and psychological growth. In J. Gackenbach & S. LaBerge (Eds.), *Conscious mind, sleeping brain* (pp. 67–103). New York: Plenum.

van Eeden, F. (1913). A study of dreams. *Proceedings of the Society for Psychical Research, 26,* 431–61.

Voss, U., Holzmann, R., Hobson, A., Paulus, W. Koppehele-Gossel, J., Klimke, A., & Nitsche, M. (2014). Induction of self awareness in dreams through frontal low current stimulation of gamma activity. *Nature Neuroscience, 17,* 810–812.

Voss, U., Holzmann, R., Tuin, I., & Hobson, J. A. (2009). Lucid dreaming: a state of consciousness with features of both waking and non-lucid dreaming. *Sleep, 32,* 1191–1200.

Watanabe, T. (2003). Lucid dreaming: Its experimental proof and psychological conditions. *Journal of International Society of Life Information Science (Japan) 21,* 159–162.

Wegner, D. M. (1994). Ironic processes of mental control. *Psychological Review, 101,* 34–52.

Zadra, A. L., & Pihl, R. O. (1997). Lucid dreaming as a treatment for recurrent nightmares. *Psychotherapy and Psychosomatics, 66,* 50–55.

17

REALITY

Waking, Sleeping, or Virtual?

*Jayne Gackenbach, Hannah Stark,
Arielle Boyes, and Carson Flockhart*

MACEWAN UNIVERSITY

Merging of realities has been the focus of our research program thus far as we have examined the dreams of video game players who have played approximately 10,000 hours since childhood. In other words, we have been studying the dreams of expert video game players. The content of video gamers' dreams show incorporation of game content, consistent with the continuity hypothesis, which suggests that there is a continuum between waking activities and dreamt activities (Shredl, 2003). Often, however, such content is not limited to a game being represented but rather the entire dreamt sequence is thought to be a game (Gackenbach, Sample, & Mandel, 2011). Thus, the dreamers' choices are affected by the attribution of "this is a game." In one gamers' dream, for instance, he wondered what it would be like to burn to death and subsequently chose to stay in a burning car to find out (Gackenbach & Hunt, 2014). While virtual gaming dreams are often lucid, meaning the gamers know they are in a dream, what is more consistent in our research is the felt sense by the gamers that they can control the events and outcomes of the dreamt scenario (Gackenbach, 2012a). One consequence of confidence in personal dream control is nightmare protection. This automatic response to threats is developed when a gamer fights threats for many hours over many years in a video game. For example, chases and attacks in dreams are more likely to result in fight rather than the flight response (Boyes & Gackenbach, 2014). In addition, although the dreamt chases and attacks may remain frightening and threatening, gamers also report that they are fun and empowering. Nightmares, consequently, are viewed as less threatening and thus not as psychologically damaging as they are for non-gamers who do not experience such empowerment.

To begin, we explain the impact of virtual worlds on dreams by examining virtual reality. Next, we consider how lucidity and dream control are affected by virtual reality as well as the theoretical and empirical underpinnings of this association. Finally, we discuss the nightmare protection research. In this chapter we go beyond previous summaries of our work (Gackenbach, 2012a) and explore current projects, applications, and future directions.

What Is Virtual Reality?

Virtual reality (VR) technology is a computer-simulated environment that replicates the experience of being present in another location. The extent to which one feels present in another location depends on how well the VR technology creates immersion. *Immersion* refers to the degree to which a virtual environment submerges the perceptual systems of the user in computer-generated stimuli. While relatively new in computer-mediated communications, the idea of *presence* is long-standing in the VR literature as well in the arts. What is changing is the quality of the replication of reality and its fully interactive nature (Biocca, Kim, & Levy, 1995).

The newest way to capture these experiences is by wearing a quality pair of VR goggles that once were only available at a high cost to specialist laboratories. However, with the development of the Oculus Rift, a state-of-the-art VR technology, many more people will be experiencing enhanced VR. Therefore, we expect that there will be greater immersion into dreams and the experience of dream lucidity, control, and nightmare protection (summarized in Gackenbach, 2012b).

Theoretical Basis for Lucidity/Control in Dreams Associated With Gaming

Our inquiries into the dreams of gamers began when we observed that both lucid dreamers (Snyder & Gackenbach, 1988) and gamers (Greenfield, Brannon, & Lohr, 1996) had superior spatial skills. Thus, we set out to explore lucidity in dreams and immersion in VR gaming, noting that they had similar characteristics with potentially the latter affecting the former (Gackenbach, 2008). Hunt (1995) pointed out that meditators have more lucidity, control, and bizarreness, and less threat in their dreams than non-meditators. Therefore, it may be that gaming enhances the experience of lucidity along the lines of meditators' experiences with lucidity. Gackenbach (2008) argued that video game play specifically—and more generically all electronically mediated interactions—can become a sort of meditative experience. Gackenbach's argument was built by tracing parallels between game play and meditation. These include improved attention skills, deep absorption, flow experiences, improved spatial skills, and increased lucid dreaming, all of which are characteristic of both meditation and video game play (for a review of each of these areas see Gackenbach, 2012b). While the effects of gaming are certainly not as profound or far reaching as meditation (Gackenbach, 2008), the base of our argument is that gaming allows access to the states of consciousness typically accessed by meditators. The notion that virtual worlds enable the high absorption characteristic of higher states of consciousness claimed by meditators was originally put forth by Preston (1998).

Directly related to this thesis is an experimental manipulation from our laboratory that examined how gaming effects dreams. Gackenbach and Rosie (2011) reported that gamers tended to experience a sense of presence that paralleled what they experienced in dreams. In short, in both the dream and game, individuals are totally absorbed into their environment and feel that they are really there experiencing the dream/game. When gamers are experiencing high levels of presence their attention is fully focused on the game. Such game play has been shown to enhance gamers' attentional abilities (Wright, Blakeley, & Boot, 2012). One outcome of meditation, similarly, is improved attentional abilities (MacKillop & Anderson, 2007). When information is multimodal it allows a greater sense of presence in an immersive virtual reality. Video games exploit these modalities in the virtual world by providing an opportunity for people who do not generally experience presence in alternative states of consciousness to do so at a level akin to that experienced in meditation (Preston, 1998). Consequently, since video games can elicit high levels of absorption, they may also have an effect on mindfulness through the enhancement of attentional skill. We have found some tentative support for this thesis (Gackenbach & Bown, 2011).

Psychological absorption is another way to view presence. According to Hölzel and Ott (2006), waking experiences of absorption predict meditative depth better than years of meditation practice. Meditation depth is a predictor of mindfulness, a widely held primary element of well-being. The high attention and absorption reported by gamers (Glicksohn & Avnon, 1997–98) and gaming research (Gackenbach, 2008) is reminiscent of the qualities associated with meditation (Weinstein & Smith, 1992). Thus, video game play has the potential to alter a broad range of human mental functioning, including making possible significant advances in attention and cognitive ability in both the long- and short-term (Boot, Kramer, Simons, Fabiani, & Gratton, 2008; Green & Bavalier, 2003). Dream changes include lucid and control dreaming.

In a quasi-experimental study from our laboratory, which directly examined the similarities between gaming and meditation, Swanston and Gackenbach (2011) reported that the highest levels of lucidity were found in those who often meditate or engage in meditative prayer. However, gamers were significantly higher on lucidity than the control group. In addition, when it came to dream control it was gamers who reported significantly more control than the meditative and control groups. Thus, we might speculate that as gaming and similar virtual immersive experiences become widely spread throughout society the associated meditative-type experiences may also increase.

The ability to lucid dream can be classified as a learned skill, and it can be enhanced through suggestion (LaBerge, 2004), drugs (LaBerge, 2014), and gamma stimulation (Voss, et al., 2014). Lucid dreaming has the potential to enhance treatment options for depression, anxiety, posttraumatic stress disorder (PTSD), physical pain, and attention deficits (Jones & Stumbrys, 2014; Holzinger, 2014). Lucid dreaming appears to be a commonality between meditation and video game play. In addition, the potential of virtual technologies to facilitate psychological well-being can be linked to their similar cognitive effects on lucidity and dream control (Zadra & Pihl, 1997) through meditation.

Nightmare Protection Thesis

Given these associations between lucidity/control dreaming and gaming, it is not surprising that one of the most fruitful areas of inquiry into gamers' dreams has been the hypothesis that gaming may protect gamers against nightmares. The nightmare is one of the most studied topics in dream research because of its disturbing nature (Hartmann, 1984; Levin & Nielsen, 2009). During REM sleep a person is paralyzed, which prevents them from acting out their dreams, yet a nightmare subjects a sleeper to a state of autonomic arousal so that they are forced awake, often in a state of panic. During the course of our initial inquiries into the impact of gaming on dreaming, we noticed that nightmares were either not reported or were reported as "fun" (Gackenbach & Kuruvilla, 2008). This led us to hypothesize that video game play during the day may act as protection from threats and fearful stimuli in a subsequent dream state.

Several studies have been conducted on the Nightmare Protection Thesis using participants in a non-threatening university setting (Gackenbach, Darlington, Ferguson, & Boyes, 2013) from high-threat occupations, such as military personal (Gackenbach, Ellerman, & Hall, 2011), and first responders (Gackenbach & Flockhart, 2013). The research has shown that males who play a high amount of combat-centric video games report fewer nightmares or a more positive response to self-identified nightmares. Such responses might include "I always wonder why my dreams are so fun"; admissions of not experiencing any nightmares; or if nightmares are acknowledged, being able to fight back in the dream without the common victim stance found in typical nightmares.

The nightmare protection research suggests that—consciously or unconsciously—the act of video game play in a virtual combat environment allows the gamer to better deal with negative experiences during sleep. The Nightmare Protection Thesis was born out of the research that conceptualizes long-term defensive rehearsals in combat-centric video games as resulting in well-learned defensive responses. These rehearsals should generalize to other virtual/altered realities as it is very similar in process to the imagery rehearsal technique used for treating nightmares (Krakow, Kellner, Neidhardt, Pathak, & Lambert, 1993). Most of the nightmare protection work in our laboratory has been correlational. In a recent experimental manipulation designed to elicit the nightmare protection effect; however, Flockhart, Gackenbach, and Ditner (2014) found support for high-end male gamers exclusively. Conversely, when males who rarely game were exposed to a stressful film stimulus and then played a video game (versus a control condition with a computer search task), they had more stressful dreams than those who gamed frequently. While gaming may facilitate the nightmare protection effect this may only be the case for high-end male gamers.

The concept of nightmare protection may have another important application in addition to the obvious benefit of not experiencing nightmares. PTSD is a debilitating experience that afflicts many individuals who fight on the front lines to defend us and can also affect first responders to threats on home soil. One of the symptoms of PTSD is severe nightmares that retraumatize sufferers (Barrett, 2001). On the surface it may seem that video game play may serve to inoculate those who face real trauma in the line of their work (i.e., military personnel and first responders). However, the extant research on the Nightmare Protection Thesis has been conducted with subjects not suffering from PTSD. For instance, in the military study and first responders studies (Gackenbach, Ellerman, & Hall, 2011; Gackenbach & Flockhart, 2013) potential research respondents were screened and subsequently omitted if they reported PTSD symptoms in the six months prior to the survey. Despite the lack of research, there is now clinical work that employs video game–type simulations (i.e., Virtual Iraq) to treat veterans with PTSD (Gerardi, Rothbaum, Ressler, Heekin, & Rizzo, 2008).

Female Gamers: One Exception to Nightmare Protection

While evidence supporting the Nightmare Protection Thesis has been found for males with repeated gaming exposure (Gackenbach, et al., 2011), this has not been the case for high-end female gamers (Gackenbach et al., 2013; Gackenbach & Flockhart, 2013). Unlike male gamers, female gamers report more frequent nightmares, feel their nightmares as more threatening, and/or feel less empowered by them. Boyes and Gackenbach (2015) explored several reasons for this discrepancy: genre of games typically played, state and trait coping styles, and susceptibility to stereotype threat. While stereotype threat was not found to affect the female nightmare finding, there was evidence for differences in genre preferences. We found that males are more likely to pick games that are "hard-core" (i.e., first-person shooters), while females are more likely to choose casual games (i.e., match-three type). These genre preferences may be confounding the difference in nightmare protection between males and females. High-end male gamers who primarily choose hard-core or combat-centric games practice defense techniques for threatening stimuli. Conversely, females who generally choose casual games[1] do not appear to get this practice. Thus, it is the rehearsal of reactions to threatening stimuli that may create this nightmare protection in males, such that the protection is only seen in males who are high-end gamers (Flockhart et al., 2014).

State coping, similarly, was examined in terms of dream actions to avoid threat in self-identified nightmares. Although flight from the dreamt threat was the most frequent response among informants, fighting back was unique to high-end male gamers. This finding verifies our conceptual understanding that practicing fighting back repeatedly over a long period of time translates to protection from into nightmares for male gamers. Thus, while there may be clinical implications for the Nightmare Protection Thesis, it needs to be further explored.

Cultural Influences in the Study of Media Use and Dreams

Previous research has shown that there is a difference between cultures dreams. Such differences have been examined by assessing self-construal (independent versus interdependent) and dream content. Independent self-construal was significantly related to the dreamer friendliness while interdependence was more associated with total acts of aggression and total social interactions (King & DeCicco, 2007).

Accordingly, our laboratory has been exploring the question "is there a differential influence of media use on dreams as a function of culture in China versus Canada?" Early results from Taiwan were recently presented from 451 Canadian and 205 Taiwanese respondents; data collection from three universities in China is nearly complete (Gackenbach, Lee, Gahr, & Yu, 2014). As expected, interdependent self-construal was higher among the Taiwanese students than among the Canadians. However, there was no difference in their independent self-construal scores, which speaks to the possible westernization of Taiwan. Further, while the Taiwanese reported playing video games more frequently than the Canadians, the Canadians reported higher incidence in other gaming variables. Specifically, video game play and social media use groups were formed and compared on selected responses to the Dream Intensity Scale, or DIS (Yu, 2010). These included self-reports of the incidence of lucid dreams, control dreams, and nightmares. Gaming was found to interact with culture for lucid dream frequency when controlling for dream recall. In Canada, consistent with previous research, high-end gamers reported more lucid dreams, but in Taiwan the opposite was true: Taiwanese low-end gamers reported more lucid dreams. This suggests that the virtual environment exposure may not be influential in developing lucid skills as we had previously thought.

There was a three-way interaction for culture, gaming group, and social media use group on dream control. The highest dream control in Canadians was reported by high-end gamers who were also high-end social media users. In Taiwan, the highest dream control was found in high-end gamers who had low social media use. In both cases it was gaming that was associated with dream control while social media use differed as a function of culture. This makes sense as social media use may more directly tap the essential difference between individualistic and collectivist societies. Relatedly, we have found that social media use and gaming were reflected in dream content differences and may be mediated by psychological boundaries (Gackenbach & Boyes, 2014).

Summary and Conclusions

The forthcoming release of Oculus Rift, a state-of-the-art VR technology for consumers, as well as the projected worldwide saturation of the Internet, may revolutionize the online world as we know it (Zuckerberg, 2014). Thus, it is important to understand how VR-type experiences are currently affecting mental health as expressed through dreams. For more than a decade our laboratory has been investigating the relationship between immersive virtual reality type media use and dreams. Beginning with inquiries into high-end video game players, we have expanded to explore social media users as it has become increasingly apparent that immersion in virtual worlds is no longer exclusively occurring in gaming. Cirucci (2013) hypothesized that video game players would display similarities to social media users. So too culture and gender have become important mediating variables in our inquiries. More detailed summaries of our work have appeared in several books (Gackenbach, 2012a; 2012b; Gackenbach & Hunt, 2014).

Beyond simple dream incorporation, as per Schredl's (2003) continuity hypothesis, there is some indication that virtual immersion may also be associated with increased recognition during lucid dreaming and the often associated dream control. One potential benefit of the increasing appearance of these qualities in dreams is nightmare protection. Although nightmare protection is strongest for high-end male gamers, it still offers some potential for imagery rehearsal type techniques via virtual reality immersion when dealing with clinically distressing dreams.

Acknowledgements

We would like to thank Allison Ditner, Sarah Gahr, and Ann Sinyard for their help in preparing this manuscript.

Note

1. Casual games take less time, are easy to learn, are less complex, and are less likely to be combative.

References

Barrett, D. (2001). *Trauma and dreams*. Cambridge, MA: Harvard University Press.
Biocca, F., Kim, Y., & Levy, M. R. (1995). The vision of virtual reality. In F. Biocca (Ed.), *Communication in the Age of Virtual Reality* (pp. 3–14). Hillsdale, NJ: Erlbaum.
Boot, W. R., Kramer, A. F., Simons, D. J., Fabiani, M., & Gratton, G. (2008). The effects of video game playing on attention, memory and executive control. *Acta Psychologica, 129*, 387–398.
Boyes, A., & Gackenbach, J. I. (2014, June). *Nightmare Protection Hypothesis and Female Gamers*. Paper presented at the annual meeting of the International Association for the Study of Dreams, Berkeley, CA.

Boyes, A. & Gackenbach, J. I. (2015). An inquiry into the lack of the nightmare protection associated with video game play by female gamers. Paper under editorial consideration *CyberPsychology*.

Cirucci, A. M. (2013). First person paparazzi: Why social media should be studied more like video games. *Telematics and Informatics, 30*(1), 47–59.

Flockhart, C., Gackenbach, J. I., & Ditner, A. (2014, June). *Video Game Nightmare Protection: An Experimental Inquiry*. Poster presented at the annual meeting of the International Association for the Study of Dreams, Berkeley, CA.

Gackenbach, J. I. (2008). Video game play and consciousness development: A transpersonal perspective. *Journal of Transpersonal Psychology, 40*(1), 60–87.

Gackenbach, J. I. (2012a). Video game play and dreams. In D. Barrett & P. McNamara (Eds.), *Encyclopedia of Sleep and Dreams* (pp. 795–800). Santa Barbara, CA: ABC-CLIO.

Gackenbach, J. I. (2012b). Dreams and video game play. In J. I. Gackenbach (Ed.), *Video Game Play and Consciousness*. New York: NOVA Science Publishers.

Gackenbach, J. I., & Bown, J. (2011). Mindfulness and video game play: A preliminary inquiry. *Mindfulness, 2*(2), 114–122. Retrieved from Meditative: www.springerlink.com/content/p26n3h1uq1w00771/.

Gackenbach, J. I., & Boyes, A. (2014). Social media versus gaming associations with typical and recent dreams. *Dreaming, 24*(3), 182–202.

Gackenbach, J. I., Darlington, M., Ferguson, M. L., & Boyes, A. (2013). Video game play as nightmare protection: A replication and extension. *Dreaming, 23*(2), 97–111.

Gackenbach, J. I., Ellerman, E., & Hall, C. (2011). Video game play as nightmare protection: A preliminary inquiry in military gamers. *Dreaming, 21*(4), 221–245.

Gackenbach, J. I., & Flockhart, C. (2013, June). *Nightmare Protection Thesis of Video Game Play in First Responders*. Proceedings of the International Association for the Study of Dreams: 6, *International Journal of Dream Research*: Supplement (pdf). DOI: http://dx.doi.org/10.11588/ijodr.2013.0.10874.

Gackenbach, J. I., & Hunt, H. (2014). A deeper inquiry into the association between lucid dreams and video game play. In K. Buckeley & R. Hurd (Eds.), *Lucid Dreaming Cross Cultural Understandings of Consciousness in the Dream State*. New York: ABC-CLIO.

Gackenbach, J.I., & Kuruvilla, B. (2008). The relationship between video game play and threat simulation dreams. *Dreaming, 18*(4), 236–256.

Gackenbach, J., Lee, M. N., Gahr, S., & Yu, G. (2014, June). *The Relationship Between Self-Construal, Media Use and Dreams: A Cross Cultural Study*. Paper presented at the annual meeting of the International Association for the Study of Dreams, Berkeley, CA.

Gackenbach, J. I., & Rosie, M. (2011). Presence in video game play and nighttime dreams: An empirical inquiry. *International Journal of Dream Research, 4(2),* 98–109.

Gackenbach, J. I., Sample, T., & Mandel, G. (2011). The continuity versus discontinuity hypotheses: A consideration of issues for coding video game incorporation. *International Journal of Dream Research, 4*(2), 63–76.

Gerardi, M., Rothbaum, B. O., Ressler, K., Heekin, M., & Rizzo, A. (2008). Virtual reality exposure therapy using a virtual Iraq: Case report. *Journal of Traumatic Stress, 21*(2), 209–213.

Glicksohn, J., & Avnon, M. (1997–98). Explorations in virtual reality: Absorption, cognition and altered state of consciousness. *Imagination, Cognition, and Personality, 172*, 141–151.

Green, S., & Bavalier, D. (2003). Action video game modifies visual selective attention. *Nature, 423*, 534–537.

Greenfield, P. M., Brannon, C., & Lohr, D. (1996). Two-dimensional representation of movement through three-dimensional space: The role of video game expertise. In P. M. Greenfield, & R. R. Cocking (Eds.), *Interacting with Video. Advances in Applied Developmental Psychology* (pp. 169–185). Norwood, NJ: Ablex Publishing.

Hartmann, E. (1984). *The Nightmare: The Psychology and Biology of Terrifying Dreams*. New York: Basic Books.

Hölzel, B., & Ott, U. (2006). Relationships between meditation depth, absorption, meditation, practice, and mindfulness: A latent variable approach. *The Journal of Transpersonal Psychology, 38*(2), 179–199.

Holzinger, B. (2014, June). *Lucid Dreaming: A Technique in Psychotherapy?* Paper presented at the annual conference of the International Association for the Study of Dreams, Berkeley, CA.

Hunt, H. (1995). *On the Nature of Consciousness: Cognitive, Phenomenological, and Transpersonal Perspectives*. New Haven, CT: Yale University Press.

Jones, S.M.R., & Stumbrys, T. (2014). Mental health, physical self and lucid dreaming: A correlational study in sport students. *International Journal of Dream Research, 7*(1), 54–60.

King, D., & DeCicco, T. L. (2007). The relationship between dream content and physical health, mood and self construals. *Dreaming, 17,* 127–139.

Krakow, B., Kellner, R., Neidhardt, J., Pathak, D., & Lambert, L. (1993). Imagery rehearsal treatment of chronic nightmares: With a thirty month follow-up. *Journal of Behavior Therapy and Experimental Psychiatry, 24*(4), 325–330.

LaBerge, S. (2004). *Lucid Dreaming: A Concise Guide to Awakening in Your Dreams and in Your Life*. Boulder, CO: Sounds True.

LaBerge, S. (2014, April). *Pre-sleep Treatment with Acetylcholinesterase Inhibitors Enhances Memory, Cognition and Metaconsciousness (Lucidity) during Dreaming*. Paper presented at Towards a Science of Consciousness, Tucson, AZ.

Levin, R., & Nielsen, T. A. (2009). Nightmares, bad dreams, and emotional dysregulation: A review and new neurocognitive model of dreaming. *Current Directions in Psychological Science, 18*(2), 84–88.

MacKillop, J., & Anderson, E. J. (2007). Further psychometric validation of the mindful attention awareness scale (MAAS). *Journal of Psychopathological Behaviour Assessment, 29,* 289–293.

Preston, J. (1998). From mediated environments to the development of consciousness. In J.I. Gackenbach (Ed.), *Psychology and the Internet* (pp. 255–291). San Diego: Academic Press.

Schredl, M. (2003). Continuity between waking and dreaming: A proposal for a mathematical model. *Sleep and Hypnosis, 5*(1), 26–39.

Snyder, T. J., & Gackenbach, J.I. (1988). Individual differences associated with lucid dreaming. In J.I. Gackenbach and S. P. LaBerge (Eds.), *Conscious Mind, Sleeping Brain: Perspectives on Lucid Dreaming* (pp. 221–255). New York: Plenum.

Swanston, D., & Gackenbach, J. I. (2011, June). *Morning After Dreams of Video Game Play versus Meditation/Prayer*. Paper presented at the annual meeting of the International Association for the Study of Dreams, Kerkrade, The Netherlands.

Voss, U., Holzmann, R., Hobson, A., Paulus, W., Koppehele-Gossel, J., Klimke, A, & Nitsche, M. A. (2014). Induction of self awareness in dreams through frontal low current stimulation of gamma activity. *Nature Neuroscience, 17,* 810–812.

Weinstein, M., & Smith, J. (1992). Isometric squeeze relaxation (progressive relaxation) vs. meditation: Absorption and focusing as predictors of state effects. *Perceptual & Motor Skills, 75,* 1263–1271.

Wright, T., Blakeley, D. P., & Boot, W. R. (2012). The effects of action video game play on vision and attention. In J. I. Gackenbach (Ed.), *Video Game Play and Consciousness* (pp. 71–88), New York: NOVA.

Yu, C. K.-C. (2010). Dream Intensity Scale: Factors in the phenomenological analysis of dreams. *Dreaming, 20,* 107–129.

Zadra, L., & Pihl, R. O. (1997). Lucid dreaming as a treatment for recurrent nightmares. *Psychotherapy and Psychosomatics, 66*(1), 50–55.

Zuckerberg, M. (2014, 03 25). [Web log message]. Retrieved from www.facebook.com/zuck.

INDEX

Notes are indicated by *n* and tables by *t*.

Adler, A. 8, 63
Adlerian dream literature ix
advice dreams 86–7
affect valance 10, 109–11, 114–16, 119
aggression: dream reports 5–6, 34, 58, 60–2, 64; male schizophrenics 70–1; psychological well-being 72
alcohol-use disorders, nightmares and 153
Ali, K. 139
Allen, D. N. 141
American Academy of Sleep Medicine (AASM) 150, 153
American Psychiatric Association (APA) 175, 185
antidepressants, dream content and 68, 75
anxiety: dream reports 75–6; nightmares 142, 149
Aristotle 174, 189, 199
Artemidorus ix, 14, 27
artistic personalities *see* creative personalities
Aserinsky, E. ix, 1, 27
avoidance behavior 33
avoidance symptoms 142

Babson, K. 142
Babylonian Talmud ix
"back to life" dreams 86–7
bad dreams, vs. nightmares 176
Baker, R. C. 57, 59
Banting, F. 81

Barrett, D. 39, 80–92
baseline dream content 96–101
Beatty Papyrus ix
Beck Depression Inventory 82
behavior: avoidance 33; covert 28; overt 28
Behbehani, J. 84
Belicki, K. 31
Beowulf 169
Beratis, S. 111
bereavement 175; dreams and 86–7, 185
Bergmann, I. 32
bizarreness scales 90
"Black Stars, The" (Levi) 184
Blank, Y. 136–7
Boarts, J. M. 136
Bollacker, K. 96
Bommaritto, M. 141
Bootzin, R. R. 136
Boronat, C. 182
Bosch, H. 169
Boss, M. 14
Bowdle, B. 182
Boyes, A. 219
brain damaged patients, dream reports 6
bridging 21–4, 39, 44; linking 46; testing the strength of the bridge 46
Bryant, R. A. 137
Buckley, K. 169
Bulkeley, K. 77, 95–6, 189
Burstein, A. 141
Busink, R. 178

Campbell, C. 184
Cartwright, R. ix, 39
Cartwright, R. D. 185
cassette theory of dreams 200
Celan, P. 183–4
centaurs of dream interpretation 104–5
Chen, S. 126
child molester, dream reports of 73–4
children: dream diaries 139; dream reports 63; posttraumatic nightmares 139–40
chronic nightmare disorder 149–53
Cirucci, A. M. 221
clairvoyant dreams 190; example of 193
Cleckley, H. M. 86
clients 133; attitudes towards dreams 127–9; involvement in dream work 126; therapist partnerships 38
clinical improvement: affect and 119; cognitive-experiential dream model (CEDM) 126–8, 133; dream narratives and 119–20; manifest dream reports (MDR) and 106–10, 114–15, 118–20
clinicians *see* therapists
cognitive behavioral therapy 17, 27, 138
cognitive-experiential dream model (CEDM) 32; action stage 125–6; client involvement 126; cultural factors 129–30; DRAW steps 124, 126, 131–2; exploration stage 124, 126; goals 127–8; insight stage 124–6; nightmares 130–3; outcomes 127–30; session quality 127; stages of 123–6; therapist factors 126–7; therapist training 130
Cohen's *h* 69
Coleridge, S. T. 169, 183–4
Content Analysis of Dreams, The (Hall and Van de Castle) ix
continuity hypothesis 29; clinical implications of 32–3; defined 28; emotional intensity 30; extraordinary dreams 188; lucid dreams 30; measuring 28–30; nightmares 31–2, 140; personality traits 30; psychopathological symptoms 31; time and 30
coping strategies 33
covert behavior 28
creative dreams 170, 190; example of 192–4; historical 80–1; incubation 81; interviews of 81; problem-solving 81–2
creative inspiration 32, 80–2
creative nightmares 168–71
creative personalities: dream recall 170–1; nightmares and 169–71

Critique of Judgment (Kant) 184
Crook-Lyon, R. E. 20
Cue Card questions 47–9
cultural differences: aggression in dreams 62, 64; cross-cultural dreams 189–95, 220; dream reports 57–62, 64
cultural psychologists 63

Dali, S. 32, 169
Davis, J. L. 139
Davis, L. 81
daydreams 90
day-residue 28–30
"Death Fugue" (Celan) 184
death in dreams 89
deconstruction of nightmares 131–2
Dekkers, T. 141
Delahanty, D. L. 136
Delaney, G. M. 14, 42, 44
Dement, W. 81, 200, 207
denial 24
depressed patients: dream recall 68; dream reports 5–6, 31, 71, 82; friends/friendly interactions 71; nightmares 138, 149, 168
description in dreams 46–8
desensitization techniques, nightmares and 150, 157
Diagnostic and Statistical Manual of Mental Disorders, Fifth Edition (DSM-5) (APA) 175, 177–8, 185
diary dreams 29; study of 30
digital analysis 95–7, 103–5
digital dream journaling 103, 105
Dijk, J. van 136
Dilthey, W. 9
Dimensions of Dreams (Winget and Kramer) ix
dissociative identity disorder (DID): dream content 85–6; hallucinations 86; hysterical conversion symptoms 85; nightmares 85; repressed memories 85; trauma-related hallucinations 85
Ditner, A. 218, 221
Dohnt, H. K. 140
Domhoff, G. W. 56–7, 63–4, 80, 96, 102–3, 175
DRAW steps 124, 126, 131–2
dream analysis: digital tools 95, 97, 103–5; word searching tools 96–105
DreamBank 77, 96
dream categories: monothetic approaches 176; polythetic approaches 176–81

dream content: age and 4, 6; anxiety 4; baselines 96–101; cultural factors 137; digital analysis 95–7; emotional preoccupations 7; experimental manipulation 28–9; gender and 3–5, 56–7; individual differences 63; latent 106; mental illness and 5; positional differences 6–7; posttraumatic 136–7; psychopathological symptoms 31; psychotropic medications and 67–8
dream content scoring systems 3; bizarreness scales 90; Hall-Van de Castle system 3–6, 56–62, 68–70, 72–3, 75–7, 88, 90, 96, 102; *h-profile* 70, 77; research for 103; Sleep and Dream Database (SDDb) 98–101, 104
dream control 220
dream diaries: gender differences 56; trauma-exposed children 139
dreamer-as-character 90
dreamers: bridging 21–3; dying in dreams 89; engagement of 20; memory 28; motivation 38–9, 41; self-interpretation 15–18, 20, 43–6; spatial skills of 216
Dream Experience, The (Kramer) 1
dream incubation 38–9, 81; clinical implications of 92; group therapy 52–3; historical interest 39; hospice/end-of-life care 54; individual therapy 49–52; notes 41; Phrase-Focusing 38–42; topic choice 52
dream-initiated lucid dreams 204–5
Dream Intensity Scale 220
dream interpretation 10; bridging 39, 44; centaurs 104–5; challenges of 20; cognitive-experiential 32; by dreamers 15–18, 39; Dream Interview method 40, 42–8; effectiveness of 32; historical interest ix, 14, 27; listening to the dreamer approach 34–5; model for 33–4; nightmares 152; teaching of 14–17
dream interviewing 15–17; bridging 21–4; interpretive shortcuts 22–3; medical practices 53; pivotal images 23; self-help dream groups 24; steps for 44–9; therapist/interviewer role 43–53; training in 17–25
Dream Interview method 40, 42–3; actions/plots 53; bridge and test 46, 49; Cue Card questions 47–9; description 45–9; group therapy 52–3; linking and summary 46, 49; recapitulation 45; steps for 44–9

dream journals 72, 76, 103, 105
dream lag effect 30
dream length, gender differences 57
dream metaphor 182–3
dream narratives 116–17, 119–20
dream recall 3, 32, 41, 163, 170–1
dream rehearsal therapy 83
dream reports x, 1; aggression 4–6, 34, 58, 60–2, 64; of an anxious patient 75–6; brain damaged patients 6; of a child molester 73–4; children 63; cultural differences 57–62, 64; cultural psychologists 63; cycles 2; defined 27–8; demographic variables 3–5; depressed patients 82; dissociative identity disorder (DID) 85–6; emotion 4, 62; extraordinary dreams 190–6; friends/friendly interactions 68–71, 75, 77; gender differences 3–5, 29, 56–64; group data 6; hysterical conversion symptoms 85; interpretation of 8–9; mental illness variables 3, 5–6, 31, 70–1; of a neurotic patient 74–5; reliability of 2–3; repressed memories 85; settings 62; sexual interactions 4, 62, 73; socioeconomic class 4–5; validity 28
dream research ix, 1, 27; blind analysis 72–3; consistency of 67–8; dream content patterns 103; dream series 72, 76; inference-and- response methodology 73; Most Recent Dream method 76; psychiatric populations 76–7; psychophysiological studies 205–8; quantitative studies 72, 76; stimuli 28
dreams: actions/plots 48–9; affect and 119; attitudes towards 127–9; of the bereaved 86–7, 185; cassette theory 200; clairvoyant 190; classification of 178, 182; clinical implications of 91–2; collection of 2; continuity hypothesis 28–30; coping strategies 33; cultural factors 129–30; day notes 41; day-residue 28–30; dream within a dream 190; of dying 89; existential 178–83; as experiences 2, 10, 28; extraordinary 188–95; of flying 89; focused thinking 30; folk beliefs 84; function of 91; hyperarousal in 175; initial 110–12; initiation 190; laboratory 29; long-term memory and 130; lucid 30, 87–90, 190, 198–210; magnitude 174–5, 177–8; meaning of 8–10, 124–5; media use and 220; as metaphors 39–40, 42;

mood-regulatory functions 11; mundane 178, 181; mutual/shared 190; as narratives 9–10; negative 162, 171; non-lucid 199, 208; orderliness of 7–8; out-of-body 190; past-life 190; personality tests and 73; poetry and 184–5; posttraumatic 136; precognitive 190; of prisoners 88; recent 29; reenactments 140–1; spirituality and 128, 130; telepathic 190; as threat simulations 91; transcendent 178–83; turning point 106; visitation 191; waking life and 27–35, 72–3, 123–5, 170
dreams, impactful *see* impactful dreams
DreamSAT 77
dream seminars 190
dream series 72, 74
dreamsigns 205
dream translation method 8–10
dream within a dream 190; example of 193
Duke, L. A. 141
Dunn, K. 82
Duval, M. 137

Ellis, H. 199–200
emotional intensity 178
emotional processing 166–8, 171
emotions 1, 4, 176; dream content and 7, 30; existential dreams 180; negative 31, 58, 62; nightmares 179–80; transcendent dreams 180–1
Encel, J. S. 140
Eng, T. 178
existential dreams 178–9; effects of 182–3; emotions in 180; sublime feeling 183–5
experience, language and 63
"Exposure" (Owen) 184
extraordinary dreams: clinical implications of 194–5; continuity hypothesis and 188; cross-cultural 189–96; gender differences 191; historical interest 189; research on 189–92, 194; types of 188–94

Fabio, S. 81
Faith, L. 189, 191, 195
Field, N. P. 137
"First Duino Elegy" (Rilke) 184
Fischmann, T. 137
Fisler, R. 141
flashbacks 141, 144
Flockhart, C. 218
Flowers, L. K. 42
flying dreams 89
focused thinking 30

folk belief dreams 84
Fosse, M. J. 138, 140
Fosse, R. 138
Foulkes, D. 182–3, 204
Frankenstein (Shelley) 80
Freud, Sigmund ix, 8, 14, 16, 27–8, 31, 91, 106, 166, 169, 189, 198–9
Freudian dream literature ix
Freudian psychoanalysis 95
friends/friendly interactions 70; dream reports 68–71, 74–5, 77; psychopathological symptoms 70–1
"Frost at Midnight" (Coleridge) 184
Fussili, J. H. 169

Gabbard, G. 23
Gackenbach, J. I. 217–19
Gahr, S. 221
gamers *see* video game players
Gardner, S. E. 145
Gassendi, P. 199–200
gender differences: dream length 57; dream reports 3, 5, 29, 56–64; historical interest 56; manifest dream reports (MDR) 113
gender roles, cultural 56
Gentner, D. 182
Gerhart, J. I. 138
Germain, A. 136, 176
Gilgamesh myth ix, 161
Giordano, A. 76
Glicksohn, J. 194
Glucksberg, S. 182
Glucksman, M. 106–19
Goates, M. K. 32, 125
Goya, F. 169
Gratton, N. 54
grief, lucid dreams and 211
group therapy, dream incubation 52–3

Hall, C. 56, 58–62, 68–70, 73, 75–7, 80, 88, 90, 96, 102, 107
Hall, C. S. ix, 3, 5, 27–8, 32–3, 57
hallucinations 85–6, 162
Hall-Van de Castle system of dream content 3–6, 56–62, 68–70, 72–3, 75–7, 88, 90, 96, 102
Harb, G. C. 138
Hartmann, A. 58
Hartmann, E. 39, 64, 96, 169, 175, 179, 185n
Hasler, B. P. 176
Hau, S. 137
Haynes, P. L. 136
healing dreams 190; example of 193

Helminen, E. 139
herald dreams 111
Hill, C. E. 17, 32, 125–7
Hillman, J. 169
Hill's Cognitive-Experimental Model 17
Hinton, D. E. 137, 144
Hippocrates 23
Hobson, A. 90
Hobson, J. A. 138
Holen, A. 135
Hölzel, B. 217
Holzinger, B. 209
Hopkins, K. 88
Horowitz, P. 81
hospice/end-of-life care, dream incubation 54
hostility 5
h-profile 70, 77
Hummel, A. 131
Hunt, H. 200
Hunt, H. T. 182
hypnotic dreams 90
hysterical conversion symptoms 85

Imagery Rehearsal Therapy (IRT) 27, 33, 130, 138; children and 140; evidence base 138; nightmares and 150–4; randomized controlled trials 139; sexual assault survivors 150; therapeutic principles of 151*t*
images 45
immersion 216, 221
impactful dreams 174–5, 177–8; aesthetic effects of 183–5; classification of 177–8; effects of 182; emotions in 178, 179*t*, 180–1; existential 178–80, 184–5; literary theory and 183–4; nightmares 178–80; transcendent 178–81
individual therapy: client involvement 126; dream incubation 49–52
initial dreams 110–20
initiation dreams 190; example of 194
insomnia 154–5; nightmares and 163–5
International Association for the Study of Dreams (IASD) 14, 84
Interpretation of Dreams, The (Freud) ix, 14, 32
Irma dream 9
Ismahil, K. H. 139

James, W. 198
Johns, J. 81
Johnson, D. C. 130
Jovic, V. 137

Jung, C. 8, 14, 16, 157, 174–5, 182, 189
Jungian dream literature ix

Kahan, T. 96
Kant, I. 183–4
Kasparov, G. 104
Kekulé, F. A. 80, 82
Kelly, M. 136
King Lear (Shakespeare) 174–5
Kleijn, W. C. 136
Kleitman, N. ix, 27
Kline, K. V. 126
Knox, S. 125
Kobayashi, I. 136
Korde, S. 81
Köthe, M. 31
Kozak, M. 142
Kradin, R. 111
Krakow, B. 83, 185
Kramer, M. ix, 1, 67, 96, 106–19
Krippner, S. 57–9, 62, 189–91, 195
Krischner, N. 75
Kuiken, D. 177–8, 182, 184–5
Kwiatkowski, C. F. 171

LaBerge, S. 189, 202, 207, 210
laboratory dreams 29
Lamberg, L. 39
Langston, T. J. 139–40
language, experience and 63
Lansky, M. R. 142, 145
latent dream content 106, 119
leave-taking dreams 86–7
LeDoux, J. E. 130
Lee, M-N. 178
Levi, P. 184
Levin, R. 140, 175
Levitan, L. 203
Life on the Mississippi (Twain) 188
Lin, C. 126
listening to the dreamer approach 34–5
Loeffler, M. 82
Loewi, O. 81
loss 175
lucid dreaming therapy 211
lucid dreams 30, 87–90, 190; absence of sensory input 203; clinical implications of 208, 217–18; defined 88, 198–9; dream-initiated 204–5; dreamsigns 205; example of 193; flying and 89; grief and 211; meditation and 217–18; physiological characteristics of 203–5; positive effects of 208–11; psychophysiological studies 205–8;

REM sleep and 200–5; self-integration and 210; signal-verified 201–3, 206–8; in sleep cycle 204–5; spatial skills of dreamers 216; terminally ill and 211; trained subjects 205–8; video game players and 217–18, 220; wake-initiated 204–5; working memory 205
Lyons, J. 156
Lyotard, J.-F. 183

McCartney, P. 32
McGowan, K. 200
McGregor, D. 90
Macnish, R. 161
magnitude, dreams with *see* impactful dreams
Mallarmé, S. 183
manifest dream reports (MDR) 10, 106; affect and 109–11, 114–16, 119; association themes 113, 115–16; clinical improvement and 106–10, 114–15, 118–19; dream narratives 116–17; gender differences 113; initial dreams 111–14, 116–20; last dreams 114–19; psychodynamic formulation of 117–18, 120; transference 112–13, 115, 118–20
Marc, I. 155
Martinez, J. 137
media use, dreams and 220
medical practices, dream interviewing 53
medications: antidepressants 68, 75; dream content and 67–8, 75–6; nightmares and 82; Prazosin 154, 157; psychotropic 67–8
meditation 216–18
Mellman, T. A. 137
men: aggression in dreams 4, 61–2, 64, 70–1; dream recall 63; dream reports 57–64; dream work and 129; extraordinary dreams 191; negative emotions 58; video game players 218–20
mental control 141–2
mental disorders: dreams and 30; nightmares and 167–8, 171; sleep-oriented treatment 154, 156
Merckelbach, H. 141
metaphor 182–3
military personnel: nightmare protection 219; posttraumatic stress disorder (PTSD) 153–4, 156, 168; prisoner-of-war veterans 135–6, 141; suicidality 168; video game players 219
mindfulness 217

Minnesota Multiphasic Personality Inventory (MMPI) 70, 72
Monfils, M. J. 130
"Mont Blanc" (Shelley) 184
Most Recent Dream method 76
Mukarovský, J. 183
mundane dreams 178; emotions in 181
mutual/shared dreams 190; example of 193

Nagel, L. 207
narcissistic injury 142
negative dreams 162, 171
neurotic patient, dream reports of 74–5
Neylan, T. C. 137
Nickerson, A. 137
Nielsen, T. A. 140, 175
nightmare art 169
Nightmare Deconstruction and Reprocessing (NDR) 131–3
Nightmare Protection Thesis 215–16, 218–21
nightmare recall 163–5
nightmares xi; alcohol-use disorders 153; avoidance symptoms 142; vs. bad dreams 176; causes of 149; characteristics of 83; children 139–40; classification of 178; cognitive behavioral therapy 138; confabulated 1–2; creative process and 168–71; deconstructing 131–2; defining 175–7; depressed patients 138, 149, 168; desensitization techniques 150, 157; diagnostic criteria for 175–6; dissociative identity disorder (DID) 85; effects of 182–3; emotional intensity 178–9; emotional processing 166–7, 171; emotions 179–80; evolutionary function 166; experienced 2; folk beliefs 84; historical interest 161, 168–9; imagery rehearsal 27, 33, 130, 138–40, 150, 157; incidence of 135, 162–4; insomnia and 154–5; long-term memory and 130; lucidity during 208–11; medications and 82; nontraumatic 141; posttraumatic 83–5, 130–1, 135–8, 141, 149, 152, 156–7; quality of sleep and 163–4; reconsolidating 130–2; REM sleep and 162–5, 167; sleep apnea and 153–7, 164–5; sleep quality 136, 138; stress and 82–3; of suffocation 164; suicidality 153; treatment of 150–7; waking life and 31–2
Nightmare Triad Syndrome 154–5

night terrors 162
non-lucid dreams 199, 208
non-REM sleep 8; posttraumatic stress disorder (PTSD) 136
Nordby, V. J. 28, 32–3
Nuutinen, J. 139

obstructive sleep apnea (OSA) 156 ; see also sleep apnea
Oculus Rift 216, 221
Ogilvie, R. 200
Oneirocritica 14
Oppenheim, A. L. ix
Ørner, R. J. 145
Ott, U. 217
out-of-body dreams 190; example of 193
overt behavior 28
Owen, W. 184

Paley, K. S. 189
PAP devices *see* positive airway pressure therapy (PAP)
Parker, J. D. 156
past-life dreams 190; example of 193
personality tests, dreams and 73
personality traits 30; thin boundaries 32
Pesant, N. 126
Phelps, E. A. 130
Phrase-Focusing dream incubation 38–9, 42; steps for 40–1
Picasso, P. 169
Pietrowsky, R. 31
Pigeon, W. R. 137
pivotal images 23
Plato ix
Poe, E. A. 169
poetry, dreaming and 184–5
polysomnography 163
positive airway pressure therapy (PAP) 155–6
posttraumatic dreams: mixed 136; nonreplicative 136; replicative 136–7, 140
posttraumatic nightmares 135–7, 141, 175; anxiety 142; children 139–40; content of 136–7; diagnostic value 143–4; flashbacks 141, 144; imagery rehearsal 138; nonreplicative 140; psychopathological symptoms 137–8; reexperiencing 137; replicative 138, 140–2, 145; as screening tools 143; as screen memories 142; shame 142; treatment of 138

posttraumatic reenactments 140–1, 143, 145
posttraumatic stress disorder (PTSD) 83; diagnostic criteria for 177; flashbacks 141; imagery rehearsal 130, 154; insomnia 155; military personnel 153–4, 156, 168; nightmare protection 219; nightmares 84–5, 130–1, 135–8, 140, 143–5, 149, 151–2, 154–7, 162, 166–8, 176; reexperiencing 137; REM imagery 86; sexual assault survivors 150; sleep apnea 155–6; sleep quality 136
Prazosin 154, 157
precognitive dreams 190; example of 193–4
prefrontal cortex 82
presence 216
Preston, J. 217
prisoner dreams 88
prisoner-of-war veterans: flashbacks 141; nightmares 135–6, 141
problem-solving: creative dreams and 80–2; during sleep 39–40, 106
Profet, M. 81
psychiatric populations: aggression 70–2; blind analysis 73; dream content 67–70; dream research 76–7; friends/friendly interactions 70–2, 74–5; medications 67–8, 75–6; vs. nonpatient populations 67–8, 70
psychodynamic psychotherapy 17, 23, 124
psychological well-being (PWB) 72
psychopathological symptoms 70–1
psychophysiological studies 205–8
psychotherapy: cognitive-experiential dream model (CEDM) 123–33; dream content 67–8; dream interpretation 14–16, 27, 32, 38, 95; dream interviewing 15–17; dream reports and 9–10, 75; imagery rehearsal 139; improvement in 10; initial dreams 110–20; last dreams 114–19; latent dream content 106; manifest dream reports (MDR) 106–20; Nightmare Deconstruction and Reprocessing (NDR) 131–3; posttraumatic nightmares 143–4; training in dream interpretation 15–25; transference 144
psychotropic medications, dream content and 67–8
Punamäki, R.-L. 139

Raio, C. M. 130
Ramanujan, S. 81
recall of dreams *see* dream recall

recapitulation 45
reconsolidating nightmares 130–2
Reed, H. 39, 81
reenactments 140–1, 145
reexperiencing 137
REM sleep ix, x; cycles 1; dream content intensity 1–2; dream reports 3–7; dreams outside 162; emotional processing 166–8; lucid dreams and 200–5; medications suppressing 168; nightmares during 162–5, 167; posttraumatic stress disorder (PTSD) 136; secondary visual cortex 82; signal-verified lucid dreams (SVLDs) 201–3; sleep talking 90; stimulus during 2
replicative nightmares 138, 140–2, 144–5
repressed memories 85
resistance 24
Revonsuo, A. 91
Rilke, R. M. 184
Roe, C. A. 189
Roefs, A. 141
Rosenbaum, B. 137
Rosie, M. 217
Ross, 86
Roth, T. 67
Roy, N. 155
Rozee, P. D. 141
Rubinstein, K. 58

Saint-Denys, H. D. 208
Salis, P. 67
Saul, L. 111
Sawicki, C. 200
Schatzman, M. 81
Schiller, D. 130
schizophrenic patients: dream reports 3, 5–6, 31, 70–1; friends/friendly interactions 70–1
Schliermacher, F. 9
Schneider, A. 77, 96
Schredl, M. 29, 33, 140, 221
Schreuder, B. 136
secondary visual cortex 82
Séguin, M. 54
self-help dream groups 24
separation anxiety disorder, nightmares and 176
separation distress 175
Series, F. 155
sexual assault survivors, nightmare treatment 150
sexual interactions, dream reports 4, 62, 73

Shakespeare, W. 174–5
Shelley, M. 80, 169, 184
signal-verified lucid dreams (SVLDs) 205–8; REM sleep and 201–3
Sikora, S. 177–8, 182
Simon, N. 137
Singh, T. 178
Sinyard, A. 221
Sizemore, C. 86
sleep: brain activity 28; nightmares 136–8; poor quality 163–5, 171; problem-solving during 39–40
Sleep and Dream Database (SDDb) 96–101, 104
sleep apnea: nightmares and 153–7, 164–5; suffocation nightmares 164; treatment of 155–7
sleep disorders: chronic nightmare disorder 149–50, 152–4, 156–7; insomnia 154–5, 163–5; nightmares 156, 163; sleep apnea 155–7, 164–5
Sleep Dynamic Therapy model 153
sleep medicine 149–50, 152
sleep records 3
sleep talking 90
sleep-wake transition 28
Smarter Than You Think (Thompson) 104
social media users, dreams and 221
somniloquies *see* sleep talking
Sopčák, P. 184
Spiritual Dreaming (Bulkeley) 189
spirituality, dreams and 128, 130
state of death dreams 86–7
States, B. 174–5
Stekel, W. 111
stereotype threat 219
Stevenson, R. L. 32, 80, 169
Stickgold, R. J. 138
Strange Case of Dr. Jekyll and Mr. Hyde, The (Stevenson) 32, 80
stress: nightmares and 82–3; posttraumatic stress disorder (PTSD) 83; waking life 30
stress-reduction techniques 131–2
Subjective Units of Distress Scale (SUDS) 132
sublime feeling 183–5
suffocation nightmares 164
suicidality: among military personnel 168; nightmares and 153
Sundance Filmmaker Studies 169–70
Suzuki, Y. 191
Swanston, D. 217
Swopes, R. M. 139

Tamanna, S. 156
Tartz, R. S. 57, 59
Taytroe, L. 38–9
Tedlock, B. 64
telepathic dreams 190; example of 193
terminally ill, lucid dreams and 211
testing the strength of the bridge 46
therapist/interviewer role 50
therapists: client partnerships 38; cognitive-experiential dream model (CEDM) 123–33; dream work 91–2; as interviewer 43–4; professional development 24–5; training in dream interpretation 15–25, 27, 123, 130; use of manifest dream content 106, 119
Thigpen, C. H. 86
thin boundaries 32
Tholey, P. 208–10
Thompson, C. 104
threat simulation dreams 91
Three Faces of Eve, The (Thigpen and Cleckley) 86
Tien, H. S. 126–7
Tonay, V. 57
Total Recall (film) 200
training in dream interpretation 15–25, 27, 123, 130
transcendent dreams 178–9; effects of 182–3; emotions in 180–1
transference 112–13, 115, 118–20, 144
trauma; *see also* posttraumatic stress disorder (PTSD): dreams and 83–5; emotional processing 167; hallucinations 85–6; mental control 141–2; nightmares 83–5, 130–1, 135–41, 166, 168
Trauma and Dreams (Barrett) 83–4
turning point dreams 106
Twain, M. 188

Ullah, M. I. 156
Ullman, M. 14, 16, 53, 191
unfocused activity 30

validity 28
Valli, K. 139
Van de Castle, R. ix, 3, 5, 56–62, 68–70, 75–7, 88, 90, 96, 102, 107, 169
Van der Kolk, B. A. 141, 145

Varvin, S. 137
Vaughan, A. 191
video game players: coping strategies 219–20; cross-cultural 220; dream control 220; dreams of 215; females 219; genre preferences 219; lucid dreams and 217–18, 220; males 218–20; military personnel 219; mindfulness and 217; nightmare protection 218–21; presence 217; spatial skills of 216; state of consciousness 216–17; stereotype threat 219
virtual reality technology: defined 216; dreams and 215, 221; immersion 216, 221; Oculus Rift 216, 221; presence 216; social media users 221; video game players 215–21
visitation dreams 191; example of 194

wake-initiated lucid dreams 204–5
waking life: covert behavior 28; dreams and 27–35, 72–3, 123–5, 170; long-term memory and 130; nightmares and 31–2; overt behavior 28; stress 30
Warner, S. L. 106
Wegner, D. M. 141–2
Weinhold, J. 57, 62
Wellcome Medical Collection 88
Wenzlaff, R. M. 142
Wessel, I. 141
White, G. L. 38–9
Wild Strawberries (film) 32
Winget, C. ix
Wittmann, L. 138
Wolff, P. 182
women: aggression in dreams 61–2; dream recall 63; dream reports 57–64; extraordinary dreams 191; negative emotions 58; nightmares 162; video game players 219
Woolf, V. 183
word searching tools 96–105
working memory 205

"Yesterday" (McCartney) 32

Zadra, A. 126, 137
Zamore, N. 90
Zarcone, V., Jr. 207